HARRY'S COSMETICOLOGY 9TH EDITION

FOCUS BOOKS

The Skin: Structure, Biochemistry, Function and Testing for Cosmetic Formulators

ISBN: 978-0-8206-0403-9

Harry's Cosmeticology

9th Edition

Volume One - ISBN: 978-0-8206-01762
Volume Two - ISBN: 978-0-8206-01779
Volume Three - ISBN: 978-0-8206-01786
eBook - ISBN: 978-0-8206-01793

First Edition

Chemical Publishing Company

www.chemical-publishing.com

Printed in the United States of America

A Note from the Publisher:

The new 9th edition of Harry's Cosmeticology is available as a 3 volume set containing over 2600 pages of new information on the recent changes in the cosmetic and personal care products industry.

Chemical Publishing is now offering key parts of the title for those interested in a particular subject area covered in the book.

Harry's Cosmeticology 9th Edition has developed a new line of titles called "Focus Books" for this purpose.

"Focus Books" are a series of selected chapters that can be used as a reference guide for partial subject areas covered in the parent text.

Because the chapters have been taken from the original individual volumes, the reader will find that the pages have not been renumbered in standard order starting from page one, moving forward, but rather they have been left in the original format so that the information will flow chronologically, although the pages may in fact not be numbered as so.

The benefit of leaving the page numbers as they were taken from the original text is that the reader will be able to use the Table of Contents and page numbers referenced within the Focus Book to find the desired content and we have tried to keep the chapter segments in the same order in which you would find them in the master text.

The full 3 volume Trilogy of Harry's Cosmeticology 9th Edition can be purchased through Chemical Publishing Company at www.chemical-publishing.com or through any major online retailer. It is also available in Ebook format through Kindle or as mobi, or ePub available directly from the publisher.

www.chemical-publishing.com

Our webpage featuring Authors, Reviews and other information about the 9th edition:

www.harryscosmeticology.com

About the Editor-in-Chief

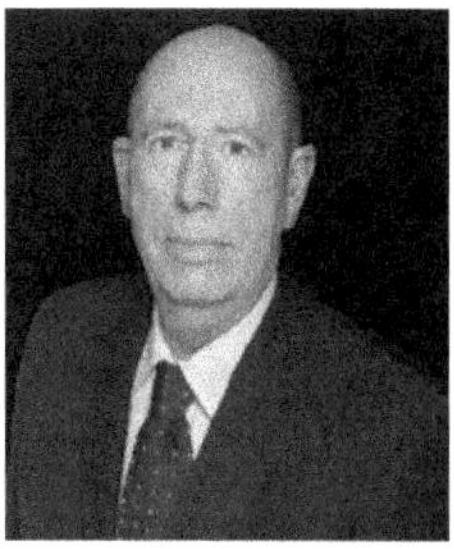

Meyer R. Rosen

CChem, CPC, CChE, CFEI, DABFE, DABFET, FAIC

Meyer R. Rosen is President of Interactive Consulting, Inc. (www.chemicalconsult.com). He is a Thought-Leader and expert in the field of Technical Marketing and multi-industry Technology Transfer Applications including, but not limited to: cosmetics and personal care, applied rheology, applied surface and interfacial chemistry, polymers, organosilicones, professional editing and custom preparation of Mind-Maps® for the organization and presentation of complex information.

Mr. Rosen is a Chartered Chemist and Fellow of the Royal Society of Chemistry (London); a Fellow of the American Institute of Chemists and both a Nationally Certified Professional Chemist and Certified Professional Chemical Engineer. He is a member of the U.S. Society of Cosmetic Chemists (SCC) & the American Institute of Chemical Engineers. Meyer serves as an Advisor for David Smith, Executive Director of the SCC Advisory Committee. He is also Editor for U.S. & Canada and Editor-in-Chief for North and Latin America for Euro Cosmetics Magazine in Germany. Mr. Rosen is Editor of the Delivery System Handbook for Personal Care and Cosmetic Products and Editor-in-Chief of Harry's Cosmeticology, 9th Ed.

Meyer served for six years as the Chief Scientific Advisor and Director of Technical Programming for United Business Media's (UBM) HBA Technical Conferences. He a former Director of the American Institute of Chemists, past Vice President of the Association of Consulting Chemists and has served on the Scientific Advisory Board of Supply Side West/East: Virgo Publications. Mr. Rosen is also the Founder, Organizer and co-moderator for HBA's Annual International Safety, Regulatory and Certification Symposia.

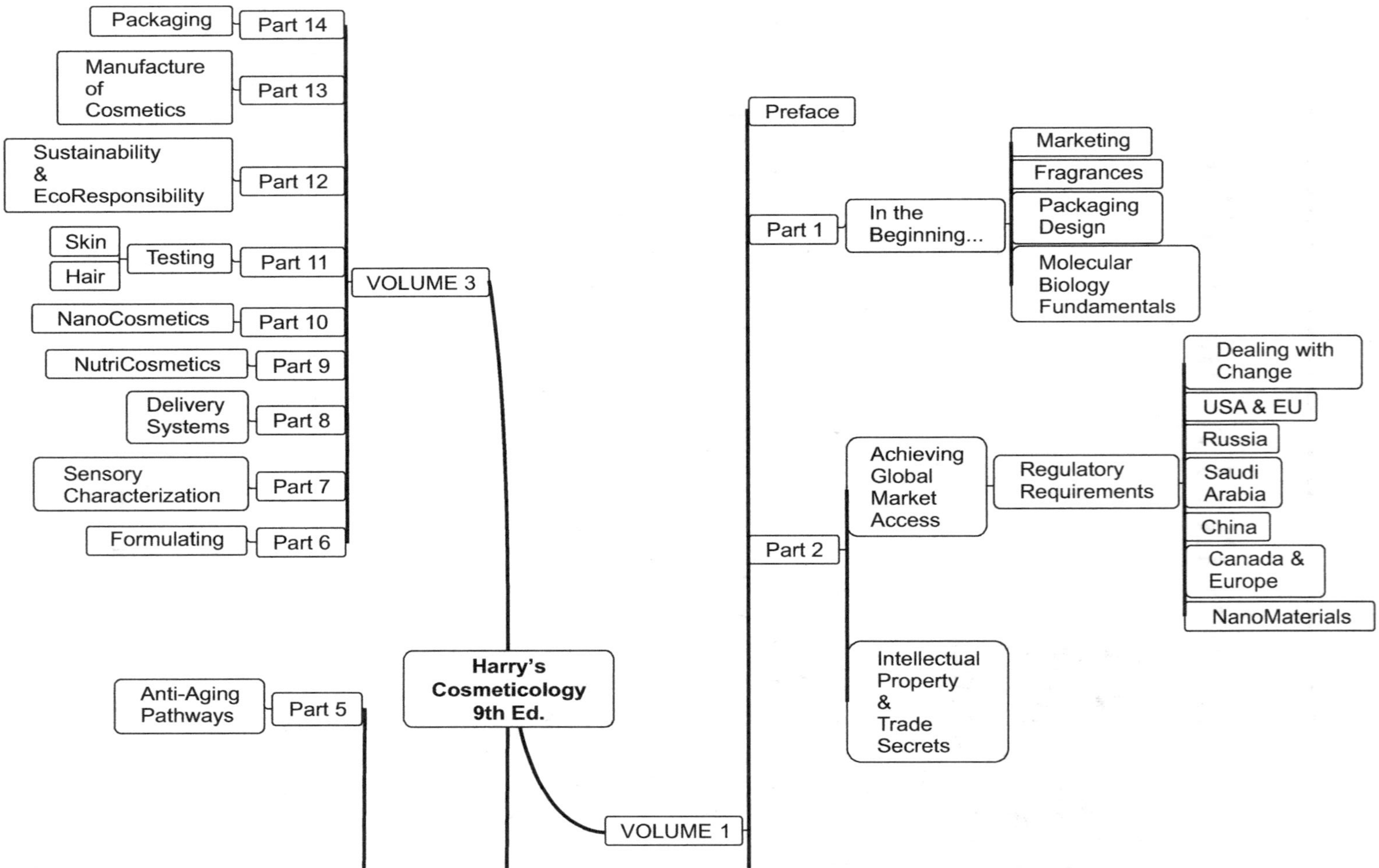
Harry's Cosmeticology 9th Ed.
VOLUME 1
Preface
Part 1
In the Beginning...
Marketing
Fragrances
Packaging Design
Molecular Biology Fundamentals
Part 2
Achieving Global Market Access
Regulatory Requirements
Dealing with Change
USA & EU
Russia
Saudi Arabia
China
Canada & Europe
NanoMaterials
Intellectual Property & Trade Secrets
VOLUME 3
Part 14
Packaging
Part 13
Manufacture of Cosmetics
Part 12
Sustainability & EcoResponsibility
Part 11
Testing
Skin
Hair
Part 10
NanoCosmetics
Part 9
NutriCosmetics
Part 8
Delivery Systems
Part 7
Sensory Characterization
Part 6
Formulating
Part 5
Anti-Aging Pathways

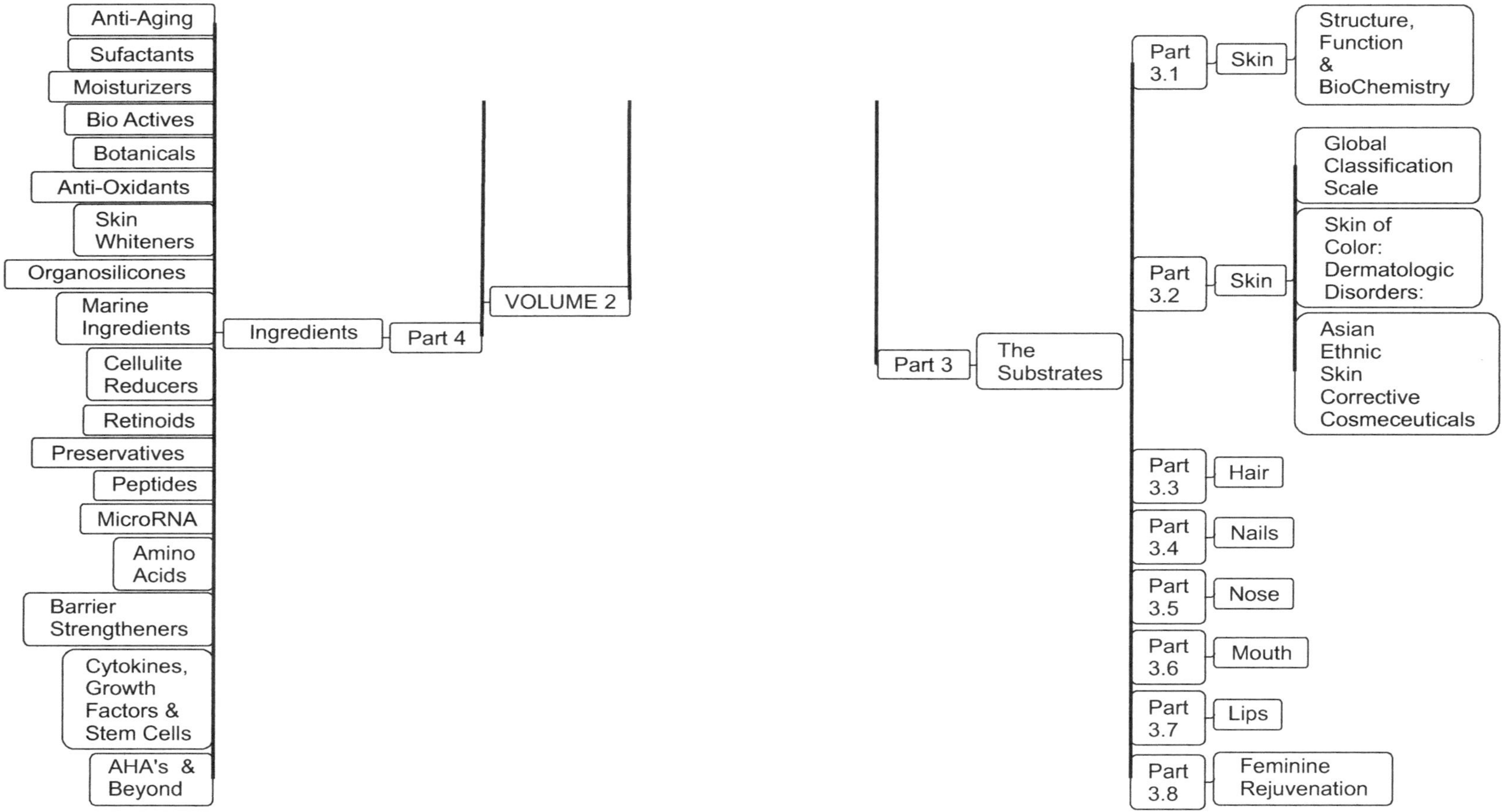
VOLUME 2
Part 4
Ingredients
Anti-Aging
Sufactants
Moisturizers
Bio Actives
Botanicals
Anti-Oxidants
Skin Whiteners
Organosilicones
Marine Ingredients
Cellulite Reducers
Retinoids
Preservatives
Peptides
MicroRNA
Amino Acids
Barrier Strengtheners
Cytokines, Growth Factors & Stem Cells
AHA's & Beyond
Part 3
The Substrates
Part 3.1
Skin
Structure, Function & BioChemistry
Part 3.2
Skin
Global Classification Scale
Skin of Color: Dermatologic Disorders:
Asian Ethnic Skin Corrective Cosmeceuticals
Part 3.3
Hair
Part 3.4
Nails
Part 3.5
Nose
Part 3.6
Mouth
Part 3.7
Lips
Part 3.8
Feminine Rejuvenation

AUTHORS

THE SKIN: STRUCTURE, BIOCHEMISTRY, AND FUNCTION

Editor: Bozena B. Michniak-Kohn, Ph.D., M.R. Pharm. S.

Contributors:
Amy S. Pappert, M.D.
Philip Wertz, Ph.D.
Nripen Sharma, Ph.D.
Anna Langerveld, Ph.D.
Ada Polla
Barbara Polla, M.D.
Anne Pouillot, MS
Karen E. Burke, M.D., Ph.D.
Gopi Menon, Ph.D.
Nava Dayan Ph.D.

CLASSIFICATION SCALE FOR SKIN COMPLEXIONS AROUND THE WORLD

Eva Patel

DERMATOLOGIC DISORDERS IN SKIN OF COLOR

Aanand N. Geria, MD

ASIAN ETHNIC SKIN: SPECIALTY CORRECTIVE COSMECEUTICALS FOR ASIAN ETHNIC SKIN CARE

Eva Patel

COMPROMISED SKIN IN THE ELDERLY

R. Randall Wickett, Ph.D.,
Martha Tate, Ph.D.

AUTHORS

METHODS TO ASSESS SKIN BARRIER INTEGRITY

Authors:
Guojin Lu,
Roger L. McMullen,
David J. Moore

IMAGING TECHNIQUES AND ANALYSIS FOR QUANTIFICATION OF SKIN APPEARANCE

Roger L. McMullen, Ph.D.

BIOPHYSICAL MEASUREMENT AND EVALUATION OF SKIN ELASTICITY AND TOPOGRAPHY

Authors:
Stefanie Luebberding, Ph.D.
Nils Krueger, Ph.D.

CLINICAL TESTING OF COSMETICS AND SKIN CARE PRODUCTS: METHODS AND INSTRUMENTATIONS

Iqbal Sadiq, M.Phil.

PART 3 THE SUBSTRATES

PART 3.1

THE SKIN: STRUCTURE, BIOCHEMISTRY, AND FUNCTION

Editor of The Skin, Structure, Biochemistry, and Function:
Bozena "Bo" B. Michniak-Kohn, Ph.D., M.R. Pharm. S.
Professor of Pharmaceutics
Ernest Mario School of Pharmacy

Director & Founder
Center for Dermal Research (CDR)
NJ Center for Biomaterials, Life Sciences Building
Rutgers—The State University of New Jersey
145, Bevier Road,
Piscataway, NJ 08854.
www.michniaklab.org

Contributors:
1. Amy S. Pappert, M.D.
Assistant Professor, Department of Dermatology
UMDNJ—Robert Wood Johnson Medical School
1 World's Fair Drive, Suite 2400Somerset, NJ 08873

2. Philip Wertz, Ph.D.
Professor Department of Oral Pathology, Radiology, and Medicine
N450 DSB, Dows Institute
University of Iowa
Iowa City IA 52242

3. Nripen Sharma, Ph.D.
Clinical Scientist/Project Manager/Technical Support
Salvona Technologies LLC
65 Stults Rd., Dayton, NJ 08810

4. Anna Langerveld, Ph.D.
President and CEO
Genemarkers
4717 Campus Drive, Suite 1800
Kalamazoo, MI 49008

5. Ada Polla
Alchimie Forever, The Polla Beauty Group
1010 Wisconsin Avenue NW, Suite 201
Washington, DC 20007
Online: www.alchimie-forever.com

6. Barbara Polla, M.D.
Medical Doctor
Alchimie Forever, The Polla Beauty Group
1010 Wisconsin Avenue NW, Suite 201
Washington, DC 20007

7. Anne Pouillot, MS
Director of Science of Alchimie Forever
Alchimie Forever, The Polla Beauty Group
1010 Wisconsin Avenue NW, Suite 201
Washington, DC 20007

8. Karen E. Burke, M.D., Ph.D.
Dermatologist
429 East 52nd Street
New York, New York 10022

9. Gopi Menon, Ph.D.
Senior Science Fellow
Ashland Specialty Ingredients
1361 Alps Road
Wayne, NJ

10. Nava Dayan Ph.D.
President
Dr. Nava Dayan LLC

PART 3.1 SUBSTRATE:

THE SKIN: STRUCTURE, BIOCHEMISTRY AND FUNCTION

TABLE OF CONTENTS

PART 3.2.1

CLASSIFICATION SCALE FOR SKIN COMPLEx IONS AROUND THE WORLD

Eva Patel
Skin Rx Inc.
Founder & CEO

TABLE OF CONTENTS:

PART 3.2.2

DERMATOLOGIC DISORDERS IN SKIN OF COLOR

Aanand N. Geria, MD

TABLE OF CONTENTS:

PART 3.2.3

ASIAN ETHNIC SKIN: SPECIALTY CORRECTIv E COSMECEUTICALS FOR ASIAN ETHNIC SKIN CARE

Eva Patel
Skin Rx Inc.
Founder & CEO

Gurpreet (Gogi) Sangha
G.S. Cosmeceutical USA Inc.
Founder & CEO

TABLE OF CONTENTS

COMPROMISED SKIN IN THE ELDERLY

Authors:
R. Randal Wickett, Ph.D., Martha Tate, Ph.D.

Randall Wickett, Ph.D.
Emeritus Professor
Pharmaceutics and Cosmetic Science
Univ. Cincinnati College of Pharmacy

Martha Tate, Ph.D.

TABLE OF CONTENTS

PART 11 TESTING

PART 11.1

METHODS TO ASSESS SKIN BARRIER INTEGRITY: EFFECTS OF CLEANSING PRODUCTS

Authors:
Guojin Lu,
Roger L. McMullen,
David J. Moore
Ashland Specialty Ingredients

TABLE OF CONTENTS:

PART 11.2

IMAGING TECHNIQUES AND ANALYSIS FOR QUANTIFICATION OF SKIN APPEARANCE

Author:
Roger L. McMullen, Ph.D.
Principal Scientist
Materials Science Department
Ashland, Inc.
Bridgewater, NJ 08807

Adjunct Professor
School of Natural Sciences
Fairleigh Dickinson University
Teaneck, NJ 07666

TABLE OF CONTENTS:

PART 11.3

BIOPHYSICAL MEASUREMENT AND EVALUATION OF SKIN ELASTICITY AND TOPOGRAPHY

Authors:
Stefanie Luebberding, PhD
Nils Krueger, PhD

IRosenpark Research
Wilhelminenstrae 13
64283 Darmstadt (Germany)

TABLE OF CONTENTS:

PART 11.5

CLINICAL TESTING OF COSMETICS AND SKIN CARE PRODUCTS: METHODS AND INSTRUMENTATIONS

Author:
Iqbal Sadiq, M.Phil.
Director Research and Technology
Product Investigations, Inc.
151 East Tenth Ave., Conshohocken, PA 19428, USA

TABLE OF CONTENTS:

PART 3.1

SKIN MORPHOLOGY

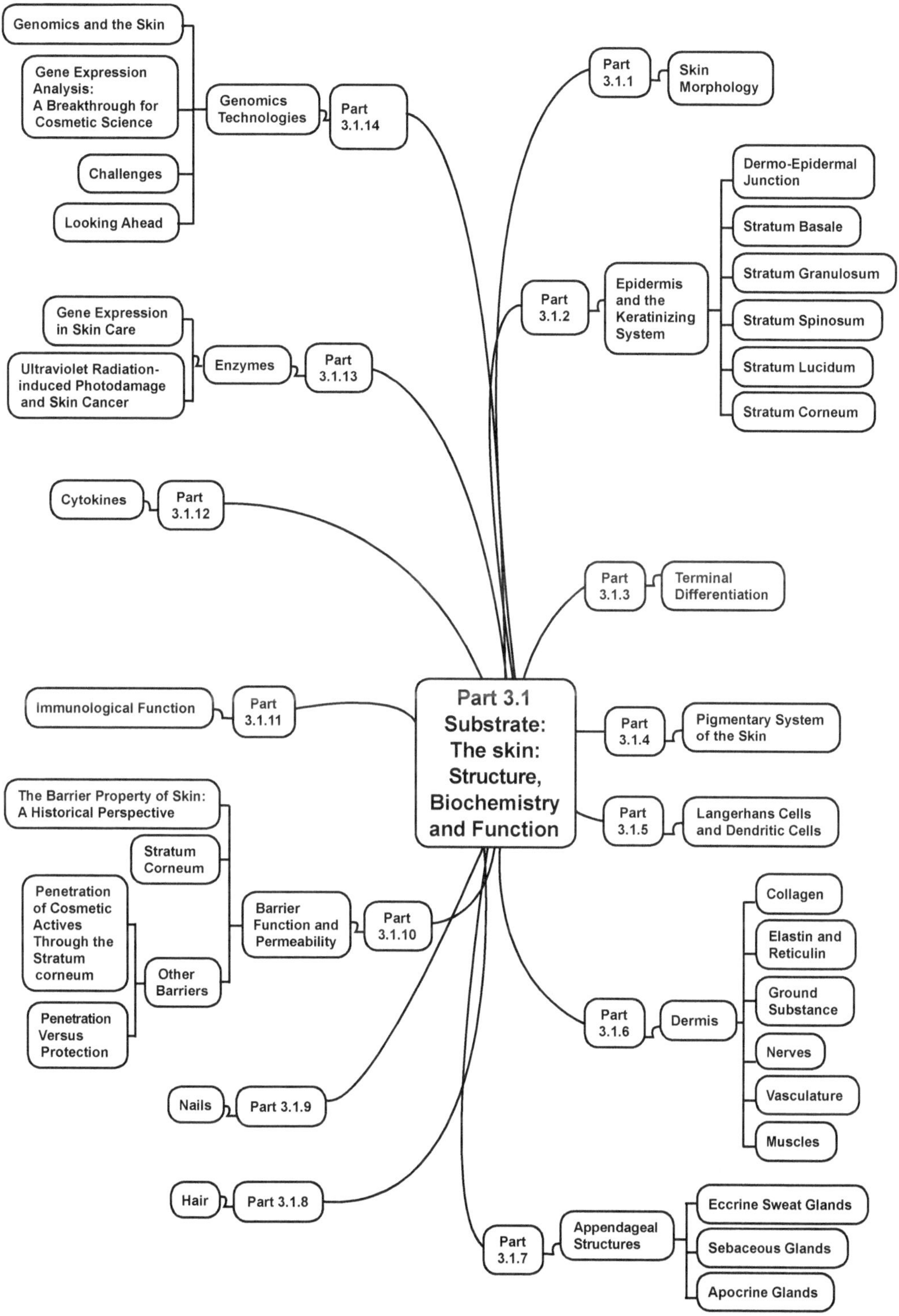

PART 3.1

THE SKIN: STRUCTURE, BIOCHEMISTRY, AND FUNCTION

Editor of The Substrates:

Bozena "Bo" B. Michniak-Kohn, Ph.D., M.R.Pharm.S.
Professor of Pharmaceutics
Ernest Mario School of Pharmacy

Director & Founder
Center for Dermal Research (CDR)
NJ Center for Biomaterials, Life Sciences Building
Rutgers—The State University of New Jersey
145, Bevier Road,
Piscataway, NJ 08854
www.michniaklab.org

CONTRIBUTORS:

1. Amy S. Pappert, M.D.
   Assistant Professor, Department of Dermatology
   UMDNJ—Robert Wood Johnson Medical School
   1 World's Fair Drive, Suite 2400 Somerset, NJ 08873

2. Philip Wertz, Ph.D.
   Professor Department of Oral Pathology, Radiology, and Medicine
   N450 DSB, Dows Institute
   University of Iowa
   Iowa City IA 52242

3. Nripen Sharma, Ph.D.
   Clinical Scientist/Project Manager/Technical Support
   Salvona Technologies LLC
   65 Stults Rd., Dayton, NJ 08810
   www.salvona.com

4. Anna Langerveld, Ph.D.
President and CEO
Genemarkers
4717 Campus Drive, Suite 1800
Kalamazoo, MI 49008
www.genemarkersllc.com

5. Ada Polla
Alchimie Forever, The Polla Beauty Group
1010 Wisconsin Avenue NW, Suite 201
Washington, DC 20007
www.alchimie-forever.com

6. Barbara Polla, M.D.
Medical Doctor
Alchimie Forever, The Polla Beauty Group
1010 Wisconsin Avenue NW, Suite 201
Washington, DC 20007

7. Anne Pouillot, MS
Director of Science of Alchimie Forever
Alchimie Forever, The Polla Beauty Group
1010 Wisconsin Avenue NW, Suite 201
Washington, DC 20007

8. Karen E. Burke, M.D., Ph.D.
Dermatologist
429 East 52nd Street
New York, New York 10022

9. Gopi Menon, Ph.D.
Senior Science Fellow
Ashland Specialty Ingredients
1361 Alps Road
Wayne, NJ

10. Nava Dayan Ph.D.
President
Dr. Nava Dayan LLC

ABSTRACT

The skin is the organ that forms the border between the organism and the environment. Skin prevents dehydration, stops the penetration of noxious foreign materials and microorganisms, cushions against mechanical shock, helps to maintain a constant body temperature, and transduces incoming stimuli. In order to perform these functions, skin must be maintained in good condition, an important objective for cosmetic formulators. For cosmetic and personal care scientists, whether they are concerned with the improvement of the skin by pharmacology or cosmeceuticals, with the prevention or repair of damage, an understanding of skin structure and function is essential. As such, this section has a primary focus upon these issues.

Further, the impact of light on skin and on skin aging has become so important in cosmetics that it too requires a complete discussion. This chapter is carefully and thoroughly designed to provide a basic knowledge of skin structure and function, thereby forming a sound foundation for the reader to understand key issues and provide stimulation towards the generation of new ideas and novel approaches for new ingredients, addressing the global quest for advanced cosmetic and personal care products.

TABLE OF CONTENTS

Part 3.1 Substrate:
The Skin: Structure, Biochemistry and Function

PART 3.1.1 SKIN MORPHOLOGY

The skin is divided into three layers: the epidermis, the dermis, and the subcutaneous tissue. The epidermis is the outermost layer of the skin and consists of a stratified squamous epithelium. Its thickness varies, depending on location, and varies from 0.05 mm to 1.5 mm. The epidermis is made up primarily of keratinocytes, whose basic function is to produce a filamentous protein, keratin, to serve as a protective barrier in combination with various lipid components. These cells also produce several other proteins, for example, cytokines, which play a role in the cutaneous inflammatory response. Separated from the epidermis by the basement membrane, the dermis is composed primarily of the so-called ground substance, which includes glycosaminoglycans (GAGs) and the structural protein collagen. Its thickness also varies with location from 0.3 mm to 3.0 mm. The dermis is divided into two layers: the papillary layer, which interdigitates with the epidermal rete ridges, and the reticular layer, which extends to the subcutaneous tissue. This deepest layer of the skin, also known as the subcutis or hypodermis, is composed primarily of lipocytes with fibrous septae providing structure and support (Fig. 1.1).

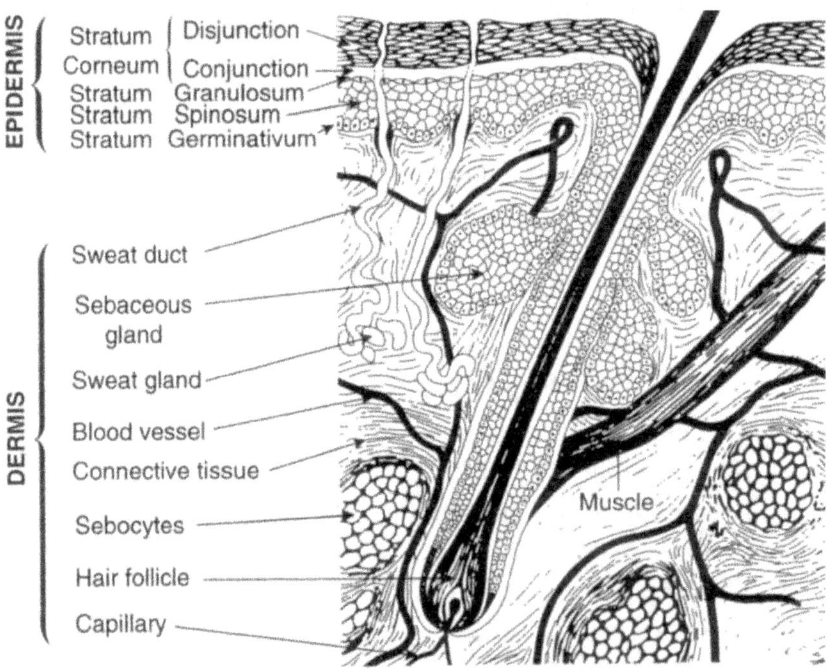

Figure 1.1 Diagram of normal human skin
(Reprinted from Harry's Cosmeticology 8th Ed.2000)

PART 3.1.2 EPIDERMIS AND THE KERATINIZING SYSTEM

The epidermis measures approximately 100 micrometers in thickness and consists of a number of layers: the innermost basal layer (*stratum basale* or *stratum germinativum*) which attaches to the basement membrane at the dermoepidermal junction, the prickle layer (*stratum spinosum*), the granular layer (*stratum granulosum*), the clear layer (*stratum lucidum*) and the horny layer (*stratum corneum*). Together the basal layer and the prickle layer comprise the Malpighian layer. The viable epidermis (the basal, prickle, and granular layers) consists of about 10 biologically active keratinocytes. The stratum corneum is located on top of the viable epidermis. The stratification into the layers is the result of changes in the keratinocytes as they mature and move outward from the basal layer, in which they are continuously formed by the mitosis of self-renewing progenitor cells, which lose their nuclei and are shed from the skin surface (Fig. 1.2).

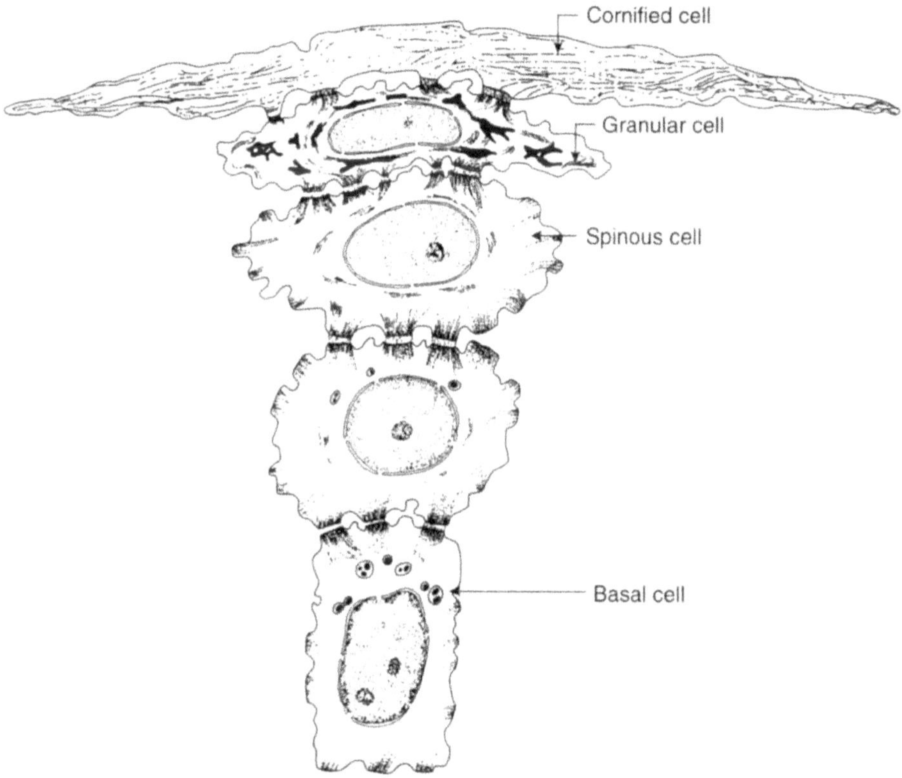

Figure 1.2. Conversion of individual basal keratinocytes into the flat cells of the stratum corneum (*Reprinted from Harry's Cosmeticology 8th Ed.2000*)

The replacement time for the whole epidermis is about 42 days and it is about 14 days for the *stratum corneum*. While the process of keratinization remains incompletely understood, in normal skin the desquamation of keratinocytes is in equilibrium with the generation of keratinocytes by mitosis of the proliferating cells. The importance of this equilibrium is best understood by studying examples of those skin diseases with abnormal keratinization. Abnormally rapid transformation of basal cells into horny cells of the *stratum corneum* occurs in psoriasis. *Ichthyosis vulgaris*, on the other hand, is a genetic disorder that results from abnormal retention of keratinocytes.

Three other cell types are present in the epidermis: melanocytes, the dendritic pigment-synthesizing cells; Langerhans cells, which are colorless and dendritic in form and perform functions related to immunology; and Merkel cells, which are concerned with sensation. The melanocytes and the Merkel cells are confined mainly to the basal layer, while the Langerhans cells are distributed in the basal, spinous, and granular layers.

a. Dermo-Epidermal Junction

The basement membrane zone forms the junction between the epidermis and the dermis. Under the electron microscope, it is seen to be composed of four components, listed from the outermost layer: the plasma membrane of the basal keratinocytes, the clear lamina lucida, the electron-dense basal lamina, and the dermal fibrils and bundles of fine filaments [1]. Some details of the components of this junction are provided in a later segment of this section.

b. Stratum Basale

The basal layer is a continuous layer of cells that gives rise to all the keratinocytes through mitotic activity. It is usually described as being one cell thick, but in thick normal or in pathological epidermis it appears that mitosis may not only be confined to cells in contact with the basement membrane. A portion of the basal cells is proliferative; these are the cells that differentiate and move up through the epidermis, eventually to become the components of the *stratum corneum* (essentially "dead" cells that are anuclear) and later desquamate at the top of the skin.

Cells of the *stratum basale* are cuboidal and have a basophilic cytoplasm and dark-staining, elongated nuclei; under the electron microscope their cytoplasm reveals many ribosomes, mitochondria, and in some cases smooth membranes. In addition, they contain numerous fine tonofilaments, about five nm in diameter, which form the developing cytoskeleton. The basal cells also often contain melanin, transferred from adjacent melanocytes. Intercellular bridges, or desmosomes, connect basal cells with one another and with the overlying squamous cells. Modified desmosomes, or hemidesmosomes, connect the basal cells to the underlying basement membrane zone.

c. Stratum Spinosum

The *stratum spinosum* is so called because the cells are given a spiny appearance by the numerous desmosomes. These desmosomes, or specialized attachment plates for the cellular tonofilaments, correlate with the intercellular bridges between keratinocytes. The glycocalyx is the intercellular cement between keratinocytes and is composed of glycoproteins. In the upper region of the stratum spinosum, lamellar granules, also known as keratinosomes or Ödland bodies, make their appearance. These are ovoid bodies about 100–500 nm long. In the *stratum granulosum* they ultimately migrate toward the periphery of the cell and are discharged into the intercellular spaces. Their appearance there correlates with the degradation of keratinocytes. Their lipid contents act to establish a barrier to water loss and may participate in *stratum corneum* cellular cohesion. Water loss, as is well known, is a critical phenomenon that is measured in the development of new skin care products and relates to some aspects of skin aging.

d. Stratum Granulosum

The thickness of the granular cell layer is usually proportional to the thickness of the *stratum corneum*. It may be only one cell layer thick in thin skin and up to ten layers in the thicker skin found on the palms and soles of the feet. The cells contain basophilic granules of a material called keratohyalin, a material thought to be responsible for keratin filament aggregation. The "hard" keratins of hair and nail lack these keratohyalin granules.

e. Stratum Lucidum

The *stratum lucidum*, not seen in most formalin-fixed sections, is located at the deepest portion of the *stratum corneum*. It can be recognized only in palmar and plantar skin.

f. Stratum Corneum

In the *stratum corneum* the keratinocytes have lost their nuclei and virtually all of their cytoplasmic organelles and contents, including the keratohyalin granules. This layer of cells is about 10–15 cells thick (approximately 10 micrometers) and is located on top of the viable epidermis. The corneal cell layer stains eosinophilic with the hematoxylin and eosin stain due to the absence of basophilic nuclei. The cells are flattened and completely filled with keratin. The keratin is in the form of bundles of filaments embedded in an opaque interfilamentous material. They align into disulfide cross-linked macrofibers under the influence of filaggrin, the protein component of the keratohyalin granule responsible for keratin filament aggregation [2].

The structure of the *stratum corneum* has been compared to that of a brick wall, with the corneocytes as bricks and the intercellular lipids as mortar [3]. Horny cells are continuously shed from the skin surface. *Stratum corneum* lipids have been characterized and consist of phospholipids, glucosylceramides, cholesterol, cholesterol sulfate, cholesterol esters, ceramides, and fatty acids [4]. The makeup of lipids suggests that hydrophilic lipids are excluded from the *stratum corneum* to provide a hydrophobic surface on the skin.

PART 3.1.3 TERMINAL DIFFERENTIATION

Terminal differentiation describes the change of the cuboidal keratinocytes (on the basement membrane) to the flat cellular remnants that are shed from the skin surface. The progressive changes of keratinocytes as illustrated in Figure 1.2 are accompanied by biochemical changes, formation of keratins, formation and hydrolytic changes in lipids, loss of water, and cross-linking of cell envelopes. The formation of keratins proceeds from the intermediate filaments present in keratinocytes. Intermediate filaments of more than 50 types are synthesized in human tissues. In skin, two types (I and II) are specifically expressed in epithelial cells. In this classification, acidic keratins (cytokeratins K9–K20) are identified as type I, while the basic keratins (cytokeratins K1–K8) are classified as type II. In skin, the keratins are customarily dimers of one type I and one type II. The fundamental structure of the intermediate filaments includes coil-coil alpha-helical segments bonded to each other by nonhelical linker segments. Both ends of the rod-shaped filament are terminated by peptides. The exact modus of attachment of these filaments to each other to form the keratins within the keratinocytes is still under investigation. As noted, epithelial cytoskeletal filaments generally belong to one of two keratin (acidic or neutral-basic) groups ranging in molecular weight from about 40 to 70 kDa. Fillaggrin has been identified as one of the keratohyalin proteins forms in differentiating keratinocytes. Filaggrin is involved in the aggregation of keratin filaments to form the keratins found in mature keratinocytes or corneal cells. After filaggrin has served its function as a matrix between intermediate filaments, it is hydrolyzed enzymatically to create various free amino acids that form part of the natural moisturizing factor (NMF).

The hydrolytic changes of the epidermal lipids are also controlled by keratinocytes, which discharge lipids into the intercellular space after forming the lamellar granules. These lipids are distinctly different from the sebaceous lipids secreted by the sebaceous glands. In the process of terminal differentiation, which requires about three to four weeks, the basal keratinocyte generates a remarkable set of complex lipids (e.g., ceramides). During the cells' passage outward, these lipids are modified (become more hydrophobic) to contribute to the biphasic structure commonly called *stratum corneum*.

During their ascent to the skin surface, the keratinocytes shrink, primarily through loss of water. The fate of this water is not known, but one may safely assume that it becomes part of the evaporating water generally described as trans-epidermal water loss. The loss of water during the maturation of keratinocytes is an important phenomenon that must be considered in studies of skin moisture levels (Fig. 1.3) and the impact of ingredients used in cosmetic and personal care products to improve the skin's ability to retain its moisture. The level of water in the basal layer is about that found in internal tissues, that is, about 80–85%. The water level drops stepwise to about 35% at the border between the *stratum granulosum* and the *stratum corneum*. The water level in the topmost layers of the skin is variable and is under the control of the environment and the evaporative flux from lower skin layers.

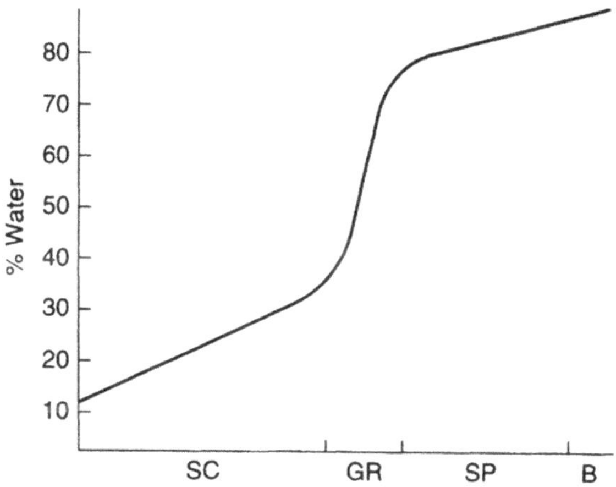

Figure 1.3. Water concentration profile in epidermal layers [SC—stratum corneum; GR—stratum granulosum; SP—stratum spinosum; B—basal layer (stratum germinativum. (*Reprinted from Harry's Cosmeticology 8th Ed.2000*)

Finally, the proteins in the cell membranes of the maturing keratinocytes undergo drastic changes due to cross-linking. This provides the terminally differentiated corneal cell with a rigid cell envelope that is chemically resistant and acts as a protective coating. The most important enzymes that play a role in this process are transglutaminases that catalyze epsilon- (gamma-glutamyl) lysine crosslinking. Involucrin is the primary cytoplasmic precursor to the protein making up the cell envelope. Other cross-linked proteins are present and have been identified—for example, loricrin.

Biologists have further identified some layers within the *stratum corneum*. The desquamating layer at the surface is frequently called the *stratum corneum* disjunction, while the layer below it is known as *stratum corneum* conjunction. To complete this highly simplified discussion of the skin, it is important to note that the latter is frequently identified as viable epidermis. Cells from this layer can be cultured and are commonly used to study the release of cytokines and the like as well as the impact of drugs and/or cosmetic ingredients. In contrast, the nonviable epidermis includes only the dead cells of the *stratum corneum.*

Before leaving the life history of the epidermis, the process of differentiation should be considered as proceeding from the inside to the exterior. The outward movement of biological debris, water, and lipids directly opposes human efforts to drive ingredients/drugs into and through the skin unless special efforts are made to create molecules that are shaped and manipulated to permeate.

PART 3.1.4 PIGMENTARY SYSTEM OF THE SKIN

Melanocytes are dendritic cells that produce and secrete melanosomes, which contain melanin. Melanin is the major determinant of skin color. The number of melanocytes in the epidermis is the same—regardless of skin color; it is rather the number and size of melanosomes produced that determine the color of one's skin. Melanosomes in dark skin are nonaggregated, whereas they are smaller and form membrane-bound complexes in light skin. Melanocytes are derived from the neural crest in the embryo and are seen in the basal layer of the epidermis by the eighth week of gestation. They differ from the other cells of the *stratum basale* by the possession of dendritic processes, by which they transfer pigment to a group of keratinocytes; the whole forming the "epidermal melanin unit" [5]. Typically each melanocyte is associated with about 36–40 keratinocytes in the human epidermis. Melanocytes have no desmosomes and thus, when stained with hematoxylin and eosin, appear to have a halo due to the separation from adjacent keratinocytes. The concentration of melanocytes, though, does vary in different areas of the skin, with the highest concentration on the face and the male genitalia and the lowest concentration on the trunk.

The characteristic feature of melanocytes is a special cytoplasmic organelle known as a melanosome in which the melanin is formed by the action of the enzyme tyrosinase. The melanosomes arise as spherical, membrane-bound vesicles in the zone of the Golgi apparatus and eventually appear as densely pigmented granules [6].

Melanins consist of two kinds of quinoid polymers: pheomelanins and eumelanins. Pheomelanins are yellow or red in color, and eumelanins produce the brown or black color. Both are formed by the same initial steps, which involve oxidation of tyrosine to 3,4-dihydroxyphenylalanine (DOPA) and its dehydrogenation to DOPAquinone. The formation of eumelanins then involves several further steps to produce indole-5,6-quinone, which polymerizes and becomes linked to protein. It is now believed that eumelanin is not a homopolymer composed solely of indole-5,6-quinone units but rather a poikilopolymer that includes several intermediates. Pheomelanins are formed by a different route. The DOPA-quinone interacts with cysteine to form 5-S- and 2-S-cysteinyldopa, and these isomers are further oxidized to a series of intermediates that then polymerize [7].

The formation of melanin depends on the generation of free radical species. The biochemical pathways leading to the formation of melanin pigments *in vivo* were described by Raper [8] and more recently by Prota [9, 10]. This information can be found in most textbooks of biochemistry and is not repeated here. Once formed, melanin has been identified as a (stable?) free radical that can react with superoxide.

The significance of melanin as a purported photoprotectant and the response of skin to ultraviolet (UV) irradiation are critically important to skin appearance and health, especially with regard to sun exposure.

PART 3.1.5 LANGERHANS CELLS AND DENDRITIC CELLS

The skin provides the first line of immune surveillance against biologic pathogens and chemical irritants through a network of sophisticated and specialized antigen-presenting cells. These include Langerhans cells (LCs) in the epidermis and several distinct types of interstitial dendritic cells (DCs) in the dermis. LCs and DCs are the sentinels that recognize certain antigens as well as recognizing tumors. For example, they recognize foreign environmental antigens such as irritating chemicals (thereby inducing contact hypersensitivity), microorganisms (thus protecting through antimicrobial immunity). They also recognize tumors (providing antitumor immunity) and allogeneic markers (causing skin graft rejection).

The extended dendrites of these unique cells form a network within the epidermis and in the dermis they create an immunologic barrier primed to recognize, capture, and process pathogens and foreign antigens for presentation to naïve and memory T-lymphocytes, thereby initiating and then modulating the subsequent immune response. Furthermore, the LCs and DCs play a significant role in inducing peripheral immunologic tolerance to innocuous environmental proteins and to self-antigens, thus helping to prevent autoimmune disease.

LCs are the epidermal resident dendritic cell population. They make up about 3–5% of the suprabasal, *stratum spinosum* layer of the epidermis [11] including the mucosal epithelia lining the ocular oral and vaginal surfaces [12]. LCs are scattered without desmosomal connections between keratinocytes. In light microscopic sections, LCs cannot be detected by routine histologic staining, but only by staining with gold chloride (for human LCs).

LCs are characteristically stellate with extensive dendritic fibers stretching in all directions, forming a network within the *stratum spinosum* layer. When viewed by phase contrast microscopy, the DCs extend delicate flower-like projections that bend, retract, and reextend. This shape and motility enable them to accomplish their function of capturing antigens and of selecting and processing the antigens for specific T-cells [13]. By means of high-powered electron microscopy, LCs have been shown to be a folded nucleus and are identified by their distinctive, intracytoplasmic *Birbeck granules* that (when mature) are rod shaped with a vacuole at one end, resembling a tennis racquet. Antigen capture seems to be a consequence of binding to langerin, a calcium-dependent lectin that specifically binds mannose as well as other sugars and is found only in LCs and some dermal DCs [14]. This binding actually induces formation of Birbeck granules and then routes the antigen into the Birbeck granules for further processing.

Langerin is a recognition receptor for carbohydrates on the surfaces of pathogens that routes antigens to different cellular compartments involved in antigen presentation in order to promote recognition by different specific T-cells [15].

In addition to LCs, the skin has at least four other subclasses of DCs in the dermis. The characterization of these DCs is quite complex because DCs can arise from several types of progenitor cells, and different functional phenotypes of DCs can be generated from the same precursor cell (as determined by function required, generating a sequential encounter with specific cytokines). Furthermore, as the LCs and DCs encounter a foreign antigen and migrate, they mature, and their surface markers as well as their functional interactions change. Thus, the steady-state population is different from the inflammatory response populations.

Langerhans cell function is impaired by UVB radiation, resulting in a decrease in the antigen-presenting capacity and in the production of cytokines. This UV suppression leads not only to adverse consequences by impairing endogenous antimicrobial activity and tumor recognition and suppression, but also to possible advantageous therapeutic treatments for skin allergy and inflammatory disease.

PART 3.1.6 DERMIS

The dermis is a tough and resilient tissue that cushions the body against mechanical injury and provides nutrients to the epidermis and cutaneous appendages [16]. It consists of an association of protein fibers within an amorphous ground substance containing glycosaminoglycans (GAGs), previously known as mucopolysaccharides. There are few cells in this matrix; most of them are fibroblasts, which secrete the dermal constituents. Fibroblasts are derived from the mesenchyme. The mast cell, also of mesenchymal origin, houses granules that contain heparin, histamine, and other active substances. The mast cell is an active participant in skin inflammation and irritation, as well as in several other skin disorders. The dermis also houses blood, contains lymphatic and nervous systems, and surrounds the invaginated epidermal appendages. The GAGs in the dermis can hold copious amounts of water and tend to surround the other constitutents of the matrix. Together with the fibrous portion of the matrix, these substances account for the skin's flexibility and resistance to deformation.

a. Collagen

The major fibrous constituent of the dermis, accounting for 75% of the dry weight and 18–30% of the volume, is collagen [17]. Under the light microscope, collagen fibers appear as eosinophilic branching wavy bands. Collagen fibers are loosely arranged in the papillary dermis and are tightly bundled in the reticular dermis. Pilosebaceous units, eccrine glands, and apocrine and dermal blood vessels are surrounded by a thin meshwork of collagen. Collagen fibers display characteristic cross-striations with a periodicity of 60–70 nm. Collagen is rich in the amino acids hydroxyproline, hydroxylysine, and glycine. The fibroblasts produce a precursor known as procollagen, which includes 300–400 additional amino acids in each of its chains; these extensions are removed after secretion, which results in the conversion to the collagen molecule. Collagen fibrils form by the association of collagen molecules. Vitamin C and copper are two of several cofactors required in the biosynthesis of collagen. Collagen production is a dynamic process that involves continual synthesis by fibroblasts and degradation by collagenases.

b. Elastin and Reticulin

Elastic fibers make up only 4% of the dry weight and 1% of the volume of the dermis. They are delicate, straight, freely branching fibers that prove very resilient. These fibers are thicker in the lower portion of the dermis and become thinner as they approach the epidermis. Elastin differs from collagen not only structurally but also chemically. Desmosine is an amino acid unique to elastin. About 0.4% of the dry weight of the dermis is made up of fine branching fibers that, unlike collagen, stain black with silver stains and are known as reticulin. Their axial periodicity is identical to that of collagen. Reticulin fibers in the papillary dermis serve to anchor the basal lamina [17].

c. Ground Substance

The amorphous ground substance in which the fibers and cells lie contains acidic GAGs. In dermis the major forms are hyaluronic acid, chondroitin sulfate, and dermatan sulfate.

d. Nerves

The skin is supplied with both sensory and autonomic nerves. It is innervated with about one million afferent nerve fibers; most terminate in the face and extremities, and relatively few supply the back. The sensory nerves, unlike autonomic nerves, possess a myelin sheath up to their terminal ramifications.

The papillary dermis is heavily innervated with unmyelinated nerve fibers that transmit the sensations of temperature, pain, and pruritus. Three types of special nerve end organs also exist in the dermis. Vater-Pacini corpuscles are large end-organs that are located in the deeper portions of the dermis and subcutis and mediate a sense of pressure. They measure up to 1 mm in diameter and have their greatest concentration at the tips of the fingers and toes. A few are present in the nipple and anogenital regions. Meissner corpuscles are located in the dermal papillae and mediate the sense of touch. They occur only on the ventral aspects of the hands and feet and are most concentrated in the fingertips. The mucocutaneous end-organs are found in the papillary dermis of the modified hairless skin of the glans, the prepuce, the clitoris, the labia minora, the perianal region, and the vermilion border. The autonomic nervous system supplies fibers to the arrector pili muscles, the blood vessels, and the eccrine and apocrine glands. The sebaceous glands are not innervated, and their functioning depends on endocrine stimuli. The autonomic nervous system controls vasoconstriction, contraction of the arrector pili muscles, and glandular secretion.

e. Vasculature

The dermal vasculature consists of intercommunicating plexuses. The subpapillary plexus lies within the papillary dermis and runs parallel to the epidermis to furnish a supply of capillaries, arterioles, and venules to the dermal papillae. The deeper plexuses are composed of larger vessels and surround hair follicles and eccrine glands. The dermal lymphatics are associated with the vascular plexuses.

f. Muscles

Smooth muscle occurs in the skin as the arrector pili muscles of the hair to pull the follicle upward with contraction. There are also smooth muscles fibers in the scrotum and the areolas. Striated muscle occurs in the skin within the neck as the platysmas and in the muscles of expression of the face. Special aggregates of smooth muscles are found between the arterioles and the venules in the skin. These serve to shunt blood from the arterial to the venous system directly and thus bypass the capillary system.

PART 3.1.7 APPENDAGEAL STRUCTURES

a. Eccrine Sweat Glands

Humans have several million eccrine sweat glands distributed over most skin sites, but they are more concentrated in the axilla, forehead, palms, and soles. In some areas they number as many as 600 glands per square cm. Eccrine sweat glands are the most numerous skin appendages and are responsible for the production of sweat. They have a cylindrical spiral duct lined with epidermal cells extending from their visible opening in the epidermis down into the deep dermis, where the duct becomes coiled and convoluted into a ball [18]. This secretory coil manufactures the odorless sweat, which rises up the duct to be released on the skin surface. It is thought that the duct of the gland has the ability to modify the sweat as it flows upward by removing salts or water.

The sweat glands control both body temperature and excretion, and they are under the control of the cholinergic nervous system. The evaporation of sweat has a cooling effect. The glands respond to environmental temperature but also to other stimuli, such as UV light, emotional stress, and increases in body temperature. On the palms and soles, the secretion from the glands serves to increase surface friction.

Sweating appears to involve activation of myoepithelial cells, which line the ducts of the glands. Although sweating is considered to be a continuous process, it seems that sweat is ejected in small bursts, suggesting a peristaltic action by the ducts. The composition of eccrine sweat is similar to that of plasma, although more dilute, and was documented about 40 years ago. It includes, in decreasing relative concentration (mg %): Cl^- (320), Na^+ (200), lactic acid (35), K^+ (20), urea (15), ammonia (5), Ca^{++} (2), glucose (2), Mg^{++} (1), amino acid (1), and creatinine (0.3).

b. Apocrine Glands

The apocrine glands are tubular glands attached to the hair follicle and, like the sebaceous glands, develop in association with it [19]. Although rudiments are found covering the entire surface of the fetus, the glands become canalized and functional almost exclusively in selective areas including: the axillae, the anogenital regions, the areola, the external auditory canal, and the eyelids. In humans, apocrine gland secretions are milky and viscous but without odor. Odor production is related to bacterial action on apocrine secretions at the skin surface.

After puberty, apocrine gland secretion is in response to emotive stimuli. Adrenergic nerves control secretory activity, in contrast to the cholinergic control of eccrine function. The function of the glands in the human species has been much debated; studies have demonstrated that the apocrine skin glands of mammals produce various glycoconjugates and antimicrobial substances, which may serve as a nonspecific defense on the skin surface [20]. In other mammals the glands serve a sexual function.

c. Sebaceous Glands

Sebaceous glands [18] secrete sebum, which forms the majority of the lipid that covers the skin and hair. They are found in all areas of human skin except the palms, soles, and dorsum of the feet. Sebaceous glands are usually associated with hair follicles, except for those on the nipples, areola, and labia minora. The greatest concentrations (reportedly as high as 400–900/cm) are found on the scalp, face, upper chest, and shoulders.

The glands are holocrine and thus form their secretion by decomposition of their cells. New cells are formed continually from the lining of the gland by cell division to replace those lost. No motor innervation has been demonstrated in humans. During the generation of sebum, cells at the periphery of the lobule undergo division. As the daughter cell moves toward the center of the lobule, it synthesizes lipids. As the sebum accumulates, the cell increases in volume as much as 150-fold. When synthesis is complete cell rupture occurs. This process from cell division to rupture requires approximately 14 days. The relatively long delay must be taken into consideration when designing drugs, cosmeceuticals, and therapies aimed at altering sebum.

Sebaceous gland activity is under hormonal control. It is stimulated by androgens of both gonadal and adrenal origin. In human males the glands are minute during the prepubertal period but undergo vast enlargement at puberty, when their output increases more than fivefold. Eunuchs secrete about half as much sebum as normal males but substantially more than boys; it seems that the secretion is dependent on adrenal androgens. Adult women secrete only a little less than men; their sebaceous activity appears to be maintained by androgens from the ovary and the adrenal cortex. Estrogens and anti-androgens, such as cyproterone acetate, inhibit sebaceous secretion in humans. On the other hand, relatively small doses of potent androgens can cause enlargement of the glands and an increase in sebum production.

Human sebum is composed of triglycerides (57.5%), wax esters (26.0%), squalene (12.0%), free fatty acids (10%), and, to a minor extent, cholesterol and cholesterol esters. Epidermally derived lipids differ in lacking wax esters and squalene and having much higher proportions of cholesterol esters and cholesterol. There are marked differences in sebum composition among species. The origins of sebaceous lipids and their composition are different from those of the epidermal lipids [21]. The purpose of sebum is not entirely understood, but sebum has been shown to have thermoregulatory functions, and plays a role in the regulation of immunological functions and inflammatory processes. In addition, sebum contains lipids with antimicrobial activity [22]. While excessive sebum production has been associated with the development of acne vulgaris, lack of sebum production in prepubertal children is not associated with any skin abnormalities.

PART 3.1.8 HAIR

The hair follicle is quite variable, depending on its location. In adults, deep terminal hairs are found on the scalp and male beard area. Hair on the extremities and trunk is located more superficially in the skin. Vellus hairs are present on the female face and on the nonbearded areas of the male face. Lanugo is soft fine hair that covers the fetus and is shed prior to birth.

In general, the cross-sectional shape of terminal Caucasian scalp hair is round and somewhat curly; African American scalp hair is oval, sometimes flattened, and usually kinky; hair in Asians is round in cross-section and straight. These relationships do not apply to pubic hair, beard hair, and eyelashes, which have similar features in all races and are typically oval.

Hair color is due to the distribution of melanosomes within the hair shaft produced by melanocytes in the hair bulb. These are transferred to cells of the hair matrix similar to the transfer from melanocytes to keratinocyte in the epidermis. Three types of melanosomes are present in hair. Eumelanins are seen in dark hair, and pheomelanins predominate in blond hair. The intensity of color is related to the number of fully melanized melanosomes produced. Gray hair and white hair are due to a decreased number of melanocytes that produce fewer melanosomes.

Despite the vast body of knowledge regarding the anatomy, biology, and function of hair, humans are still unable to induce hair regrowth in the many disorders that result in hair loss, or to induce permanent hair removal in states of excessive hair. The cost of hair care in terms of time and money spent is huge in many cultures, and the psychological impact of hair disorders should not be underestimated.

PART 3.1.9 NAILS

The nail plate is composed of keratinized cells that originate in the nail matrix. As discussed previously, there are no keratohyalin granules. The proximal nail fold forms the cuticle. The nailbed does not contribute to the development of the nail plate but serves as a base for the adherent keratinous nail plate.

PART 3.1.10 BARRIER FUNCTION AND PERMEABILITY

For the cosmetic industry, by and large, the skin has been synonymous with the epidermal permeability barrier, located in the *stratum corneum*. This is a somewhat restricted view, but nevertheless remains in place due to the fact that skin moisturization—a function that is of prime interest to the industry—is dependent on a functional permeability barrier. As the saying goes, a good moisturizer is not necessarily a barrier product, but all barrier products are good moisturizers. The two-compartment, "brick and mortar" organization of the healthy *stratum corneum*, with its organized lipid membranes, do "lock in" moisture and prevent dry, chapped skin. However, the significance of other types of barriers in the skin, i.e., UV barrier, antioxidant, and antimicrobial defenses have all begun to be appreciated and emphasized, as evidenced by the proliferation of active ingredients targeted to them. This growing recognition, in concert with an improved understanding of the other areas of the skin, is critically important to novel thinking leading to new functional ingredients for this important cosmetic and personal care category.

a. The Barrier Property of Skin: A Historical Perspective

The barrier property of skin against influx and efflux of water was acknowledged as early as the 1800s, but the conclusive evidence was provided by the work of Irvin Blank and Scheuplein, who convincingly demonstrated its location in the *stratum corneum* (horny layer) [23]. The barrier properties are of interest to different scientific disciplines and industry; especially the pharmaceutical and personal care sectors that are interested in delivering drugs transdermally or active ingredients for topical delivery to improve the skin conditions (anti-aging, moisturizers, skin lighteners, etc.) respectively. For the dermatologists, inherited and acquired skin diseases such as various types of ichthyosis, atopic dermatitis, and psoriasis all have a compelling barrier dysfunction associated with it [24]. Extensive damage to the barrier, as in third-degree burns, can be lethal; attesting to the significance of a functional permeability barrier to prevent life-threatening dehydration of the body.

Details of barrier (and *stratum corneum*) formation, its structural complexity, and chemical characterization

Early investigators interpreted what appeared as a "basket weave" structure of the SC in routine histological studies as an indication that it is a passively occluding structure on the skin surface—a more or less uniform membrane functioning like "Saran wrap." Investigators who followed them have dispelled the notion of the SC as a "basket weave" structure passively occluding the surface. A battery of investigative techniques (electron microscopy, laser confocal microscopy, two-photon microscopy, as well as biochemical characterization of lipids and proteins) have led to the understanding first of a "brick and mortar" organization of SC, and a later concept of the SC as being a composite material with several characteristics of a "smart" material [24]. In this latest model, the bulk of the SC is made up of corneocytes, which are the "bricks."

Before discussing the secretion of the lamellar lipids (pro-barrier lipids) and the further processing of the lipids in the SC extracellular domains (the "mortar"), a brief description of a multiplicity of the phenomena that occur in the SC is warranted.

These phenomena include: a description of the keratinocyte differentiation, synthesis of proteins (keratins, filaggrin, involucrin, loricrin, desmosomal components, enzymes involved in cornification) and lipids (which are packaged with lipid metabolizing enzymes and anti-microbial peptides within secretory organelles) in the form of lamellar bodies (Odland bodies, keratinosomes).

Keratinocytes (keratinizing epithelia) account for about 95% of the stratified epidermis (other cell types are melanocytes, Langerhans cells, Merkel cells), and based on its position within the strata as well as its progressive differentiation, is designated as belonging to several layers including: the basal layer (*stratum basale*), the spinous layer (*stratum spinosum*), the granular layer (*stratum granulosum*), and the cornified layer (*stratum corneum*). Epidermal stem cells that usually contribute to the maintenance of the interfollicular epidermis are located within the stratum basale. Their division (either symmetric or asymmetric) replenishes the keratinocyte population as cells from the basal layer move to the suprabasal layers and progressively undergo differentiation.

Stratum basale is made up of one layer of columnar basal cells attached to the basement membrane via hemidesmosomes. These cells display a high nucleo-cytoplasmic ratio, cell organelles like mitochondria and RER, as well as keratin filaments inserting into the hemidesmosomes. The cells also connect to the adjacent cells as well as those of the suprabasal cells via desmosomes. Biomarker proteins for the basal cells are keratins K14 and K5.

The *spinous* or prickly layer (*stratum spinosum*) above the *stratum basale* is named for its characteristic histological appearance due to the large numbers of desmosomes. In addition to the typical cell organelles, these cells often display a few lipid-enriched epidermal lamellar bodies (Odland bodies, keratinosomes, membrane coating granules). These will be described later in this section.

The biomarkers that distinguish this layer from the basal layer are keratins K1 and K10. *S.spinosum* also shows an increase in keratin filament content compared to *S.basale*. In the upper layers of *S.spinosum*, the cells begin to elongate and become slightly flattened. Above this layer is the *stratum granulosum*, a few layers of cells that are characterized by the presence of distinct, darkly staining (histological preparations) keratohyalin granules (KHK), composed of profilaggrin, loricrin, and a cystine-rich protein as well as keratins 1 and 10. The filaggrin subunits of profilaggrin play the role of matrix molecules to aggregate and align the keratin filaments.

In the upper granular layers of *stratum spinosum*, the keratin filaments are highly phosphorylated and have an extensive population of disulfide bonds compared to the cell layers below. As the cells of *stratum granulosum* stratify and differentiate, both the protein and lipid synthesis is ramped up, as evidenced from the boost in involucrin, KHKs, and LBs. In fact, the uppermost SG cells show an abundance of LBs (about 20% of the cell volume), which are apically polarized and poised to be secreted out. These details are not seen in histological preparations, but electron microscopy reveals both the internal structure of LBs, as well as tortuous and complex invaginations of the apical cell membrane at the *stratum granulosum–stratum corneum* interface. Secreted contents of LBs fill the interstices between the SG, and the overlying layer of *stratum corneum*, which still remain connected by means of desmosomes. The transition between the granular cell and the corneocyte presumably occurs within the span of a few hours, in response to several signals that involve but are not limited to an influx of calcium ions. The calcium signaling activates Ca++ dependant transglutaminase, which catalyzes the cross-linking of involucrin and loricrin. This process then forms a toughened "cornified envelope" immediately subjacent to the cell membrane. The phenomenon is also accompanied by dissolution of the nucleus, as well as cytosolic organelles, mediated by caspases, especially caspase 14. In fortuitous sections, electron microscopy captures the images of the "transitional cell," while the images primarily display an abrupt transition between the nucleated SG and the non-nucleated, flattened, organelle-depleted and keratin-filled corneocytes (Figure 1).

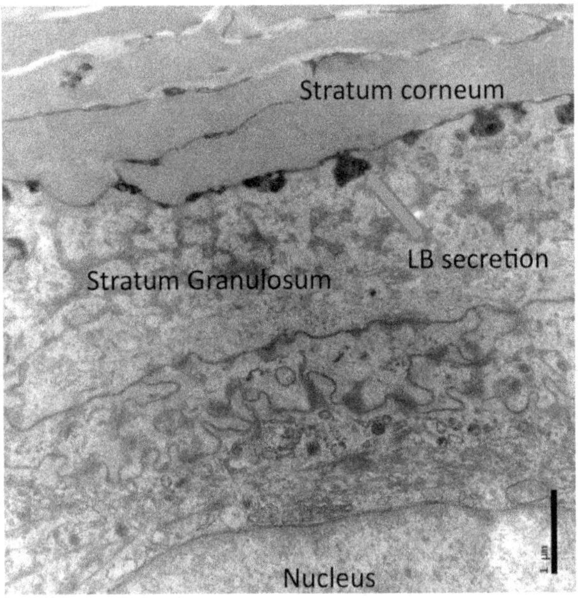

Figure 1 (Conventional TEM shows terminal differentiation of nucleated keratinocytes to keratin filled, non-nucleated corneocytes)

Conventional electron microscopy has illustrated the nature of the SC organization (Reference Fig 1), which consists of the secretion of epidermal lamellar bodies (enriched in cholesterol, sphingolipids, fatty acids, and a battery of enzymes and antimicrobial peptides) at the *stratum granulosum–stratum corneum* interface. Hydrophilic tracers (such as colloidal lanthanum) injected subcutaneously have been used to visualize its efflux (and hence of water) through the epidermis. This efflux is blocked at the SG–SC interface where the LB contents occlude the extracellular space [25].

The lamellar bodies are organelles, ranging from 0.2 to 0.5 microns in diameter, which originate from the Golgi apparatus, and begin to appear from the *stratum spinosum* and increase in numbers towards the upper *stratum granulosum*. In the uppermost SG, they occupy nearly 20% of the cell volume, and are polarized towards the apical surface. A recent proteomic investigation [26] identified up to 985 different proteins within the LBs. Freeze fracture studies [27] as well as ruthenium tetroxide post-fixation techniques [28, 29] have unraveled the sequence of events that follow the secretion of epidermal lamellar bodies (Figure 2) (i.e., the fusion of disk-like contents of the LBs into multiple lamellae that occlude the intercellular spaces of the SC). Cytochemical localization, as well as experimental studies with various enzyme inhibitors, delineated the role of enzymes (lipases, phospholipase, sphingomyelinase, B glucocerebrosidase, cholesterol sulfatase) in conversion of these disks into compact lamellar structures that surround the corneocytes akin to the mortar in a brick (corneocytes) wall [4, 30-35]. Investigations on animal models with specific gene defects or knockouts further extended the knowledge on enzymes such as B glucocerebrosidase [36], stearoyl CoA desaturase (SCD) [37], and Elov 14, which are involved in elongation of long-chain fatty acids crucial for ceramides [38, 39] as critical to barrier competency. In addition, proteolytic enzymes like kallikreins that lead to progressive dissolution of the corneodesmosomes for orderly desquamation of corneocytes [40, 41] and antimicrobial peptides such as beta defensins and cathelicidins [42] are co-localized to the lamellar bodies and within the extracellular matrix of SC, linking the formation of permeability barrier with an antimicrobial barrier [43] and innate immunity.

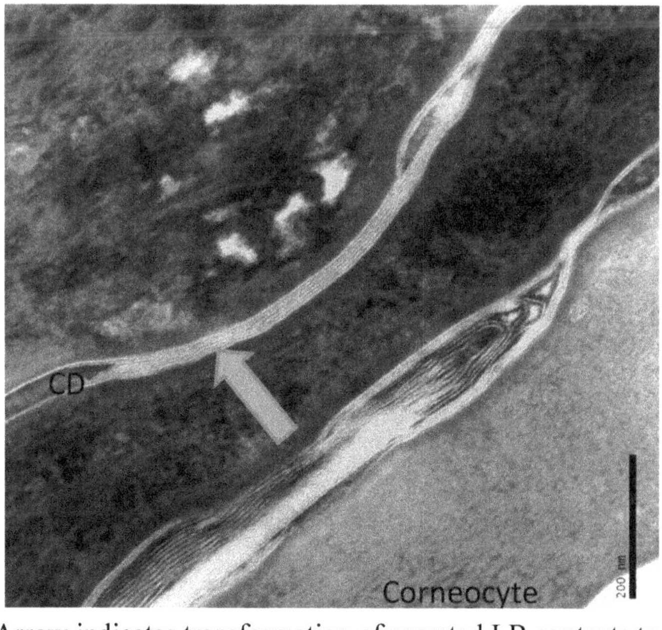

Figure 2 (Arrow indicates transformation of secreted LB contents to tight lamellae in upper SC)

The epidermal lamellar bodies initially considered to be discrete organelles (0.2 to 0.5 micrometers in diameter) were later found to form an interconnected network within the cells of the *stratum granulosum* [44], enabling a well-coordinated secretion in response to acute barrier disruption, as in tape stripping. Conventional TEM of a lamellar body in perfect cross-section shows the disc structures well, but not all LBs show such crisp morphology, a fact thought to reflect the plane of sectioning (oblique sections or grazing sections along the outer surface). LBs deficient in internal contents ("motheaten appearance") characterize a variety of skin dysfunctions [25], which correlate with permeability barrier defects and increased TEWL. Lamellar bodies are also crucial to the formation of "acid mantle" of the SC, which is of considerable interest to the cosmetic and personal care industry. These fascinating organelles consist of something resembling a cross between a lysosome and a secretory vesicle. They transport and secrete a diverse variety of molecules including: lipids, lipases, proteases, protease inhibitors, beta-glucocerebrosidase, antimicrobial peptides, etc.). An exhaustive proteomic and immunocytochemical analysis of lamellar-body enriched fractions and skin [26] identified about 985 proteins from the LB-enriched fraction: some secreted proteins, those with potential roles in desquamation, lysosomal proteins, related to transport and secretion of LBs, as well as proteins with putative roles in sorting of the LB cargo. It is possible that several subpopulations of LBs exist, and that the morphological diversity seen in electron micrographs may indeed reflect the pleomorphism of LBs, relating to either their contents or functional status. For example, hBD-2, which is virtually absent in normal skin keratinocytes, is induced when stimulated by cytokines or bacteria, and are localized to LB [45]. Most probably, some LBs synthesized in response to the bacterial challenge (LBS designed for microbial barrier?) must have a disproportionate content of the antimicrobial peptide (AMP), and it was speculated that pro-barrier lipids may not be the predominant components of this subpopulation [46]. They also may look different (deficient in lipids) or imperfect under the electron microscope. Could this be the basis of some of the abnormal, deficient LBs seen in various skin diseases such as psoriasis where keratinocytes show a high expression of AMPs? The study by Raymond et al. [26] showing 31 LB proteins corresponded to lysosomal components suggest that LBs are a new class of secretory lysosomes. Hence on a broad biological basis, they could be considered as "exolysosomes" involved in the matrix remodeling of the SC, or its exfoliation (the same way that lysosomes function in the molt of crustacean integument).

b. Stratum corneum

As the major barrier to flux of chemicals, water and other molecules into the skin, SC penetration pathways have attracted considerable attention. Since the SC is a two-compartment, composite system, three different routes of penetration have been proposed: transcellular, intercellular, and trans-appendageal (follicular) pathways (see for more details in the next section of this chapter). Much of the experimental results support the follicular and the intercellular pathway models. The intercellular pathway through the lipid domains is a tortuous path, and possibly both nonpolar and polar pathways are localized to this region. A true transcellular pathway (envisioned as a network of micro- or nano-channels) may only be opened up with the aid of microneedles or power-jet (gene gun) types of devices. The polar pathway may be located intercellularly and comprises aqueous regions surrounded by polar lipids, which create the walls of such microchannels as surmised by results of experiments designed to elucidate the contribution of extracellular lipids and intracellular keratin to the structure of this pathway. This has been demonstrated by means of using baclofen, a model zwitterion, *in vitro* using human cadaver skin [47]. This contention is in conformity with the morphological characterization of a "pore pathway" through the mortar lipids, as proposed by Menon and Elias [48].

c. Other Barriers:

Other effective barriers in skin are antimicrobial barriers (AMP-mediated), immune barriers (innate and adaptive) mediated by Langerhans cells, oxidant barriers (keratinocyte and sebocyte derived antioxidants), and barrier to UV radiation (melanin-mediated). These diverse barriers are interdependent components of the skin barrier, as exemplified by facts that the permeability barrier recovery is faster/more efficient in darkly pigmented skin; the Langerhans cells are affected by a breach in the permeability barrier; and antimicrobial peptide synthesis is also upregulated by challenges to permeability barrier.

As the tight junctions are also crucial for epidermal permeability barrier (the knockout models develop defective epidermal lipid synthesis and secretion), it is interesting to note that the Langerhans cells have been reported to extend their dendrites through the TJs, during the "search" mode when they scan the sub-SC domains for any sensitizers that have crossed the primary barrier. Such phenomena have only recently gained the attention of scientists and the appreciation of the cosmetic and personal care industry.

d. Penetration of Cosmetic Actives Through the Stratum Corneum

One of the most recurring debates in cosmetics has to do with the penetration of ingredients. How do manufacturers ensure optimal and targeted penetration of ingredients for efficacy at specific locations within the structure? What is the optimal penetration? How do water, lipophilic molecules, liposomes, or nanoparticles penetrate (if at all) through the *stratum corneum*, deep in the epidermis and below? From a scientific point of view, these questions are imperative towards the industry's goals of achieving improvements in compromised skin or anti-aging effects. We point out that the (global) regulatory definitions and distinctions drawn between "drugs" and "cosmetics" are carefully excluded in this scientific discussion and merely note that if one is to actually impact the multiplicity of biological phenomena occurring in the skin, then, inevitably, the schism between the legal definitions of "drug" and "cosmetic" must merge into a single "zone," and the difficulties in defining the zone are indeed a challenge for all concerned.

In this section, we will take a somewhat different approach to exploring the question of penetration. We will focus on the *stratum corneum*, the outermost layer of human skin, which optimizes the delivery and efficacy of topical products in the skin. We will investigate now only how molecules are indeed able to penetrate this outermost layer, but also focus on the fact that even if they penetrate no deeper, they play an essential role in skin health and youthfulness.

As described above, the *stratum corneum* is the outermost layer of the skin. It consists of two distinct structural components: corneocytes and the intercellular lipid matrix. The corneocytes are differentiated keratinocytes (i.e., anucleated cells without intracellular organelles such as nuclei or mitochondria). They provide the structural support for the *stratum corneum* and act as a barrier against environmental aggression. Corneodesmosomes interconnect corneocytes as desmosomes interconnect keratinocytes in the epidermis. Essential corneodesmosomal proteins include desmocollin and desmoglein. The intercellular lipid matrix is located between corneocytes. The lipid species are composed of ceramides, fatty acids, cholesterol, and glucosylceramide derivatives. These lipids are synthesized by the keratinocytes in the upper layer of *stratum granulosum*. The covalent bonds between the ceramides of the intercellular lipid matrix and the structural proteins of corneocytes membrane create, through ester bonds, a dense and impermeable network [49].

Having identified what the *stratum corneum* is, let us now turn to the question at hand, namely: How do molecules of different sizes and forms, which have different physicochemical properties, penetrate into the *stratum corneum*?

Penetration

In general:

As discussed above, there are various ways for molecules (using passive diffusion) to penetrate the *stratum corneum*: intercellular, transcellular, intrafollicular, and polar. The intercellular pathway allows for a sinuous penetration of molecules between the corneocytes, through the intercellular lipids. The gaps between the intercellular lipids, which enable for penetration of molecules, measure 0.013 μm. This intercellular pathway is how most hydrophilic and lipophilic molecules penetrate through the *stratum corneum*.

The **transcellular pathway** involves corneodesmosomes creating bridges between cells and becoming sufficiently amphiphilic to enable transportation of molecules. The transcellular pathway is how amphiphilic molecules, as well as small other molecules, penetrate through the *stratum corneum*. These substances are able to integrate at the double layer of phospholipids constituting the cell membrane and can penetrate into the corneocytes. The speed of penetration by this pathway is very slow, but it is offset by the fact that the surface area is significant.

The **intrafollicular pathway** enables penetration through hair follicles (which account for 1 to 2% of the total skin surface). As the pilosebaceous follicles are located in deep invaginations of the epidermis, in the dermis, they lead molecules to the reticular dermis. Furthermore, hair follicles do not have a highly developed *stratum corneum*, which further facilitates penetration at this level. This intrafollicular pathway is how large molecules, which are typically highly insoluble, penetrate through the *stratum corneum*.

Finally, the **polar pathway** enables penetration of molecules through the polar pores. These pores are present between cells and are surrounded by polar lipids, which generate discontinuities in the organization of the lipids. This pathway is hydrophilic by nature. For example, sucrose penetrates into the epidermis this way.

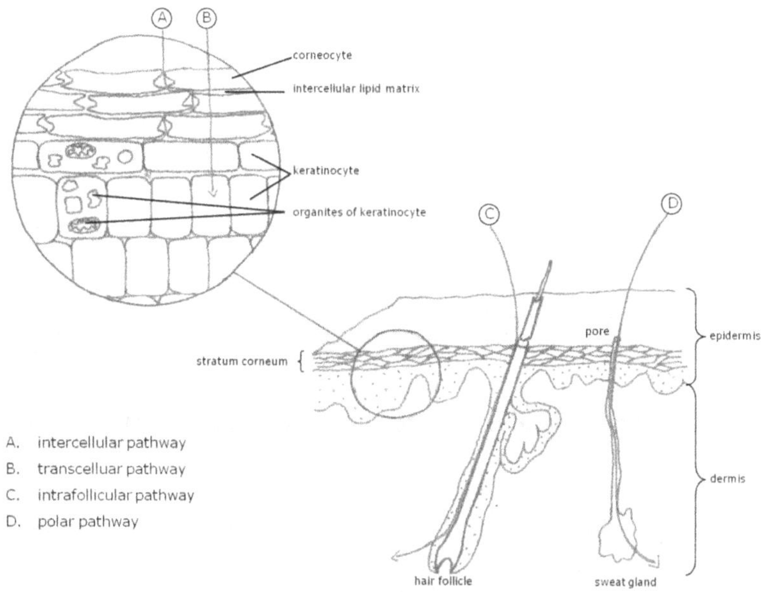

Figure 1: Various pathways of penetration through the *stratum corneum*. There are various pathways for molecules to penetrate the *stratum corneum*: intercellular (penetration between the corneocytes through the intercellular lipids), transcellular (penetration through the corneocytes), intrafollicular (penetration through hair follicles), and polar (penetration through the polar pores).

Penetration of a substance through the skin depends on many parameters that can interact with each other. These parameters are biological factors such as skin condition and age, the site of application, and skin hydration. Physicochemical factors, in particular those related to the substances themselves, also play a role, for example the size of the molecules or their attraction with the surface of the skin. These different pathways are passive diffusions through the *stratum corneum*. Only small molecules (molecular weight below 500 Da) penetrate through the pathways. It should be noted that the vehicle that carries the active ingredient can facilitate the penetration through the *stratum corneum*.

Penetration of water into the *stratum corneum*

The *stratum corneum* is virtually impermeable except for a small quantity of water that is delivered to it by the epidermis. This transferrable water hydrates the SC's external layers, helps maintain its flexibility, and enables adequate enzymatic reactions and corneodesmolysis. The passage of water in the other direction, from the body through the skin into the outside environment, is called trans-epidermal water loss or TEWL. Trans-epidermal water loss is influenced by the concentration of water in the epidermis, by cellular integrity, by relative humidity, by diffusivity of water in the *stratum corneum*, and by the thickness of the *stratum corneum*.

The ability to maintain water in the skin depends on the arrangement of corneocytes, the composition and structure of intercellular lipids, and the presence of naturally moisturizing factors. Naturally moisturizing factors are made of water-soluble compounds and absorb water from atmosphere; they are typically amino acids or other chemical substances that hold water and rehydrate the *stratum corneum*. Naturally moisturizing factors are formed during the epidermis differentiation and represent 10% of corneocyte mass.

Penetration of lipophilic molecules into the *stratum corneum*

Lipophilic molecules of low molecular mass enter the *stratum corneum* essentially by the intercellular pathway (a sinuous penetration between the corneocytes through the intercellular lipids). These intercellular spaces are composed of lipids providing the last step of epidermic differentiation (such as free or esterified sterols, free fatty acids, triglycerides, sphingolipides), arranged in oriented bilayers bounding hydrophilic and lipophilic areas. The higher the concentration gradient of cutaneous lipids in lipid bilayers, the lower the penetration speed of hydrophilic molecules will be. Hence, by increasing the fluidity of cutaneous lipids, penetration can be facilitated.

Penetration of liposomes into the *stratum corneum*

Liposomes are lipid vesicles that can be used as carriers for hydrophilic substances solubilized into aqueous domains, or lipophilic substances solubilized into lipidic membranes. These colloidal carriers are formed as concentric bi-molecular layers of phospholipids. The presence of cholesterol may improve the bi-layer characteristics of liposomes by increasing the microviscosity/interfacial rheological behavior of the bi-layer, thereby reducing the permeability of the membrane to water-soluble molecules, or stabilizing the membrane and increasing the rigidity of the vesicle.

Liposomes represent an alternative method to enhance the permeation of substances through the skin. There are five possible mechanisms for liposomes to penetrate into the *stratum corneum* [50]:

1. Liposomes release the active substances that then penetrate independently into the skin;
2. Liposomes are first absorbed and then fused with the skin's surface and constituents, then change the ultrastructure of the intercellular regions in the deeper layer of the *stratum corneum*. This decreases the impermeability of the *stratum corneum* and enhances the penetration of the encapsulated molecule [51];
3. Liposomes gravitate to the surface of the *stratum corneum*, resulting in a direct transfer of the molecule encapsulated from the liposome to the skin. Vesicles could also fuse and mix with the lipids matrix of the *stratum corneum*, increasing the distribution of molecule into the skin [52];
4. Liposomes penetrate into the skin as an intact form. Although it is now generally accepted that conventional liposomes do not penetrate directly into the skin, this penetration mechanism has been described by Cevc et al. for deformable liposomes, also known as transfersomes [53].

In view of the presence of a surfactant in their bilayer, these vesicles exhibit viscoelastic properties that allow them to deform and pass between the cells of the *stratum corneum*, thus arriving intact into the epidermis. This mechanism is similar to the deformation of red blood cells as they change shape in order to pass through narrow blood vessels whose diameters are smaller than the undeformed blood cells. This penetration is made possible by the presence of a natural trans-epidermal water gradient, which is created by the hydrophilicity of phospholipids. Furthermore, these liposomes avoid dry environments and will follow the gradient of moisture, moving into the deeper layers and more hydrated skin.

5. Liposomes penetrate into the skin via cutaneous annexes such as sweat glands and hair follicles. An excellent review of these studies is provided in a review by Knorr et al [54].

The work with liposomes suggested that carrier/vesicle size may have an influence on skin penetration as well as deposition into hair follicles. The nanosizing approach has the potential to offer increased skin deposition of compounds and also the more efficient delivery of agents to hair follicles. Recent work by the group of Michniak-Kohn et al. suggests that some nanoparticulate carriers are able to deliver various lipophilic compounds to skin fairly efficiently while making sure that no compounds traverse the skin layers (no *trans*dermal penetration occurs). Additional benefits of these carriers included high solubilization (in one case 5000-fold) and improved stability of the encapsulated compounds. There are many other such examples in the literature, and nanosized particles have been used for a long time in sunscreen formulations and facial foundations.

Penetration of nanoparticles into the *stratum corneum*

The penetration of nanoparticles occurs through two possible pathways: intercellular and intrafollicular pathways. While the transfollicular pathway plays a central role in the study of the penetration of nanoparticles [55], it is not yet clear if nanoparticles penetrate into the hair follicles, or if they are stored in the outer layer of these hair follicles.

Intelligent Targeting Carriers

Intelligent Targeting Carriers have the ability to be recognized by fibroblasts, melanocytes, or adipocytes, thus delivering anti-aging, whitening, or slimming active ingredients, directly to the cells where they have to act.

Capsules are formed by a matrix of poly (lactic-co-glycolic acid) PLGA with an outer polyvinyl alcohol (PVA) shell with the addition of N-pantothenic-peptide [56]. A proper ligand is covalently bonded to the surface of the capsule. These ligands (mostly peptides) are recognized by receptors in the surface of the target cells. The cells are thus able to uptake the particle by endocytosis, while the particles are able to escape from the endosomal compartment, then degraded and therefore able to deliver the active to the cytoplasm.

Cruz et al. suggested that the PLGA capsules used as intelligent targeting devices increase the activity of the encapsulated active ingredients by concentrating them solely in the place where they can be biologically active. This is thus of interest to personal care products (anti-aging, whitening, tanning, slimming) [57].

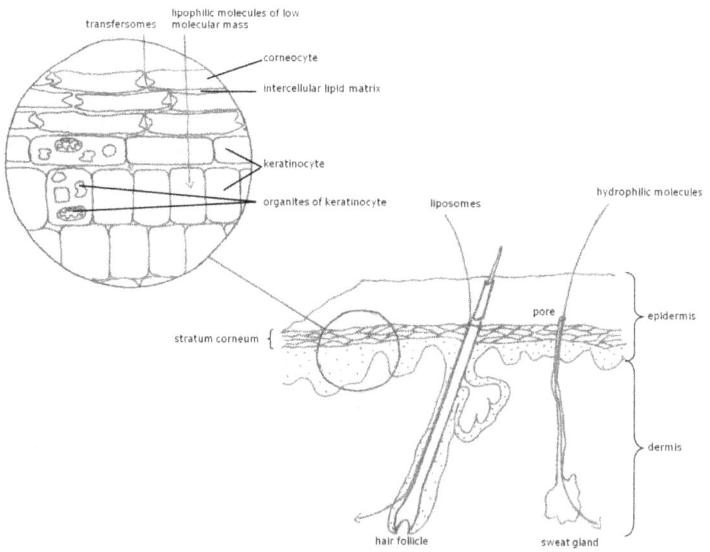

Figure 2: Examples of penetration pathways by various molecules. The lipophilic molecules of low molecular mass penetrate through the *stratum corneum* by the intracellular pathway while the hydrophilic molecules prefer the polar pathway. The liposomes may penetrate via the transfollicular pathway and the transferosomes (i.e., deformable liposomes), pass between cells, and prioritize the intercellular pathway.

e. Penetration Versus Protection

It is not clear yet whether there truly is real *in vivo* penetration of the ingredients incorporated in cosmetic and personal care formulations. While many will propose that this means cosmetic formulations lack clear efficacy, we propose rather that the lack of penetration of a product's active ingredients need not be a negative characteristic. Indeed, these ingredients still possess the ability to protect the *stratum corneum* against environmental stressors and damage. This concept is significant since the *stratum corneum* constitutes only 10% of the entire skin, yet it contributes to over 80% of the cutaneous barrier function. For example, the use of antioxidant molecules in cosmetic products can help the *stratum corneum* regenerate and protect itself and thus also regenerating and protecting the underlying epidermis and dermis from the harmful effects of UV and other environmental toxins.

In summary, while the individual penetration of water, lipophilic molecules, liposomes, and nanoparticles through the *stratum corneum* is becoming better understood when viewed through their intercellular, transcellular, intrafollicular, and polar pathways, the penetration mechanisms of cosmetic formulations remain poorly understood and are an area in need of further exploration.

In this review, we presented not only the known and various pathways of penetration through the *stratum corneum*, but also the fact that even if cosmetic formulations penetration is no deeper than the SC, their efficacy is demonstrable. Indeed, the *stratum corneum* represents the barrier function of skin, and thus needs to be protected from environmental toxins. By regenerating and protecting the *stratum corneum*, active cosmetic ingredients protect the epidermis and dermis.

PART 3.1.11 IMMUNOLOGICAL FUNCTION

The skin is the largest organ of the human body and possesses the unique function of protecting the body from allergens, chemicals, and microbial infection [58]. It is an immunoprotective organ that comprises of specialized cells called Langerhans cells in the epidermis. The dermal collagen network comprises of dendritic cells, T-cells and T-cell subtypes, B cells and mast cells. Langerhans cells are activated in response to allergen-mediated contact sensitization that elicits an immune response [59, 60]. Resident dermal dendritic cells in addition are induced in this phenomenon. As a result, the Langerhans cells migrate into the lymph nodes in response to chemokines such as CCL19. The migrated cells activate T-cells that undergo differentiation and proliferation, which results in the selective expansion of clonal populations of allergen-specific T-cells. The activation of Th1 and/or Th2 clonal T-cell populations ultimately results in allergen-specific sensitivity [61].

After first phase of infection with a pathogen, dendritic cells resident in the dermis present antigens to naïve T-cells in the skin-draining lymph node, initiating an adaptive immune response that generates central memory T-cells and effector memory T-cells. At second round of infection, dendritic cells present antigen to central memory T-cells in skin-draining lymph nodes, giving rise to another population of effector memory T-cells that migrate into skin and attempt to destroy the infection.

There is a marked decrease in number of Langerhans cells with age. This affects the ability of TNF-alpha to induce Langerhans cell migration in response to an infection. There is an overall reduced cutaneous immune function with aging, thus rendering aged skin more prone to infections. There is a reduction in dendrite formation, reduction in Birbeck granules, and reduced antigen trapping capacity. Thus, skin immune function is associated with and decreases with aging.

UV radiation results in changes in the immune response. It suppresses the immune response and results in skin cancer development [62]. In harsh circumstances, it also destroys the Langerhans cells on skin.

Psoriasis is a common skin condition characterized by immune and genetic factors. The symptoms of the disease include skin lesions, dryness, redness, and irritation associated with inflammation. The process is an inflammatory skin disorder that results in dermal infiltration of T-cells, dendritic cells, macrophages, and neutrophils [63]. Anti-TNF alpha as well as anti-IL-12 and anti-IL-23 therapy and methods to exfoliate the skin lesions including reduction of inflammation are suggested interventions to treat psoriasis. A systems biology approach to characterize the transcriptome of the diseased state versus normal skin can be indicative of suggested therapeutic options to combat the disease.

PART 3.1.12 CYTOKINES

Cytokines are small proteins or glycoproteins produced by epidermal keratinocytes, Langerhans cells, monocytes/macrophages, fibroblasts, and lymphocytes in the skin. The cytokines bind to receptors on target cells and initiate an active immune response. The cytokines produced by keratinocytes have been most extensively studied. Keratinocytes produce interleukins (IL-1, IL-3, IL-6, IL-7, IL-9, IL-10), interferons (IFN-α, IFN-β), cytotoxins (TNF-α, TNF-β), colony-stimulating factors (G-CSF, MCSF, MG-CSF), and growth factors (bFGF, EGF, KGF, MGSA, NGF, TGF-α, TGF-β, PDGF) [64]. There is a relatively low basal level of cytokine production in normal healthy skin; however, in the presence of a challenge (e.g., viral, bacterial, fungal), cytokine production increases. This is regulated by membrane proteins, known as toll-like receptors, that bind certain molecular components of pathogens [65]. Different toll-like receptors recognize different molecular components of the pathogen. The ligands include bacterial DNA, lipopolysaccharide, flagellin, β-glucan, etc. Cytokine production is altered in a variety of skin diseases.

PART 3.1.13 ENZYMES

Enzymes within the skin layers play an important role in maintaining the biochemistry of the skin, supporting the synthesis of its components and hence cell replication. This results in skin lipid production and the formation of the *stratum corneum* barrier properties that play such a crucial role in the penetration of cosmetic actives into the skin layers. In addition, the presence of enzymes influences how cosmetic actives and formulation excipients are metabolized. Also, enzymes function as skin protectors by scavenging free radicals and maintaining a pH gradient that influences the number and type of bacterial flora on the skin surface. They are one of the most essential components of the skin.

Enzymes in the dermis are responsible for continuous remodeling of the extracellular matrix [66]. In the basal layer of the epidermis, the metabolic activity of most cells is low. The exceptions are the few basal cells undergoing replication, where enzyme activity is high. As cells move up from the basal layer and enter into differentiation, there is a general increase in the enzymatic activities necessary to synthesize the components of desmosomes, keratohyalin granules, keratin proteins, and lipids [67]. In the spinous layer most energy is produced by mitochondrial activity, but as cells reach the upper granular layer, the mitochondria are degraded and energy production is dependent on anaerobic glycolysis with lactic acid as a by-product. Most of the protein synthesized during differentiation is keratin, which makes up the keratinocyte cytoskeleton [68]. Most of the lipid that accumulates with differentiation is packaged into lamellar granules [69, 70]. In the late stages of differentiation, the lamellar granules migrate to the apical end of the cell, and the bounding membrane of the lamellar granule fuses into the cell plasma membrane [71, 72]. The lipids and a battery of hydrolytic enzymes are extruded into the intercellular space. At about this time, some proteins from the keratohyalin granules are deposited on the inner surface of the plasma membrane [73]. A high-molecular-weight, histidine-rich and highly phosphorylated protein, profilaggrin, is dephosphorylated and proteolytically clipped to small filaggrin units [74]. On passage into the *stratum corneum*, the filaggrin units induce aggregation of the keratin filaments into bundles of keratin that lie parallel to the plane of the skin. The filaggrin proteins are subsequently acted upon by proteases until they are degraded to their component amino acids [75]. This results in a very high osmotic strength in the corneocytes. At about the time of the transition from the granular layer to the *stratum corneum*, a calcium-dependant transglutaminase cross-links the proteins on the inner surface of the plasma membrane through formation of isopeptide linkages [73]. There is further cross-linking of these proteins through the spontaneous formation of disulfide linkages. ω-Hydroxyceramides derived from the bounding membrane of the lamellar granules becomes ester-linked to the outer surface of this cross-linked protein layer [76]. Thus the original plasma membrane of the keratinocyte is replaced by a compound envelope consisting of a thick cross-linked band of protein with a covalently bound lipid layer on the outer surface.

The main source of carbon for epidermal lipid biosynthesis appears to be acetate from the circulation [77]. The rate-limiting enzyme for synthesis of fatty acids is acetyl-CoA carboxylase [78]. This is a biotin-dependent enzyme that converts acetyl-CoA to malonyl-CoA at the expense of one ATP. The fatty acids are incorporated into phosphoglycerides, sphingomyelin, and glucosylceramides in the viable portion of the epidermis. The rate-limiting enzyme in synthesis of sphingolipids is serine palmitoyl transferase [79], and the rate-limiting enzyme in cholesterol biosynthesis is β-hydroxymethylglutaryl-CoA reductase [80]. HMG-CoA reductase uses two molecules of NADPH to reduce HMG to mevalonate-CoA.

The lipids found in isolated lamellar granules include phosphoglycerides, sphingomyelin, glucosylceramides, and cholesterol [69]. One unusual glucosylceramide contains 30- through 34-carbon long ω-hydroxyacids amide-linked to a mixture of sphingosines and dihydrosphingosines with linoleate ester-linked to the ω-hydroxyl group and glucose β-glycosidically linked to the primary hydroxyl group of the base [81]. This unusual lipid is thought to be a major component of the bounding membrane of the lamellar granule, and is the precursor of the aforementioned covalently bound lipid of the envelope. Enzymes associated with the lamellar granules include ceramide glucosyl transferase indicating that lamellar granules arise from the Golgi apparatus, since this enzyme is considered a biochemical marker for the Golgi apparatus [82]. Hydrolytic enzymes associated with the lamellar granules include β-glucosidase, acid phosphatase, amino-glycosidases, galactosidase, aryl sulfatase, phospholipase A, sphingomyelinase, and several proteases [69, 70, 83]. The combined action of some of these enzymes converts the cholesterol-phospholipid-glucosylceramide mixture extruded into the intercellular space into the cholesterol-ceramide-fatty acid mixture of the *stratum corneum.*

A minor lipid in the *stratum corneum* is cholesterol sulfate. This lipid has been shown to be a serine protease inhibitor [84]. It is thought that this protease inhibitor protects the corneodesmosomes, until in the outer layers of the *stratum corneum,* sterol sulfatase degrades the cholesterol sulfate, and this permits the serine proteases to break down the corneodesmosomes leading to desquamation.

3.1.14 ULTRAVIOLET RADIATION-INDUCED PHOTODAMAGE AND SKIN CANCER

Photocarcinogenesis is a cosmetic concern because the UV light-absorbing agents used in cosmetic (over-the-counter) sunscreens help to lower the incidence of skin cancer.

Exposure to UV radiation causes not only photodamage with the appearance of premature aging, but also precancers and cancers of the skin. Actinic keratoses are premalignant lesions in which the epidermis proliferates, producing hyperkeratotic lesions characteristic of photodamaged skin, especially in individuals with skin types I, II, and III. These lesions have a high percentage of DNA mutations, particularly at sites p53 and p16 which are characteristic of nonmelanoma skin cancers (NMSC). Although actinic keratoses occasionally spontaneously disappear, they should be medically treated to prevent their becoming squameous cell carcinomas.

Skin cancer has been classified as nonmelanoma skin cancer, and as cutaneous malignant melanoma. NMSC has the highest incidence of any cancer, approximately one million new cases each year in the United States. One in five Americans will get a skin cancer in the course of a lifetime. Mortality from NMSC is low, but morbidity can be considerable with possible disfigurement, especially on the face and neck.

Basal cell carcinoma (BCC) is the most common NMSC (equal to about 75% of the incidence of all skin cancers). Although BCCs do not metastasize, they are locally invasive and disfiguring if not treated early. Squameous cell carcinomas

(SCC) account for about 20% of all skin cancers; approximately 2% of SCCs (particularly those originating on the head and neck) metastasize with possible mortality. Melanomas make up about 5% of all skin cancers. If excised before they become invasive, melanomas can be definitively treated; however, if allowed to invade the dermis, melanomas metastasize with high mortality.

Sun exposure (and the use of tanning beds) is linked to the skin cancer epidemic as the incidence of NMSC increases in proportion to the cumulative sunlight exposure and is highest in people with skin types I and II. In the case of melanoma, the effects of UV are not clear except in lentigo maligna melanoma (a subclass of cutaneous melanoma), for which sun exposure has been shown to increase the incidence.

UV radiation causes skin cancer by inducing mutations in DNA which lead to damaging the ability of the skin cells to control proliferation. UVB harms mainly the epidermis and UVA, the dermis. The primary damage by UVB is *via* direct absorption by DNA to generate mutations through the formation of dimers between adjacent pyrimidine residues, leading to specific UVB "signature" mutations that can accumulate over time. UVB can also indirectly induce oxidative damage by the formation of reactive oxygen species (ROS) that indirectly damage DNA. If not repaired, both the direct and indirect DNA mutations persist through subsequent subdivisions causing precancers (actinic keratoses) and skin cancers. Reactive protective mechanisms by the epidermis cause thickening of the outer layers of the skin to create a UV-protective "outer shell" that gives an unattractive leathery texture and increased pigmentation that results in mottled discoloration, both of which are characteristic of the appearance of photoaging. UVA penetrates deeper to harm the dermis. UVA damages DNA indirectly through absorption by chromophones that generate ROS which mutate DNA *via* mutagenic oxidative intermediates. UVA also activates metaloproteinases which directly break down collagen and elastic tissue and act on other transcription factors to inhibit repair, thereby causing the sagging and wrinkles of photoaged skin.

Furthermore, recent research shows that UVA in combination with common environmental pollutants is synergistic in generating oxidative damage, thereby significantly increasing visible photodamage and the risk of skin cancer [84.5]. Polycyclic aromatic hydrocarbons (PAHs) such as benzo[a]pyrene (BaP) are ubiquitous in the air, food, and water as a result of incomplete combustion of fossil fuels (from power plants, car exhaust, heaters) and from cigarette smoke (the most prevalent indoor pollutant). These chemical pollutants exist at levels below damaging or tumorigenic levels. However, when combined with UVA exposure, there is a synergistic increase in oxidative damage with the consequence of even more severe photoaging and increased incidence of skin cancer.

Thus UV radiation is a complete carcinogen; it can act alone as an initiator and a promoter in formation of cancer. UV can also act as a promoter with initiating events inside the cell, such as DNA mutations arising from DNA polymerase incorporation errors, depurination, deamination of 5-methylcytosine, or oxidative damage from free radicals. The cell can respond to the damage by repairing the DNA to avoid the effects of the mutations or, if the damage is too great, by inducing cell death through apoptosis to remove potential cancer cells from the population. Immunosurveillance aids recognition of potentially damaging mutated cells so that apoptotic mechanisms can be initiated. UVA decreases this cellular immune recognition and response.

PART 3.1.15 GENE EXPRESSION IN SKIN CARE

The Human Genome Project (HGP) was a 13-year effort that was coordinated by the U.S. Department of Energy and the National Institutes of Health. The project, which was completed in 2003, produced sequence information for the entire 3 billion base pairs in the human genome. The work cost more than one U.S. dollar per base pair, but generated over 265 times that in economic impact and job creation [85]. More importantly, the HGP gave rise to new, high-throughput technologies used to analyze genes and ultimately, a new field of science—*genomics*. From genomics, other high-throughput technologies were developed, giving rise to a suite of "omics" disciplines (e.g., proteomics and metabolomics). In combination, "omics" data provide a comprehensive view of how cells and biological systems work together in health and in disease. This information has enabled advances in dermatology and in the cosmetic and personal care industry [86]. In this section, the application of genomics-based methods to cosmetics and personal care is reviewed.

a. Genomics Technologies

Researchers have been studying the function of genes and proteins in the skin for decades using technologies such as Northern and Western blotting, and traditional polymerase chain reaction (PCR). These methods are labor intensive and only allow for analysis of a few genes or proteins at a time [87-92].

More recent technologies, including microarrays and quantitative real time PCR (qPCR), have enabled simultaneous analysis of thousands of genes and more accurate quantification. Microarrays are now the "go-to" method for screening cells and tissues to identify novel biomarkers and understanding mechanisms of action. Both microarrays and qPCR technologies are used to detect changes in the sequence of DNA (i.e., mutations), as well as gene expression (an indicator of which genes are "turned on or off") in a given cell type. When a gene is "turned on," or activated, it is transcribed from DNA into a complementary strand of RNA (ribonucleic acid)—the RNA strand serves as a template for protein synthesis, directing the ribosome as to which amino acids to put together to form specific proteins. On the other hand, when a gene is "turned off," the cell stops transcribing the DNA strand and protein synthesis is terminated. Gene expression analysis is used to determine how cells and tissues are affected by specific conditions. The methods provide information at the molecular level as to how specific cellular functions are altered from normal homeostasis. Gene expression profiles can be used as a guide for creating products or targeted treatments that will convert an aberrant profile back to homeostasis.

b. Genomics and the Skin

To date, thousands of peer-reviewed research studies have been published using high-throughput genomics methods to elucidate molecular mechanisms associated with skin biology [93, 94]. Studies have been conducted across multiple disciplines, from embryonic development to aging, as well as all areas of skin ailments [95-97]. Many studies have identified unique gene expression profiles in skin disorders such as atopic dermatitis, acne, rosacea, and psoriasis [98-102]. A large number of whole-genome sequencing studies have been conducted to elucidate genetic mutations and predisposition related to rare skin conditions [103, 104].

Molecular studies of the epidermal skin barrier provide a good example of how genomics has improved our understanding of skin biology [105, 106]. The skin barrier is our body's first line of defense against environmental insults such as chemicals, radiation, pathogens, and other stimuli. The formation and maintenance of a functionally intact epidermal barrier involves the coordination of complex regulatory networks that involve the expression and interaction of hundreds of molecules. Some of these major processes include keratinocyte differentiation, apoptosis and maturation into corneocytes, cell migration and desquamation [107]. Gene expression studies have been used to identify the expression of key molecules involved in each one of these processes [108, 109]. In other studies, microarrays have been used to identify large sets of genes [110]. For example, Taylor et al. [111] used microarrays to identify genes expressed by differentiating keratinocytes at different time intervals. The study identified 1282 genes differentially expressed; specific genes include those that code for structural molecules and innate immune molecules. Other studies have identified microRNAs that regulate genes, such as p63, in proliferating and differentiating keratinocytes [112, 113]. Again, a better understanding of how specific molecules and pathways interact will facilitate the development of high-performing topical products for cosmetics and for treating specific skin conditions.

Additional studies have identified genetic mutations associated with compromised barrier function [114, 115]. Identifying mutations in genes, such as filaggrin, may aid in creating future diagnostic tools and advanced therapies. Filaggrin is a filament-associated protein that binds keratin fibers in skin epithelial cells. In the *stratum corneum*, filaggrin monomers are incorporated into the lipid envelope that forms the skin barrier. Filaggrin undergoes further processing in the upper *stratum corneum* to release free amino acids that assist in barrier formation and water retention. These proteins can also interact with keratin intermediate filaments. Other research has shown that CYP26b1 is expressed in keratinocytes in the epidermis. CYP26b1 is a member of the cytochrome enzyme superfamily, a group of enzymes that are essential for performing metabolic functions in the cell. CYP26b1 is essential for metabolism of retinoic acid [116]. Okana et al. [115] has recently demonstrated that genetic ablation of CYP26b1 disrupts epidermal barrier formation by inhibiting retinoic acid metabolism.

c. Gene Expression Analysis: A Breakthrough for Cosmetic Science

Gene expression technologies in cosmetics and personal care are now routinely used in product development pipelines. Drawing on information produced in basic research studies that identify molecular biomarkers associated with phenotypic endpoints, cosmetics and personal care companies are performing studies to define the skin's response to topical materials and formulations [117-120]. Skin care scientists are currently utilizing gene expression methods to screen raw materials for biological effects, identify dose-response relationships, and understand how combinations of ingredients may work together—this may be additive, synergistic, or hormetic.

To date, gene expression studies have been used to:

- Demonstrate efficacy and understand mechanisms of action
- Streamline product formulations during development
- Create performance products that ultimately improve marketability, consumer confidence and brand loyalty

While most work has been conducted to improve product formulations and validate efficacy, genomics-based screening methods may also provide new and improved tools for assessing safety and toxicity [121]. This will require carefully planned studies to develop and validate improved tissue models that contain immune cells as well as sophisticated informatics and algorithms to easily analyze and interpret the datasets.

d. Challenges

Understanding how specific patterns of gene expression translate into a biological response is one of the greatest challenges in interpreting high throughput genomics data. For now, genomics data are best used as a roadmap to generate hypotheses and guide follow-on studies that utilize additional cell biology methods better suited for interrogating functional relationships.

Another challenge in conducting genomics-based studies for cosmetic science is the lack of fully representative experimental tissue models. Studies conducted for the cosmetics industry are typically carried out using *in vitro* cell cultures or artificial skin. While these models provide useful information regarding the keratinocyte and fibroblast response, they lack melanocytes, Langerhans cells, and an epidermal barrier consistent with *in vivo* human skin. *In vitro* models are an ideal tool for conducting early screening studies that should be followed up with *in vivo* clinical work.

e. Looking Ahead

Since the inception of genomics, newer, state-of-the-art technologies such as Next-Gen sequencing have been developed. These methods can rapidly sequence the entire genome in several days, perform RNA sequencing, and analyze epigenetic mechanisms (i.e., DNA methylation). While epigenetics is now a popular buzzword in cosmetic science, a greater understanding of these mechanisms in skin biology will help elucidate phenomena such as aging, photo-aging, and skin disease. Groundbreaking epigenetic research in skin biology is beginning to emerge and will soon be translated into product development.

Another emerging concept is the promise of "personalized skin care" [122]. This approach uses an individual's genetic footprint to develop skin care products to address the specific needs of an individual. Companies are beginning to explore this opportunity, and there will most likely be an increased amount of data and ultimately, product development using the "personalized medicine" approach in the next few years.

f. Recommended Reading

Contet-Audonneau, J.L., et al., A histological study of human wrinkle structures: comparison between sun-exposed areas of the face, with or without wrinkles, and sunprotected areas, *Brit. J. Dermatol.* 1999 **140,** 1038-1047.

Eller, M.S., et al., DNA damage enhances melanogenesis, *Proc. Nat. Acad. Sci., USA,* 1996 **93,** 1087-1092.

Freedberg, I.M., and Fitzpatrick, T.B., eds., 5th ed., *Dermatology in General Medicine,* McGraw-Hill, New York, N.Y., 1999.

Fuchs, E., and Weber, C, Intermediate filaments, *Ann. Rev. Biochem.* 1994 **63,** 345-382.

Fuchs, E., and Cleveland, D.W., A structural scaffolding of intermediate filaments in health and disease, *Science* 1999 **279,** 514-519.

Gilchrest, B.A., et al., Mechanisms of ultraviolet light-induced pigmentation, *Photochem. Photobiol.* 1996 **63**(1), 1-10.

Johnson, B.E., et al., Response of human skin to ultraviolet light, 139-202, in *Photophysiology: Current Topics,* Giese, A.C., ed., Academic Press, New York, 1968.

Livrea, M., and Packer, L., eds., *Clin. Photomed.,* Marcel Dekker, New York, 1993.

Rougier, A., and Schaefer, H., eds., *Protection of the Skin against Ultraviolet Radiation,* John Libbey Eurotext, Montrouge, 1998.

Urbach, F., and Gange, R.W., eds., *The Biological Effects of UVA Radiation,* Praeger Publishers, New York, 1989.

Zeise, L., et al., eds., *Melanin: Its Role in Human Photoprotection',* Proceedings of Melanin Symposium, March 11/12. 1994, Valdenmar Publishing, Overland Park, KS, 1995.

GLOSSARY

1. Epidermis - composed of the outermost layers of cells in the skin—"epi" in Greek meaning "over" or "upon," which together with the dermis forms the entire skin layer termed the cutis.
2. Dermis - a layer of skin between the epidermis and subcutaneous tissues that consists of connective tissue and cushions the body from mechanical stresses. It is divided into two layers, the area adjacent to the epidermis called the papillary region and a deeper and thicker area known as the reticular dermis.
3. *Stratum corneum* (Latin for "horned" or "horny" layer) - the outermost layer of the skin, consisting of dead cells (corneocytes) that lack nuclei and organelles. This layer is responsible for the barrier function of skin.
4. Glycoaminoglycan - any of a group of high-molecular-weight linear polysaccharides with various disaccharide repeating units and usually occurring in proteoglycans, including the chondroitin sulfates, dermatan sulfates, and hyaluronic acid. Abbreviated as GAG.
5. Collagen - protein made up of amino acids, which are in turn built of carbon, oxygen, and hydrogen. Collagen contains specific amino acids—glycine, proline, hydroxyproline, and arginine. There are many types of collagen that have been identified. Collagen is synthesized most commonly by fibroblasts.
6. Keratin - a family of fibrous structural proteins. Keratin is the key structural material making up the outer layer of human skin. It is also the key structural component of hair and nails.
7. Keratinocyte - the main cell type in the epidermis, the outermost layer of the skin. Those keratinocytes found in the basal layer (*stratum germinativum*) of the skin are sometimes referred to as "basal cells" or "basal keratinocytes."
8. Corneocyte - a terminally differentiated keratinocyte that forms part of the stratum corneum, the outermost part of the skin. The cell is regularly replaced

through desquamation and renewal from the lower epidermal layers, making it an essential part of the barrier property of the skin.

9. Fibroblast - a type of cell that synthesizes extracellular matrix and collagen, the structural framework for the skin, and plays a critical role in wound healing. Fibroblasts are the most common cells of connective tissue and in particular the dermal layer of the skin.
10. Cytokine - (Greek "cyto," cell; and "kinos," movement) are any of a variety of compounds secreted by specific cells of the immune system. They carry signals locally between cells and thus have an effect on other cells. They are a category of signaling molecules that are used extensively in cellular communication. They can be proteins, peptides, or glycoproteins.
11. Merkel cells - clear cells found in the *stratum basale* (at the bottom of sweat duct ridges) of the epidermis, approximately 10 μm in diameter. They also occur in epidermal invaginations of the plantar foot surface called rete ridges. Most often they are associated with sensory nerve endings, when they are known as Merkel nerve endings.
12. Langerhans cells - dendritic cells (antigen-presenting immune cells) of the skin, containing large granules called Birbeck granules. They are present in all layers of the epidermis, but are most prominent in the *stratum spinosum*. They also occur in the papillary dermis, particularly around blood vessels.
13. Dendritic cell - immune cell forming part of the immune system. Main function is to process antigen material and present it on the surface to other cells of the immune system. Dendritic cells are present in tissues in contact with the external environment, such as the skin (where there is a specialized dendritic cell type called Langerhans cells).
14. Birbeck granule (also known as Birbeck bodies) - rod-shaped cytoplasmic organelles with a central linear density and a striated appearance.
15. Fillagrin - a filament-associated protein that binds to keratin fibers in epithelial cells.
16. Involucrin - a protein component of human skin. In humans it is encoded by the *IVL* gene. In binding the protein termed loricrin, involucrin is involved in the formation of the cell envelope that protects corneocytes in the skin.
17. Melanin (from the Greek "melas" meaning "black") - a natural pigment in skin derived from the amino acid tyrosine.
18. Melanosome - an organelle containing melanin, the most common light-absorbing pigment found in the mammalian kingdom.
19. Pheomelanin - yellow to red-brown pigment produced by melanocytes.
20. Eumelanin - black to brown pigment produced by melanin.

21. Golgi apparatus (also known as the Golgi complex, Golgi body, or simply the Golgi) - an organelle found in most eukaryotic cells. Part of the cellular endomembrane system, the Golgi apparatus packages proteins inside the cell before they are sent to their destination; it is particularly important in the processing of proteins for secretion.
22. Macrophage - any of the large, mononuclear, highly phagocytic cells derived from monocytes that occur in the walls of blood vessels and in loose connective tissue. Macrophages are usually immobile but become actively mobile when stimulated by inflammation; they also interact with lymphocytes to facilitate antibody production.
23. Elastin - a key extracellular matrix protein that is critical to the elasticity and resilience of many tissues including skin.
24. Reticulin - name given to the chemical substance of reticular fibers, which were formerly thought to be distinct from collagen by reason of their distinctive structure and staining properties but are now regarded as type III collagen.
25. Apocrine gland - a sweat gland composed of a coiled secretory portion located at the junction of the dermis and subcutaneous fat, from which a portion inserts and secretes into the infundibular portion of the hair follicle.
26. Eccrine gland - a sweat gland that is not connected to hair follicles. It functions by responding to elevated body temperature due to heat or physical exercise.
27. Sebaceous gland - small oil-producing gland usually attached to hair follicles and releasing a fatty substance, sebum, into the follicular duct and thence to the surface of the skin.
28. Sebum - consists of a mixture of fats (triglycerides, wax esters, squalene, and cholesterol) and cellular debris, which is discharged through the sebaceous duct.
29. Kallikreins - these belong to a class of serine proteases with a high degree of substrate specificity. The enzymes are structurally related to trypsin. Kallikrein (kininogen, kininogenase = EC3.4.21.8) cleaves proteins between arginine and lysine residues.
30. Keratinosomes (otherwise known as membrane-coating granules [MCGs], lamellar bodies, lamellar granules or Odland bodies) - secretory organelles found in keratinocytes. Keratinosomes fuse with the cell membrane and release their contents into the extracellular space.
31. Androgen - a male sex hormone such as testosterone.
32. Ichthyosis - a family of genetic skin disorders characterized by dry, scaling skin that may be thickened or very thin.
33. Atopic dermatitis (eczema) - an itchy inflammation of the skin. It is usually a chronic condition that may be accompanied by other conditions such as asthma.

34. Psoriasis - a chronic skin disease that affects the life cycle of skin cells. It causes cells to build up rapidly on the surface of the skin, forming thick silvery scales and itchy, dry, red patches that are sometimes painful.
35. Transepidermal Water Loss = TEWL - This is defined as a measurement of the water amount that diffuses or evaporates from inside the body through the epidermis to the surrounding atmosphere. TEWL can increase due to disruption of the skin barrier through wounds, scratches, burns, exposure to solvents or surfactants, extreme dryness) and is affected by humidity, temperature, season, and moisture content of the skin.
36. Liposomes - nano/micro-size spherical drug carriers that can be produced from natural or synthetic phospholipids and cholesterol. They form spontaneously when phospholipids are combined with water and bi-layered spheres form, since the phospholipid molecules orient themselves according to their polarity (one end of each molecule is water soluble, while the opposite end is water insoluble).
37. Rheology - a science dealing with the deformation and flow of matter and including the measurement of viscosity.
38. Colloids - a solution that has particles ranging between 1 and 1000 nanometers in diameter and evenly distributed throughout the solution.

REFERENCES

1. Briggaman, R.A., *Biochemical composition of the epidermal-dermal junction and other basement membrane.* J Invest Dermatol, 1982. **78**(1): p. 1–6.
2. Lynley, A.M. and B.A. Dale, *The characterization of human epidermal filaggrin. A histidine-rich, keratin filament-aggregating protein.* Biochim Biophys Acta, 1983. **744**(1): p. 28–35.
3. Elias, P.M., *Epidermal lipids, barrier function, and desquamation.* J Invest Dermatol, 1983. **80**(1 Suppl): p. 44s–9s.
4. Wertz, P.W., *Lipids and barrier function of the skin.* Acta Derm Venereol Suppl (Stockh), 2000. **208**: p. 7–11.
5. Jimbow, K., et al., *Biochemistry and physiology of melanin pigmentation*, in *Physiology, Biochemistry and Molecular Biology of the Skin*, L.A. Goldsmith, Editor. 1991, Oxford University Press: New York.
6. Fitzpatrick, T.B., et al., *Sunlight and Man.* 1974, Tokyo: University of Tokyo Press.
7. Jimbow, K., et al., *Distribution of eu- and pheomelanins in human skin and melanocytic tumors and their photoprotective vs. phototoxic properties*, in *Melanin: Its Role in Human Photoprotection*, L. Zeise, Editor. 1995, Valdenmar Publishing Co.: Kansas.

8. Raper, H.S., *The Tyrosinase-tyrosine Reaction: Production from Tyrosine of 5: 6-Dihydroxyindole and 5: 6-Dihydroxyindole-2-carboxylic Acid-the Precursors of Melanin.* Biochem J, 1927. **21**(1): p. 89–96.
9. Prota, G., *Regulatory mechanisms of melanogenesis: beyond the tyrosinase concept.* J Invest Dermatol, 1993. **100**(2 Suppl): p. 156S–161S.
10. Prota, G., *Melanins, melanogenesis and melanocytes: looking at their functional significance from the chemist's viewpoint.* Pigment Cell Res, 2000. **13**(4): p. 283–93.
11. D., J.W., *The skin: basic structure and functions*, in *Andrew's Disease of the Skin: Clinical Dermatology*, R.B. Odom, et al., Editor. 2000, WD Saunders Company: New York. p. 2–3.
12. Iwasaki, A., *Mucosal dendritic cells.* Annu Rev Immunol, 2007. **25**: p. 381–418.
13. Banchereau, J. and R.M. Steinman, *Dendritic cells and the control of immunity.* Nature, 1998. **392**(6673): p. 245–52.
14. Valladeau, J., et al., *Langerin, a novel C-type lectin specific to Langerhans cells, is an endocytic receptor that induces the formation of Birbeck granules.* Immunity, 2000. **12**(1): p. 71–81.
15. Idoyaga, J., et al., *Cutting edge: langerin/CD207 receptor on dendritic cells mediates efficient antigen presentation on MHC I and II products in vivo.* J Immunol, 2008. **180**(6): p. 3647–50.
16. Montagna, W., et al., *Advances in Biology of Skin.* The Dermis. Vol. 10. 1970, New York: Century-Crofts.
17. Uitto, J., D.R. Olsen, and M.J. Fazio, *Extracellular matrix of the skin: 50 years of progress.* J Invest Dermatol, 1989. **92**(4 Suppl): p. 61S–77S.
18. Montagna, W., et al., *Advances in Biology of Skin.* Sebaceous Glands. Vol. 4. 1963, Oxford: Pergamon Press.
19. Robertshaw, D., *Apocrine sweat glands*, in *Physiology, Biochemistry and Molecular Biology of the Skin*, L.A. Goldsmith, Editor. 1991, Oxford University Press: New York.
20. Nara, T., et al., *Sialic acids and antimicrobial substances in the apocrine glands of porcine perianal skin.* Arch Dermatol Res, 2012. **304**(8): p. 609–17.
21. Rawlings, A.V., et al., *Ceramides and the skin*, in *Textbook of Cosmetic Dermatology*, R. Baran, and Maibach, H.I., Editor. 1998, Martin Dunitz Ltd.: London. p. 99–101.

22. Toth, B.I., et al., *"Sebocytes' makeup": novel mechanisms and concepts in the physiology of the human sebaceous glands.* Pflugers Arch, 2011. **461**(6): p. 593–606.

23. Menon, G.K., G.W. Cleary, and M.E. Lane, *The structure and function of the stratum corneum.* Int J Pharm, 2012. **435**(1): p. 3–9.

24. Elias, P.M.a.F., K.R., *Permeability barrier homeostatis*, in *Skin Barrier*, P.M.a.F. Elias, K., Editor. 2006, Taylor & Francis: New York. p. 337–362.

25. Menon, G. and R. Ghadially, *Morphology of lipid alterations in the epidermis: a review.* Microsc Res Tech, 1997. **37**(3): p. 180–92.

26. Raymond, A.A., et al., *Lamellar bodies of human epidermis: proteomics characterization by high throughput mass spectrometry and possible involvement of CLIP-170 in their trafficking/secretion.* Mol Cell Proteomics, 2008. **7**(11): p. 2151–75.

27. Elias, P.M. and D.S. Friend, *The permeability barrier in mammalian epidermis.* J Cell Biol, 1975. **65**(1): p. 180–91.

28. Madison, K.C., et al., *Presence of intact intercellular lipid lamellae in the upper layers of the stratum corneum.* J Invest Dermatol, 1987. **88**(6): p. 714–8.

29. Hou, S.Y., et al., *Membrane structures in normal and essential fatty acid-deficient stratum corneum: characterization by ruthenium tetroxide staining and x-ray diffraction.* J Invest Dermatol, 1991. **96**(2): p. 215–23.

30. Menon, G.K., B.E. Brown, and P.M. Elias, *Avian epidermal differentiation: role of lipids in permeability barrier formation.* Tissue Cell, 1986. **18**(1): p. 71–82.

31. Williams, M.L. and P.M. Elias, *Elevated n-alkanes in congenital ichthyosiform erythroderma. Phenotypic differentiation of two types of autosomal recessive ichthyosis.* J Clin Invest, 1984. **74**(1): p. 296–300.

32. Holleran, W.M., et al., *Processing of epidermal glucosylceramides is required for optimal mammalian cutaneous permeability barrier function.* J Clin Invest, 1993. **91**(4): p. 1656–64.

33. Madison, K.C., *Barrier function of the skin: "la raison d'etre" of the epidermis.* J Invest Dermatol, 2003. **121**(2): p. 231–41.

34. Bouwstra, J.A. and M. Ponec, *The skin barrier in healthy and diseased state.* Biochim Biophys Acta, 2006. **1758**(12): p. 2080–95.

35. Feingold, K.R., *Thematic review series: skin lipids. The role of epidermal lipids in cutaneous permeability barrier homeostasis.* J Lipid Res, 2007. **48**(12): p. 2531–46.

36. Holleran, W.M., et al., *Consequences of beta-glucocerebrosidase deficiency in epidermis. Ultrastructure and permeability barrier alterations in Gaucher disease.* J Clin Invest, 1994. **93**(4): p. 1756–64.
37. Miyazaki, M., et al., *Stearoyl-CoA desaturase-2 gene expression is required for lipid synthesis during early skin and liver development.* Proc Natl Acad Sci U S A, 2005. **102**(35): p. 12501–6.
38. Cameron, D.J., et al., *Essential role of Elovl4 in very long chain fatty acid synthesis, skin permeability barrier function, and neonatal survival.* Int J Biol Sci, 2007. **3**(2): p. 111–9.
39. Li, W., et al., *Depletion of ceramides with very long chain fatty acids causes defective skin permeability barrier function, and neonatal lethality in ELOVL4 deficient mice.* Int J Biol Sci, 2007. **3**(2): p. 120–8.
40. Milstone, L.M., *Epidermal desquamation.* J Dermatol Sci, 2004. **36**(3): p. 131–40.
41. Rawlings, A.V. and R. Voegeli, *Stratum corneum proteases and dry skin conditions.* Cell Tissue Res, 2013. **351**(2): p. 217–35.
42. Oren, A., et al., *In human epidermis, beta-defensin 2 is packaged in lamellar bodies.* Exp Mol Pathol, 2003. **74**(2): p. 180–2.
43. Braff, M.H., et al., *Keratinocyte production of cathelicidin provides direct activity against bacterial skin pathogens.* Infect Immun, 2005. **73**(10): p. 6771–81.
44. Elias, P.M., et al., *The secretory granular cell: the outermost granular cell as a specialized secretory cell.* J Investig Dermatol Symp Proc, 1998. **3**(2): p. 87–100.
45. Liu, A.Y., et al., *Human beta-defensin-2 production in keratinocytes is regulated by interleukin-1, bacteria, and the state of differentiation.* J Invest Dermatol, 2002. **118**(2): p. 275–81.
46. Menon, G.K.a.f., M., *Structural and Functional Correlations of Skin Barrier in Health and Disease: Models and Evaluation*, in *Toxicology of the Skin*, N. Montero-Riviere, Editor. 2010, Informa Healthcare. p. 110–130.
47. Sznitowska, M., S. Janicki, and A.C. Williams, *Intracellular or intercellular localization of the polar pathway of penetration across stratum corneum.* J Pharm Sci, 1998. **87**(9): p. 1109–14.
48. Menon, G.K. and P.M. Elias, *Morphologic basis for a pore-pathway in mammalian stratum corneum.* Skin Pharmacol, 1997. **10**(5–6): p. 235–46.
49. Pouillot, A., et al., *The stratum corneum: a double paradox.* J Cosmet Dermatol, 2008. **7**(2): p. 143–8.

50. El Maghraby, G.M., B.W. Barry, and A.C. Williams, *Liposomes and skin: from drug delivery to model membranes.* Eur J Pharm Sci, 2008. **34**(4–5): p. 203–22.

51. Hofland, H.E., et al., *Interactions between liposomes and human stratum corneum in vitro: freeze fracture electron microscopical visualization and small angle X-ray scattering studies.* Br J Dermatol, 1995. **132**(6): p. 853–66.

52. Kirjavainen, M., et al., *Interaction of liposomes with human skin in vitro--the influence of lipid composition and structure.* Biochim Biophys Acta, 1996. **1304**(3): p. 179–89.

53. Cevc, G. and G. Blume, *Hydrocortisone and dexamethasone in very deformable drug carriers have increased biological potency, prolonged effect, and reduced therapeutic dosage.* Biochim Biophys Acta, 2004. **1663**(1–2): p. 61–73.

54. Knorr, F., et al., *Follicular transport route--research progress and future perspectives.* Eur J Pharm Biopharm, 2009. **71**(2): p. 173–80.

55. Lademann, J., et al., *Nanoparticles--an efficient carrier for drug delivery into the hair follicles.* Eur J Pharm Biopharm, 2007. **66**(2): p. 159–64.

56. Pisani, E., et al., *Surfactant dependent morphology of polymeric capsules of perfluorooctyl bromide: influence of polymer adsorption at the dichloromethane-water interface.* J Colloid Interface Sci, 2008. **326**(1): p. 66–71.

57. Cruz, L.J., et al., *Targeted PLGA nano- but not microparticles specifically deliver antigen to human dendritic cells via DC-SIGN in vitro.* J Control Release, 2010. **144**(2): p. 118–26.

58. Di Meglio, P., G.K. Perera, and F.O. Nestle, *The multitasking organ: recent insights into skin immune function.* Immunity, 2011. **35**(6): p. 857–69.

59. Incorvaia, C., et al., *Allergy and the skin.* Clin Exp Immunol, 2008. **153 Suppl 1**: p. 27–9.

60. Beck, L.A. and D.Y. Leung, *Allergen sensitization through the skin induces systemic allergic responses.* J Allergy Clin Immunol, 2000. **106**(5 Suppl): p. S258–63.

61. Sharma, N.S., et al., *Perspectives on Non-Animal Alternatives for Assessing Sensitization Potential in Allergic Contact Dermatitis.* Cellular and Molecular Bioengineering, 2012. **5**(1): p. 52–72.

62. Ullrich, S.E. and S.N. Byrne, *The Immunologic Revolution: Photoimmunology.* Journal of Investigative Dermatology, 2012. **132**(3): p. 896–905.

63. Sweeney, C.M., A.M. Tobin, and B. Kirby, *Innate immunity in the pathogenesis of psoriasis.* Archives of Dermatological Research, 2011. **303**(10): p. 691–705.

64. Kondo, S., *The roles of keratinocyte-derived cytokines in the epidermis and their possible responses to UVA-irradiation.* J Investig Dermatol Symp Proc, 1999. **4**(2): p. 177–83.

65. Ermertcan, A.T., F. Ozturk, and K. Gunduz, *Toll-like receptors and skin.* J Eur Acad Dermatol Venereol, 2011. **25**(9): p. 997–1006.

66. Krieg, T. and M. Aumailley, *The extracellular matrix of the dermis: flexible structures with dynamic functions.* Exp Dermatol, 2011. **20**(8): p. 689–95.

67. Presland, R.B. and B.A. Dale, *Epithelial structural proteins of the skin and oral cavity: function in health and disease.* Crit Rev Oral Biol Med, 2000. **11**(4): p. 383–408.

68. Parry, D.A. and P.M. Steinert, *Intermediate filaments: molecular architecture, assembly, dynamics and polymorphism.* Q Rev Biophys, 1999. **32**(2): p. 99–187.

69. Freinkel, R.K. and T.N. Traczyk, *Lipid composition and acid hydrolase content of lamellar granules of fetal rat epidermis.* J Invest Dermatol, 1985. **85**(4): p. 295–8.

70. Grayson, S., et al., *Lamellar body-enriched fractions from neonatal mice: preparative techniques and partial characterization.* J Invest Dermatol, 1985. **85**(4): p. 289–94.

71. Landmann, L., *The epidermal permeability barrier.* Anat Embryol (Berl), 1988. **178**(1): p. 1–13.

72. Elias, P.M., N.S. McNutt, and D.S. Friend, *Membrane alterations during cornification of mammalian squamous epithelia: a freeze-fracture, tracer, and thin-section study.* Anat Rec, 1977. **189**(4): p. 577–94.

73. Kalinin, A.E., A.V. Kajava, and P.M. Steinert, *Epithelial barrier function: assembly and structural features of the cornified cell envelope.* Bioessays, 2002. **24**(9): p. 789–800.

74. Dale, B.A., K.A. Resing, and J.D. Lonsdale-Eccles, *Filaggrin: a keratin filament associated protein.* Ann N Y Acad Sci, 1985. **455**: p. 330–42.

75. Rawlings, A.V. and P.J. Matts, *Stratum corneum moisturization at the molecular level: an update in relation to the dry skin cycle.* J Invest Dermatol, 2005. **124**(6): p. 1099–110.

76. Wertz, P.W., K.C. Madison, and D.T. Downing, *Covalently bound lipids of human stratum corneum.* J Invest Dermatol, 1989. **92**(1): p. 109–11.

77. Hedberg, C.L., P.W. Wertz, and D.T. Downing, *The time course of lipid biosynthesis in pig epidermis.* J Invest Dermatol, 1988. **91**(2): p. 169–74.

78. Slabas, A.R., et al., *Pivotal reactions in fatty acid synthesis.* Prog Lipid Res, 1994. **33**(1–2): p. 39–46.

79. Radin, N.S., *Biosynthesis of the sphingoid bases: a provocation.* J Lipid Res, 1984. **25**(13): p. 1536–40.

80. Russell, D.W., *Cholesterol biosynthesis and metabolism.* Cardiovasc Drugs Ther, 1992. **6**(2): p. 103–10.

81. Hill, J.R., and Wertz, P. W., *Morphology of epidermal lipids*, in *Dermal Absorption and Toxicity Assessment*, M.S. Roberts, and Walters, K., Editor. 2008, Informa Healthcare: New York. p. 69–78.

82. Madison, K.C., et al., *Lamellar granule biogenesis: a role for ceramide glucosyltransferase, lysosomal enzyme transport, and the Golgi.* J Investig Dermatol Symp Proc, 1998. **3**(2): p. 80–6.

83. Ishida-Yamamoto, A. and M. Kishibe, *Involvement of corneodesmosome degradation and lamellar granule transportation in the desquamation process.* Med Mol Morphol, 2011. **44**(1): p. 1–6.

84. Sato, J., et al., *Cholesterol sulfate inhibits proteases that are involved in desquamation of stratum corneum.* J Invest Dermatol, 1998. **111**(2): p. 189–93.

84.5 Shyong EQ, Lu Y, Goldstein A, Lebwohl M, Wei H. Synergistic enhancement of H2O2 production in human epidermoid carcinoma cells by benzo[a]pyrene and ultraviolet A radiation. *Toxicol Appl Pharmacol* 2003:188:104–9.

85. Tripp, S. and M. Grueber, *Economic Impact of the Human Genome Project*, B.T.P. Practice, Editor. 2011, Battelle Memorial Institute. p. 1–58.

86. Blumenberg, M., *SKINOMICS: Transcriptional Profiling in Dermatology and Skin Biology.* Current Genomics, 2012. **13**(5): p. 363–368.

87. Kumar, S., A.J.T. Millis, and C. Baglioni, *Expression of interleukin 1-inducible genes and production of interleukin 1 by aging human fibroblasts.* Proceedings of the National Academy of Sciences, 1992. **89**(10): p. 4683–4687.

88. Eller, M.S., et al., *The molecular cloning and expression of two CRABP cDNAs from human skin.* Experimental cell research, 1992. **198**(2): p. 328–36.

89. Fisher, G.J. and J.J. Voorhees, *Molecular mechanisms of photoaging and its prevention by retinoic acid: ultraviolet irradiation induces MAP kinase signal transduction cascades that induce Ap-1-regulated

matrix metalloproteinases that degrade human skin in vivo. Journal of Investigative Dermatology Symposium Proceedings, 1998. **3**(1): p. 61–8.

90. Fisher, G.J., et al., *Molecular mechanisms of photoaging in human skin in vivo and their prevention by all-trans retinoic acid.* Photochemistry and Photobiology, 1999. **69**(2): p. 154–7.

91. Kono, D.H., et al., *Application of a multiprobe RNase protection assay and junctional sequences to define V beta gene diversity in Sezary syndrome.* The American Journal of Pathology, 1992. **140**(4): p. 823–30.

92. van der Rest, M. and R. Garrone, *Collagen family of proteins.* FASEB Journal, 1991. **5**(13): p. 2814–23.

93. Radoja, N., et al., *Transcriptional profiling of epidermal differentiation.* Physiological Genomics, 2006. **27**: p. 65–78.

94. Smiley, A.K., et al., *Microarray analysis of gene expression in cultured skin substitutes compared with native human skin.* The Journal of Investigative Dermatology, 2005. **125**(6): p. 1286–301.

95. Elias, P.M., Y. Hatano, and M.L. Williams, *Basis for the barrier abnormality in atopic dermatitis: outside-inside-outside pathogenic mechanisms.* The Journal of Allergy and Clinical Immunology, 2008. **121**(6): p. 1337–1343.

96. Gros, E., et al., *Expression of chemokines and chemokine receptors in lesional and nonlesional upper skin of patients with atopic dermatitis.* The Journal of Allergy and Clinical Immunology, 2009. **124**(4): p. 753–760.e1.

97. Kunz, M., *DNA microarray technology in dermatology.* Seminars in Cutaneous Medicine and Surgery, 2008. **27**(1): p. 16–24.

98. Yamasaki, K. and R.L. Gallo, *The molecular pathology of rosacea.* Journal of Dermatological Science, 2009. **55**(2): p. 77–81.

99. Paus, R., et al., *Frontiers in pruritus research: scratching the brain for more effective itch therapy.* The Journal of Clinical Investigation, 2006. **116**(5): p. 1174–86.

100. Oestreicher, J.L., et al., *Molecular classification of psoriasis disease-associated genes through pharmacogenomic expression profiling.* The Pharmacogenomics Journal, 2001. **1**(4): p. 272–87.

101. Barnes, K.C., *An update on the genetics of atopic dermatitis: scratching the surface in 2009.* The Journal of Allergy and Clinical Immunology, 2010. **125**(1): p. 16–29.e11.

102. Braconi, D., G. Bernardini, and A. Santucci, *Post-Genomics and Skin Inflammation.* Mediators of Inflammation, 2010. **2010**.

103. Goudie, D.R., et al., *Multiple self-healing squamous epithelioma is caused by a disease-specific spectrum of mutations in TGFBR1.* Nature Genetics., 2011. **43**(4): p. 365–9.

104. Kelsell, D.P., et al., *Mutations in ABCA12 Underlie the Severe Congenital Skin Disease Harlequin Ichthyosis.* The American Journal of Human Genetics, 2005. **76**(5): p. 794–803.

105. Segre, J.A., C. Bauer, and E. Fuchs, *Klf4 is a transcription factor required for establishing the barrier function of the skin.* Nature Genetics., 1999. **22**(4): p. 356–60.

106. Uchida, Y., *The role of fatty acid elongation in epidermal structure and function.* Dermatoendocrinology, 2011. **3**(2): p. 65–9.

107. Bhandari, A., et al., *Transcriptional regulation of epidermal barrier formation.* Methods in Molecular Biology, 2011. **763**: p. 51–71.

108. Mattiuzzo, N.R., et al., *A large-scale multi-technique approach identifies forty-nine new players of keratinocyte terminal differentiation in human epidermis.* Experimental Dermatology., 2011. **20**(2): p. 113–8.

109. Lee, D.D., et al., *Retinoid-responsive transcriptional changes in epidermal keratinocytes.* Journal of Cellular Physiology, 2009. **220**(2): p. 427–39.

110. Toulza, E., et al., *Large-scale identification of human genes implicated in epidermal barrier function.* Genome Biology, 2007. **8**(6): p. R107.

111. Taylor, J.M., et al., *Dynamic and physical clustering of gene expression during epidermal barrier formation in differentiating keratinocytes.* PLoS One, 2009. **4**(10): p. e7651.

112. Yi, R. and E. Fuchs, *MicroRNA-mediated control in the skin.* Cell Death and Differentiation, 2010. **17**(2): p. 229–35.

113. Banerjee, J. and C.K. Sen, *MicroRNAs in skin and wound healing.* Methods in Molecular Biology, 2012. **936**: p. 343–56.

114. Winge, M.C., et al., *Filaggrin genotype determines functional and molecular alterations in skin of patients with atopic dermatitis and ichthyosis vulgaris.* PLoS One, 2011. **6**(12): p. e28254.

115. Okano, J., et al., *Increased retinoic acid levels through ablation of Cyp26b1 determine the processes of embryonic skin barrier formation and peridermal development.* Journal of Cell Science, 2012. **125**(Pt 7): p. 1827–36.

116. Pavez Loriè, E., et al., *The involvement of cytochrome p450 (CYP) 26 in the retinoic acid metabolism of human epidermal keratinocytes.* Biochimica of Biophysica Acta, 2009. **1791**(3): p. 220–8.

117. Ohguchi, K., et al., *SIRT1 modulates expression of matrix metalloproteinases in human dermal fibroblasts.* The British Journal of Dermatology, 2010. **163**(4): p. 689–94.

118. Gopaul, R., H.E. Knaggs, and J. Lephart, *Salicin regulates the expression of functional 'youth gene clusters' to reflect a more youthful gene expression profile.* International Journal of Cosmetic Science., 2011. **33**(5): p. 416–20.

119. Tito, A., et al., *A tomato stem cell extract, containing antioxidant compounds and metal chelating factors, protects skin cells from heavy metal-induced damages.* International Journal of Cosmetic Science., 2011. **33**(6): p. 543–52.

120. Xu, Y., et al., *Baicalin modulates microRNA expression in UVB irradiated mouse skin.* Journal of Biomedical Research., 2012. **26**(2): p. 125–34.

121. Borlon, C., et al., *The usefulness of toxicogenomics for predicting acute skin irritation on in vitro reconstructed human epidermis.* Toxicology, 2007. **241**(3): p. 157–66.

122. Gilmore, S.J., *High throughput investigative dermatology in 2012 and beyond: A new era beckons.* The Australasian Journal of Dermatology. , 2013. **54**(1): p. 1–8.

Abbreviation: GAGs, glycosaminoglycans; NMF, natural moisturizing factor; DOPA, 3,4-dihydroxyphenylalanine; UV, ultraviolet; LCs, Langerhans cells; DCs, dendritic cells; SC, stratum corneum; RER, rough endoplasmic reticulum; KHK, keratohyalin granules; LBs, lipid bodies; SG, stratum granulosum; SCD, stearoyl CoA desaturase; TEM, transmission electron microscopy; AMP, antimicrobial peptide; TJs, tight junctions; TEWL, TransEpidermal Water Loss; PLGA, poly(lactic-co-glycolic acid); PVA, polyvinyl alcohol; ATP, adenosine triphosphate; NADPH, nicotinamide adenine dinucleotide phosphate; HMG, Hydroxymethylglutaryl-CoA; HGP, Human Genome Project; PCR, polymerase chain reaction; DNA, deoxyribonucleic acid; RNA, ribonucleic acid.

SUBSTRATE:
SKIN II

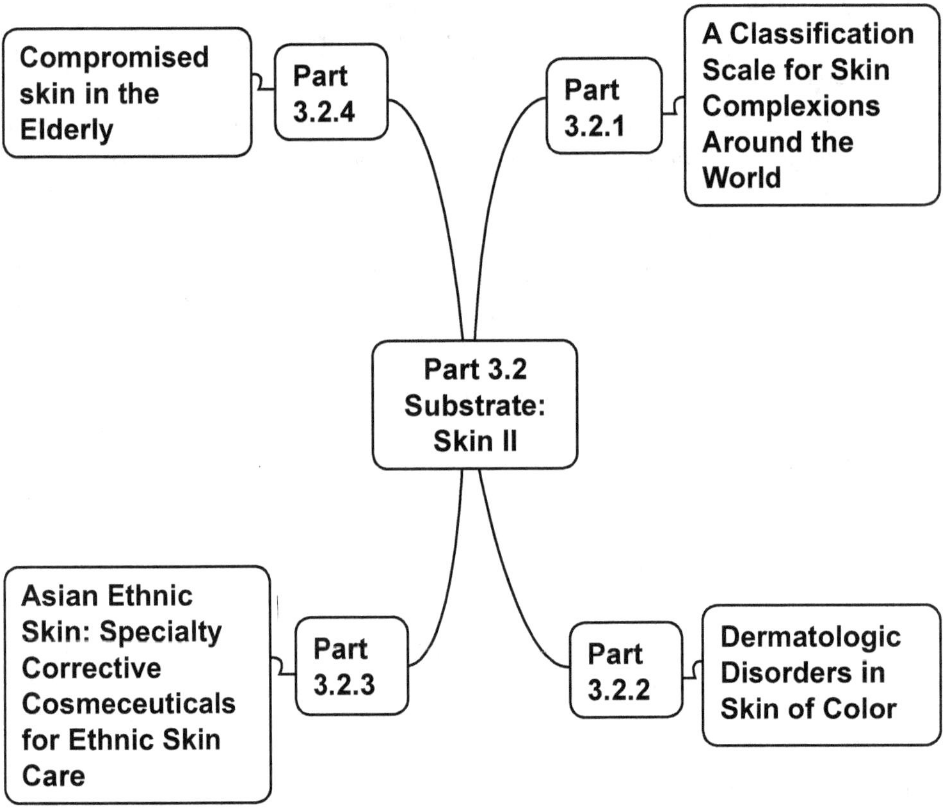

CLASSIFICATION SCALE FOR SKIN COMPLEXIONS AROUND THE WORLD

Author

Eva Patel

skin Rx **Skin Rx Inc.**
Founder & CEO
eva@skinrx.com
www.skinrx.com

ABSTRACT

Cosmetologists and aestheticians are daily faced with a wide variety of clients. In order to provide their skin with optimal health and beauty services these practitioners must accurately look at skin of different races and determine appropriate treatment protocols. Early projections of the changing global skin color landscape have now been proven to be accurate, and the main categories of skin color are no longer just Caucasian-white, but have evolved towards a dramatic escalation of brown, black, yellow, and the many shades in between.

The current scale available to the industry is the Fitzpatrick scale (Figure 4), which was developed in 1975 by Harvard dermatologist Dr. Thomas B. Fitzpatrick. The Fitzpatrick scale is described in this chapter as a custom and practice foundation for current practitioners. It is simple and easy to use; however, the method leaves a gap in the ability to classify skin in light of the evolving epidemiological landscape, and the system fails to accurately predict skin type and precautions for race, complexions, and skin characteristics.

Extensive research over the last decade reveals that beyond color alone, other key factors such as race, country of origin, and ethnicity play an important role in how the skin will respond to cosmetic and personal care products and procedures. Further, when the world is viewed as a whole, and countries are thoughtfully divided into sections, there appears to be an order that helps define how skin from similar regions acts in similar ways. This observation provides the basis for a new, more detailed skin classification scale. A proposal for this new scale is at the heart of the current chapter. The scale has been called the EP Global Skin Classification Scale (Figure 1) and is focused on an all-encompassing global approach that is comprehensive and easy to use for the skin care professional. (Figures 2 & 3 show additions to EP Global Skin Classification Scale.)

TABLE OF CONTENTS

3.2.1 WHY WE NEED AN UPDATED SKIN CLASSIFICATION SCALE

The changing of global skin color landscape is now a reality; the majority is no longer just Caucasian but Asian, with the many shades of yellow undertones and shades ranging from light to dark olive complexions. The common skin conditions among the different races also differ; therefore skin has to be diagnosed and treated according to color and race and a one-size-fits-all method of the past no longer works.

The world is divided geographically into continents:

- Asia is the most populous continent, with its 4.2 billion inhabitants accounting for over 60% of the world population. (The world's two most-populated countries alone, China and India, together constitute about 37% of the world's population).
- Africa is the second-most-populated continent, with around 1 billion people, or 15% of the world's population.

- Europe's 733 million people make up 11% of the world's population.
- Latin American and Caribbean regions are around 600 million (9%).
- Northern America, primarily consisting of the United States, and Canada, has a population of around 352 million (5%).
- Oceania, the least-populated region, has about 35 million inhabitants (0.5%).

Global Population by Continent

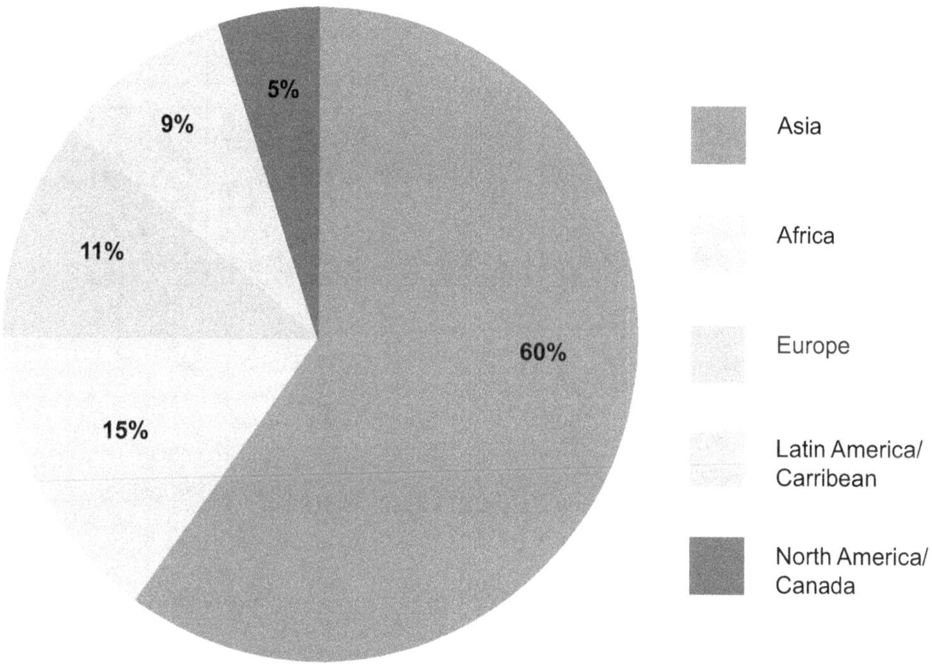

Eva Patel/Data from Wikipedia

Worlds Population by Race

East Asian 24% (Korea, Mongolia, China, Japan)
South Asian 21% (India, Sri Lanka, Pakistan, Bangladesh, Nepal)
Southeast Asian 9% (Cambodia, Burma, Philippines, Malaysia)
Black 15%
White 15%
Hispanic 8%
Middle Eastern 8%

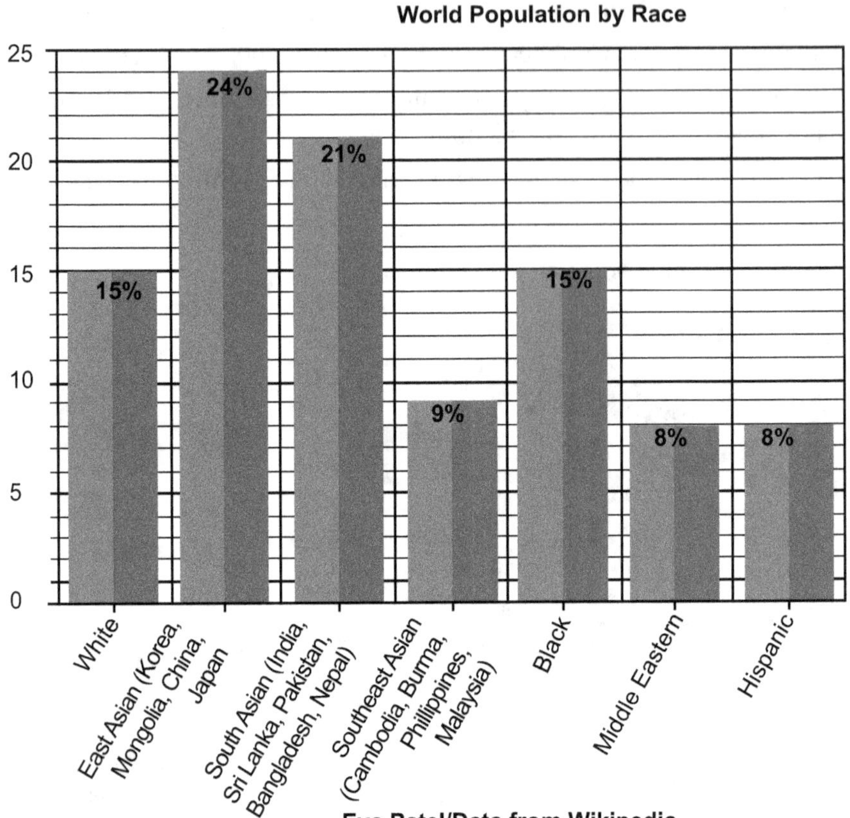

Eva Patel/Data from Wikipedia

USA

The USA is a diverse country of many races; the chart below shows the growth and census population over the past decade.

Race	Census 2010, population	Percent of population	Census 2000, population	Percent of population
Total Population	**308,745,538**	**100.0%**	**281,421,906**	**100.0%**
Single race				
White	196,817,552	63.7	211,460,626	75.1
Black or African American	37,685,848	12.2	34,658,190	12.3
American Indian and Alaska Native	2,247,098	.7	2,475,956	0.9
Asian	14,465,124	4.7	10,242,998	3.6
Native Hawaiian and other Pacific Islander	481,576	0.15	398,835	0.1

Two or more races	5,966,481	1.9	6,826,228	2.4
Some other race	604,265	.2	15,359,073	5.5
Hispanic or Latino	50,477,594	16.3	35,305,818	12.5

NOTE: Percentages do not add up to 100% due to rounding and because Hispanics may be of any race and are therefore counted under more than one category.

Source: U.S. Census Bureau: National Population Estimates; Decennial Census.

The current scale that has been industry standard for the past 38 years is the Fitzpatrick scale.

The Fitzpatrick Classification Scale was developed in 1975 by Harvard Medical School dermatologist Thomas Fitzpatrick, MD, PhD. This scale classifies a person's complexion and their tolerance of sunlight. It is used by many practitioners to determine how someone will respond or react to facial treatments, and how likely they are to get skin cancer.

Skin Type	Skin Color	Characteristics
I	White; very fair; red or blond hair; blue eyes; freckles	Always burns, never tans
II	White; fair; red or blond hair; blue, hazel, or green eyes	Usually burns, tans with difficulty
III	Cream white; fair with any eye or hair color; very common	Sometimes mild burn, gradually tans
IV	Brown; typical Mediterranean caucasian skin	Rarely burns, tans with ease
V	Dark Brown; mid-eastern skin types	very rarely burns, tans very easily
VI	Black	Never burns, tans very easily

Fitzpatrick Classification Scale (Table 1)

The method leaves a gap in the ability to classify skin in light of the evolving epidemiological landscape, and the system fails to accurately predict skin type and precautions for race, complexions, and skin characteristics.

The EP Global Skin Classification tool was designed to fill the gaps by expanding the categories and taking into consideration global skin. The following categories were implemented:

- Race
- Country of Origin
- Complexion
- Skin Characteristics
- Skin Type
- Precautions

(See Figures 1-3)

EP Global Skin Classification Scale			
EP #	**Race**	**Country of Origin**	**Complexion**
I	Caucasian I	Belgium, Denmark, Estonia, Finland, Germany, Iceland, Ireland, Latvia, Liechtenstein, Lithuania, The Netherlands, Norway, Sweden, Switzerland, United Kingdom, Canada,Greenland	Pale, Very Fair. Ruddy Freckled complexion.
II	Caucasian II	Andorra, Austria, Belarus, Bosnia & Herzegovina, Croatia, Czech Rep. France, Greece, Hungary, Italy, Kosovo, Luxembourg, Moldova, Monaco, Montenegro, Poland, Portugal, Romania, Russia, San Marino, Serbia, Slovakia, Slovenia, Spain, Ukraine, Vatican City, USA.	Fair. Light Olive undertones.
III	Caucasian III	Australia, Bulgaria, Cyprus, Georgia, Greece, Macedonia, Malta, New Zealand, Turkey, South Africa, Zimbabwe	Fair Medium Olive undertones.
IV	Hispanic/Latino	Argentina, Belize, Bolivia, Brazil, Chile, Colombia, Costa Rica, Ecuador, El Salvador, Falkland Islands (Malvinas), French Guiana, Guatemala, Guyana, Honduras, Mexico, Nicaragua, Paraguay, Panama, Peru, Suriname, Uruguay, Venezuela.	Olive undertones. Medium to Dark Olive; wide range of Olive tones.
V	Mediterranean/ Asian I	Afghanistan, Albania, Algeria, Armenia, Azerbaijan, Bahrain, Iraq, Iran, Israel, Jordon, Kazakhstan, Kuwait, Kyrgyzstan, Lebanon, Oman, Palestine, Qatar, Saudi Arabia, Syria, Tajikistan, Turkmenistan, UAE, Uzbekistan, Yemen	Medium- Dark Oliveundertones

Skin Characteristics	Skin Type	Precautions
Sensitive, thin fragile skin. Burns easily in sun, never tans, Age's rapidly. Fine wrinkling occurs early. Orange peel skin as they age. Scars usually thin. Skin tends to be dry.	Hyper-Sensitive. Environmental Damage. Acne Prone. Skin Cancer most common in this type.	Avoid excessive sun exposure and harsh, abrasive treatments. Bruising more obvious.
Sensitive, fairly thin skin. When exposed to sun will first burn then tan. Signs of aging appear early. Nominal Scarring. Dry to normal skin.	Sensitive Photo Damage Premature Aging Acne Prone Greater chance of skin cancer.	Can use certain peels and lasers with caution, Avoid harsh treatments as skin will be sensitive. Bruising obvious.
Seldom burns when exposed to sun, will tan, excessive exposure to sun will cause the skin to look leathery. Signs of aging appear later. Fine wrinkling less common. Scarring maybe thicker and darker. Normal to oily skin.	Environmental Damage Excessive Photo damage Acne Prone Skin Cancer common	May have tendencies of Hyperpigmentation with excessive sun exposure
Depending on skin tone will rarely burn; will always tan, aging process is moderate. Darker, thicker scarring. Normal to oily skin.	Photo Damage Environmental Damage Hyperpigmentation Acne Prone Skin Cancer less common	Skin color & tone varies. Use caution with Deep peels and Laser.
Seldom burns, will tan. Aging process is moderate. More advanced if over exposed to sun. Wrinkles appear later in more localized areas. Darker, thicker scarring. Normal to oily skin.	Photo Damage Environmental Damage Hyperpigmentation/ Melasma Acne Prone Post Inflammatory Hyperpigmentation (PIH) Skin Cancer rare	Hyperpigmentation tendencies and PIH with Acne, Caution with Deeper Peels and Laser.

EP #	Race	Country of Origin	Complexion
VI	Asian II	Brunei Darussalam, Cambodia, China, Hong Kong, Indonesia, Japan, Korea, Laos, Macao, Malaysia, Mongolia, Philippines, Singapore, Taiwan, Thailand, Timor Leste, Vietnam.	Medium – Dark Yellow-Olive undertones.
VII	Asian III	Bangladesh, Bhutan, India, Maldives, Myanmar (Ex-Burma), Nepal, Pakistan, Sri-Lanka, Tibet.	Light to dark Olive tones. Yellow undertones
VIII	Native Hawaiian and other Pacific Islanders	Fiji, French Polynesia, Guam, Kiribati, Marshall Islands, Micronesia, New Caledonia, New Zealand, Papua New Guinea, Samoa, Solomon Islands, Tonga, Vanuatu.	Medium-dark Olive tones.
IX	Native American Indian and Native Alaskan	There are over 70 Native American tribes and 8 Alaskan races *See attached list.	Medium Olive tones. Red undertones.
X	Black or African American	Eastern Africa, Middle Africa, Northem Africa, Southern Africa, Westem Africa, The Carribbean. *See attached list.	Medium-Dark Brown Tones.
XI	Mix of two or more races	Any combination	Varies depending on race combination.

Figure 1 (EP Global Skin Classification Scale)

Skin Characteristics	**Skin Type**	**Precautions**
Seldom burns, tans about average. Ages well, signs of aging appear late. Prone to Pigmentation changes. Scarring can be thicker and darker. Normal to oily skin	Hyperpigmentation/ Melasma Acne Prone Post Inflammatory Hyperpigmentation (PIH) Skin Cancer very rare	Sensitive to certain peels & laser treatments, Prone to Hyperpigmentation & PIH with Acne. May react to Retinoids and Hydroquinone use caution.
Rarely burns, always tans. Pigmentation changes may occur with over exposure to sun. Ages well, signs of aging appear late. Fine wrinkles do not occur. Darker thicker scars more common	Hyperpigmentation/ Melasma Active Acne/ Acne Prone Post Inflammatory Hyperpigmentation (PIH) Skin Cancer very rare.	Treat with caution concerning peels and laser. Prone to hyperpigmentation & PIH with Acne. Sensitive to Retinoids and Hydroquinone. May have tendencies to keloid.
Seldom burns, tans well, thicker skin allows better sun tolerance. Ages moderately. Thicker and darker scars. Thick Oily skin.	Photo Damage Environmental Damage Hyperpigmentation Acne Prone Skin Cancer rare	Sensitive to peels and lasers, prone to hyperpigmentation and melasma. Tendency to keloid.
Rarely burns, tans well, high sun tolerance. Skin has a tendency to turn leathery with age and excessive sun exposure. Pigmentation changes may occur. Thick dark scarring. Normal oily skin.	Environmentally Damaged Excessive photo damage Hyperpigmentation / Melasma Skin Cancer rare	Treat with caution concerning peels and laser. Prone to hyperpigmentation & PIH with Acne.
Never burns with sun exposure, tans well. Pigmentation issues common. Very little fine wrinking. Formation fo Keloids possible. Oily skin.	Hyperpigmentation/ Melasma Acne Prone Post inflammatory Hyperpigmentation Pseudo folliculitis Skin Cancer very rare	Extremely sensitive, will Hyper pigment & Keloid with certain peels and laser treatments. Use extreme caution. May react to strong topicals.
Take the predominant traits into consideration.	Treat with caution. Use milder programs to start graduating to stronger products in absence of irritation.	Use extreme caution and evaluate ancestry prior to any Peel or Laser Treatment or topical use of Hydroquinone and any Retinoid use.

EP Global Skin Classification Scale					
Race Section X (10) - Country of Origin					
Africa					
Eastern Africa	**Middle Africa**	**Northern Africa**	**Southern Africa**	**Western Africa**	**The Caribbean**
Burundi	Angola	Algeria	Botswana	Benin	Anguilla
Comoros	Cameroon	Egypt	Lesotho	Burkina Faso	Antigua and Barbuda
Djibouti	Central African Republic	Libyan Arab Jamahiriya	Namibia	Cape Verde	Aruba
Eritrea	Chad	Morocco	South Africa	Cote d'Ivoire (Ivory Coast)	Bahamas
Ethiopia	Congo (Brazzville)	South Sudan	Swaziland	Gambia	Barbados
Kenya	Congo, Democratic Republic of the	Sudan		Ghana	Bonaire, Saint Eustatius and Saba
Madagascar	Equatorial Guinea	Tunisia		Guinea	British Virgin Islands
Malawi	Gabon	Western Sahara		Guinea-Bissau	Cayman Islands
Mauritius	Sao Tome and Principe			Liberia	Cuba
Mayotte				Mali	Curaçao
Mozambique				Mauritania	Dominica
Reunion				Niger	Dominican Republic
Rwanda				Nigeria	Grenada
Seychelles				Saint Helena	Guadeloupe
Somalia				Senegal	Haiti
Tanzania, United Republic of				Sierra Leone	Jamaica
Uganda				Togo	Martinique

Zambia			Monserrat
Zimbabwe			Puerto Rico
			Saint-Barthélemy
			St. Kitts and Nevis
			Saint Lucia
			Saint Martin
			Saint Vincent and the Grenadines
			Sint Maarten
			Trinidad and Tobago
			Turks and Caicos Islands
			Virgin Islands (US)

TABLE 2 (Race Section X (10) - Country of Origin)

EP Global Skin Classification Scale

Race Section IX (9) - Country of Origin

***American Indian and Alaska Native tribes**

Alaskan Athabascan	Crow	Menominee	Puget Sound Salish	Yaqui
Aleut	Delaware	Navajo	Seminole	Yuman
Apache	Eskimo	Osage	Shoshone	
Blackfeet	Houma	Ottawa	Sioux	
Cherokee	Iroquois	Paiute	Tlingit-Haida	
Chippewa	Kiowa	Pima	Tohono O'Odham	
Comanche	Latin American	Potawatomi	Ute	
Creek	Lumbee	Pueblo	Yakama	

TABLE 3 (Race Section IX (9) - Country of Origin)

3.2.2 THE METHODOLOGY IN WHICH THE STUDY WAS CONDUCTED:

The research was carried out at Skin Rejuvenation Clinic in San Francisco during 1997–2005. All subjects were residents of USA; a total of 588 subjects, both female and male (majority female) were chosen; they were of different races.

Charts and records were followed during this period to gather the information for the study. All data were manually collected through these charts and records collected from each individual client visit. The initial consultation is where the data were collected from the client. The minimum treatment process was eight visits over a four-month period, two visits a month. Thereafter monthly maintenance visits.

During the initial visit a client filled out a three-page Skin Evaluation questionnaire that asked several questions pertaining to several different factors, which included:

Skin Evaluation

Skin Type

[ ] Very Dry	Dry all over—all the time, tight, easily irritated, sensitive
[ ] Dry/Mature	Mostly dry, tight, maturing/aging, sun/photo-damaged, loss of tone
[ ] Normal to Dry	Normal in the T-zone, dry on the sides of face
[ ] Normal	Slightly oily on the T-zone, normal on the sides of face
[ ] Normal to Oily	Oily in the T-Zone, slightly oily on sides of the face
[ ] Oily	Very oily in the T-Zone, slightly oily on the sides of the face
[ ] Very Oily	Very oily all over, all the time, prone to breakouts and acne
[ ] Blemished	Oily with tendency to active acne or acne-prone skin

History/Pigmentation

Country of origin and ancestral race

What is your ancestry? Parents:____________ Grandparents ______________

Pigmentation (How do you tan?)

How do you tan? [ ] *Burn [ ] Usually Burn [ ] Burn then Tan [ ] Usually Tan [ ] Always Tan*

Pigmentation tendencies: [ ] Even [ ] Uneven [ ] Hyperpigmented [ ] Melasma

Vascularity

Broken capillaries: [ ] Nose area [ ] Cheek area [ ] Chin area [ ] Forehead [ ] Entire face

Acne

Do you have a history of any of the following?

[ ] Acne [ ] Whiteheads [ ] Blackheads [ ] Pimples [ ] Enlarges Pores [ ] Flakiness [ ] Scars

[ ] Erythema [ ] Post-Inflammatory Hyperpigmentation [ ] Pits [ ] Cysts

Sun Exposure/Environment

Do you spend time in the sun?

[ ] Seldom [ ] Occasionally [ ] Frequently

Approximately how many hours do you spend in the sun a week? __________

Do you use a sunscreen on a daily basis? ________ What SPF? [ ] 15 [ ] 30 [ ] 30+

At what age did you start to use a sun block on a regular basis? ____________

What percentage of time do you spend in the sun?

Summer ___________ Winter ______________________________________

Where did you reside the first 20 years of your life?

Country ______________________ Region/City ______________________

Please note that most damage is accumulated during the first 18 years of your life.

Have you actively sunbathed in the past? [ ] Yes [ ] No

Do you currently sunbathe? [ ] Yes [ ] No

Do you use tanning beds? [ ] Yes [ ] No

Have you ever had skin cancer? [ ] Yes [ ] No

Do you have a family history of skin cancer? [ ] Yes [ ] No Relationship _______________

Free Radical Exposure

Do you smoke? [ ] Yes [ ] No How much? _____

Do you consume alcohol? [ ] Yes [ ] No How much?_____

Do you have a healthy diet? [ ] Yes [ ] No

Do you exercise on a regular basis? [ ] Yes [ ] No

Do you take vitamins? [ ] Yes [ ] No Which ones?_____

Lifestyle

Sleeping habits [ ] Poor [ ] Good [ ] Minimal [ ] / 6 hours [ ] 7 hours [ ] 8 hours

Stress level [ ] Minimal [ ] Moderate [ ] Excessive

Do you meditate? [ ] Yes [ ] No How often? ____________

Healing Ability

Does your skin appear fragile and thin? [ ] Yes [ ] No

Do you bruise easily? [ ] Yes [ ] No

Do you scar from cuts or burns? [ ] Yes [ ] No

Do you have a tendency to keloid? [ ] Yes [ ] No

Have you had a deep peel? [ ] Yes [ ] No Did you heal well? ___________

Do you have facial laser treatments? [ ] Yes [ ] No

When the skin evaluation was completed, the skin was further categorized and documented by complexion and skin characteristics of various skin types from different genetic backgrounds.

Complexion/ Skin Characteristics

Skin Characteristics of people with Anglo-Saxon origins

Fair, dry thin-skinned
Scars heal well
Signs of aging appear earlier
Burn easily in the sun
Bruising more obvious
Greater chance of skin cancer

Skin Characteristics of people with Southern Mediterranean origins

Oily, olive-dark complexion
Signs of aging appear later
Cartilage tends to droop
Darker, thicker scars more common
Wrinkles appear later and in more localized areas
Skin cancer rare

Skin Characteristics of people with Northern European origins / German and Scandinavian

Fair, blue-eyed, blonde
Thin skin
Scars heal well
Signs of aging appear early
Bruising more obvious
Greater chance of skin cancer

Skin Characteristics of people with Southern European origins

Dark, oily brunette complexion
Signs of aging appear later

Fine wrinkling less common
Bruising lasts longer
Scars may be thicker and darker
Skin cancers less common

Skin Characteristics of people with Northern European/Irish and Northern England

Ruddy freckled complexion
Red hair
Scars usually thin
Signs of aging appear later
Bruises easily
Pigmentation problems
Skin cancers most common in this type

Skin Characteristics of people with African origins

Signs of aging appear very late
Very little fine wrinkling
Formation of keloids is possible
Pigmentation changes may occur
Thicker cartilage hard to change
Skin cancers very rare

Genetically, this skin type is less susceptible to damage from UV radiation, although the skin can still get burned.

Skin Characteristics of people with Asian origins

Signs of aging appear late
Fine wrinkling does not usually occur
Pigmentation changes may occur
Eyelid surgery more difficult
Skin cancers very rare

The completed questionnaire was then evaluated and categorized according to primary skin condition to be treated and the secondary skin condition to be treated. A woods lamp was used during the initial consultation to further check for photo-damaged, congested skin, hyperpigmentation/melasma

This data collected gave further clarity to the client's skin type.

A UV photo was taken through the canfield polarized camera; this visually showed the UV photo damage and was documented.

3.2.3 SUMMARY, ANALYSIS

During the years of 2005 and 2011 the collected data were reviewed and the conclusions were as follows:

- Subjects from a similar geographical region or ancestral region (country of origin) had similar skin types and characteristics.
- Common skin conditions were similar.
- Complexions had similar undertones according to region (lighter complexions in northern cooler climates and darker around the equator where it's the hottest). Undertones of Asian countries were yellow/olive and undertones of Europe more ruddy, red/pink.
- Migration to another country did not change the original skin type or characteristic.
- There were many mixed races that had combined skin types.

3.2.4 WHERE METHODOLOGY MEETS RESULTS

The method in which the data were collected and notes taken during office visits showed that skin from similar races or country of origin had similar skin types and skin characteristics.

Upon completion of the review of skin evaluation data, the skin type section of the EP Global Skin Classification was based on the collective findings of skin type, with sun exposure, environment, and lifestyle data combined.

The compiled data were then assembled into an organized chart, hence creating the **EP Global Skin Classification Scale**. (Refer to Figure 1.)

PART 3.2.2

DERMATOLOGIC DISORDERS IN SKIN OF COLOR

Aanand N. Geria, MD
Private Practice Dermatology
New York, NY

TABLE OF CONTENTS

3.2.2.1 INTRODUCTION

Skin of color is sometimes referred to as pigmented or ethnic skin. It simply means having enough pigment in the skin to impart a color other than white. In general, people of African, Asian, Latin, Native American, Pacific Islander, or mixed racial origins are considered to have skin of color. The demography of the United States is predicted to shift dramatically to the point where the majority of the population will fall under this category by 2050.[1]

There are several dermatologic diseases that are more commonly encountered in this population. In particular, disorders of pigmentation such as melasma and post-inflammatory hyperpigmentation are among the top skin concerns to prompt a visit to the dermatologist.[2]

3.2.2.2 SKIN PHOTOTYPES

The Fitzpatrick classification of skin types (Table 1) is based on an individual's ability to tan and propensity to sunburn. The skin photoype is generally correlated with degree of pigmentation. For example, Type I skin is typically seen in people of Celtic origin whereas Type VI skin is mainly seen in people of Sub-Saharan African ancestry.

a. Melasma

Melasma is an acquired patchy hyperpigmentation predominantly occurring in individuals with Fitzpatrick skin phototypes III and IV. It is a common disorder affecting nearly 5 million people in the U.S. alone. Although most frequently seen in women, 10% of cases occur in men. The reported prevalence ranges from 8.8% of Hispanic women in the Southern U.S. to 40% of Southeast Asian females.[3]

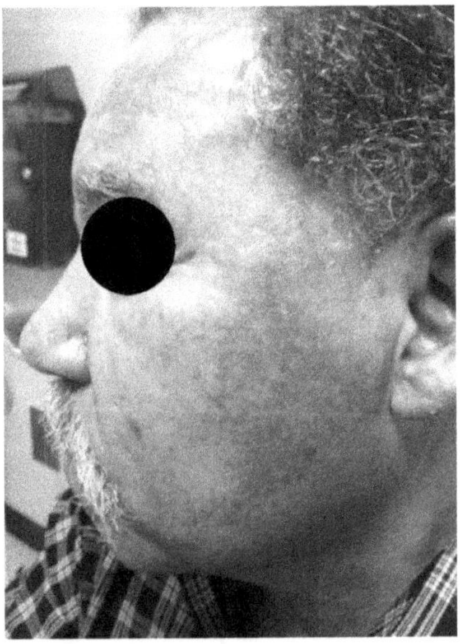

Figure 1: Melasma

Melasma occurs primarily in 3 clinical patterns: 1.) centrofacial, 2.) malar, and 3.) mandibular, although many patients have a mixture of these presentations (Figure 1). The most common is centrofacial and consists of light to dark brown patches occurring on the forehead, cheeks, nose, upper lip, or chin. The malar pattern affects the cheeks and nose, while the mandibular pattern occurs along the jawline.

The clinical manifestations of melasma are thought to result from the presence of biologically hyperactive melanocytes in the affected skin. The exact etiology of melasma remains unknown, however, several risk factors have been identified. Affected individuals frequently have a family history suggesting the influence of genetics.

In addition, sun exposure is a common exacerbating factor most likely through upregulation of melanocyte-stimulating factors. The high incidence of melasma in women, especially those who are pregnant or taking oral contraceptives, suggests an important role for estrogen.

The location of excess pigment, which can be assessed using a Wood's lamp, tends to correlate with the response to therapy. In general, involvement of the more superficial epidermis is more amenable to treatment than that of the deeper dermis.

A critical component in the treatment of disorders of hyperpigmentation is sun protection. This is most commonly achieved by wearing sun-protective clothing and a broad-spectrum sunblock. Without these measures, any treatment regimen is bound to fail. Hydroquinone 4% cream is FDA-approved for the treatment of hyperpigmentation and considered by many to be the gold standard. This medication works by inhibiting the melanin-producing enzyme known as tyrosinase. Sometimes higher concentrations are needed which must be compounded by a pharmacy. The addition of tretinoin cream may enhance efficacy. Non-FDA approved natural alternatives to hydroquinone include kojic acid, arbutin, soy, licorice extract, rucinol, mulberry, niacinamide, ellagic acid, resveratrol, and dioic acid. Other methods of treating hyperpigmentation include laser therapy and chemical peels.[4]

b. Post-inflammatory Hyperpigmentation

An increase in pigment occurring after an inflammatory event is known as post-inflammatory hyperpigmentation (PIH). This cosmetically distressful phenomenon is extremely common in people with skin of color. Frequent causes of PIH include acne, eczema, psoriasis, burns, and certain cosmetic procedures. It is of utmost importance that the underlying cause of PIH be addressed if still present. The treatment of PIH is otherwise similar to that of melasma.

c. Vitiligo

Vitiligo is an acquired disorder of depigmentation estimated to affect 0.5% to 1% of the population.[5] Although vitiligo can occur at any age, almost half present before age 20. Both sexes are affected equally and there is no difference in rates of occurrence according to skin type or race. It can be a psychologically devastating, particularly in people with darker skin, because it is more noticeable.

Vitiligo is divided into three types: localized, generalized, and universal. The generalized type is most common, resulting in widespread symmetric white macules and patches. Areas of predilection include the fingers and wrists, axillae and groin, and body orifices, such as the mouth, eyes, and genitals. There is a propensity for lesions to occur in sites of trauma, which is a process known as koebnerization. The universal type is defined as having at least 80% skin involvement (Figure 2).[5] Lesions begin insidiously and are generally slowly progressive either by centrifugal expansion of current lesions and/or the appearance of new lesions. Spontaneous repigmentation occurs in no more than 15% to 25% of cases.

Under the microscope, vitiligo is characterized by the absence of melanocytes. The exact reason behind their disappearance is unclear but several theories regarding autoimmune, genetic, oxidative stress, and neural mechanisms have been proposed. Currently, the evidence is most strongly suggestive of an autoimmune process occurring in genetically predisposed persons. Indeed, nearly 20% of people with vitiligo have at least one first-degree relative also affected by the disease.[5] Vitiligo may also be associated with other autoimmune diseases such as Addison's disease, pernicious anemia, diabetes mellitus, thyroid disease, and alopecia areata.

The treatment of vitiligo can be a frustrating process. Numerous treatment options exist but a cure remains elusive. As such, goals for treatment include halting disease progression, inducing repigmentation, and achieving an acceptable cosmetic result. It is also important to address the psychosocial impact of the disease. In general, the response to treatment is often slow and may be modest at best.

Current treatment options include topical and systemic steroids, topical calcineurin inhibitors, topical Vitamin D3 analogs, narrow-band UVB phototherapy, and excimer laser. Among these, the gold standard and most frequently used treatment is narrow-band UVB phototherapy.

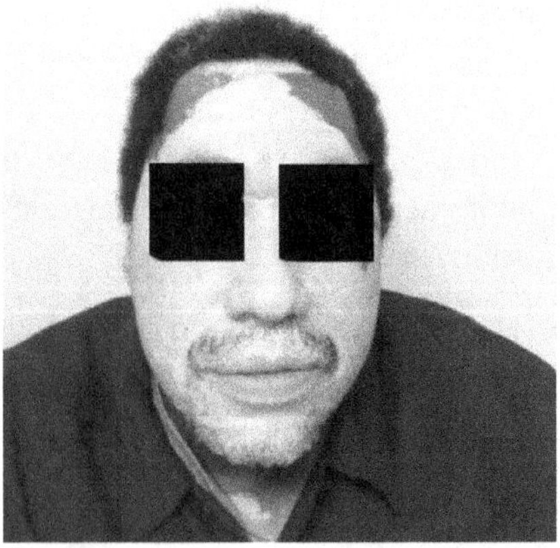

Figure 2: Extensive facial depigmentation occurring in a patient with vitiligo

Surgical therapy may be an option for people with focal nonprogressive vitiligo who have failed phototherapy. Total depigmentation with monobenzone is a last resort reserved for individuals with extensive recalcitrant vitiligo who desire a uniform skin color. Cosmetic camouflage may be helpful in concealing areas of vitiligo occurring in particularly noticeable areas such as the face and neck.

d. Idiopathic Guttate Hypomelanosis

Idiopathic guttate hypomelanosis is a common disorder affecting nearly 80% of people over age 70. Although it occurs in all races and skin types, it is more noticeable in darker skinned individuals. It presents as several, well-defined, hypopigmented 1-6 mm flat spots with a smooth surface on the forearms and shins. The etiology is unknown but sun exposure is thought to play a role. Treatment with liquid nitrogen may be beneficial but must be weighed against the risk of causing post-inflammatory hyper- or hypopigmentation in darkly pigmented skin.

e. Pseudofolliculitis Barbae

Pseudofolliculitis barbae (PFB) is otherwise known as razor bumps or ingrown hairs. The disorder is associated with shaving and is particularly common in the beard area of black men or groin area in women. It is caused by newly shaved tightly curled hairs curving back into and piercing the skin, which results in an inflammatory reaction. PFB presents clinically as inflamed bumps and pustules, which may result in post-inflammatory hyperpigmentation and keloids.

The ideal treatment is to completely stop shaving and instead use a trimmer to leave 1-2mm of stubble. If this is not feasible for personal or professional reasons, a low potency topical steroid and topical antibiotic may be used to reduce inflammation. Other options for treatment include chemical depilatories, laser hair removal, and eflornithine cream.

CONCLUSION

The study of ethnic skin is absolutely necessary to meet the demands of our shifting demographics. Tremendous progress has been made in terms of understanding the biological mechanisms behind disorders of pigmentation. This, in turn, should spur the innovation of more effective medications and cosmeceuticals.

Table 1: Fitzpatrick Skin Types

Skin type	Skin color	Sunburn and tanning history
I	White	Always burns, never tans
II	White	Always burns, tans minimally
III	White	Burns moderately, tans gradually
IV	Olive	Minimal burning, tans well
V	Brown	Rarely burns, tans darkly
VI	Dark brown	Never burns, tans darkly black

REFERENCES:

1. U.S. Census Bureau, The Older Population in the United States: 2010 to 2050.
2. Alexis AF, Sergay AB, Taylor SC. Common dermatologic disorders in skin of color: a comparative practice survey. *Cutis.* Nov 2007;80(5):387-394.
3. Sheth VM, Pandya AG. Melasma: a comprehensive update: part I. *J Am Acad Dermatol.* Oct 2011;65(4):689-697; quiz 698.
4. Konda S, Geria AN, Halder RM. New horizons in treating disorders of hyperpigmentation in skin of color. *Semin Cutan Med Surg.* Jun 2012;31(2):133-139.
5. Alikhan A, Felsten LM, Daly M, Petronic-Rosic V. Vitiligo: a comprehensive overview Part I. Introduction, epidemiology, quality of life, diagnosis, differential diagnosis, associations, histopathology, etiology, and work-up. *J Am Acad Dermatol.* Sep 2011;65(3):473-491.

PART 3.2.3

ASIAN ETHNIC SKIN: SPECIALTY CORRECTIVE COSMECEUTICALS FOR ASIAN ETHNIC SKIN CARE

Authors: Eva Patel & Gurpreet (Gogi) Sangha

Eva Patel
Skin Rx Inc.
Founder & CEO
eva@skinrx.com
www.skinrx.com

Gurpreet (Gogi) Sangha
G.S. Cosmeceutical USA Inc.
Founder & CEO
gogi@gscos.com
www.gscos.com

ABSTRACT

The darkening of skin color in larger segments of the world's population is an emerging trend according to numerous projections. Concomitant with this change is that new, specific skin care needs are an emerging opportunity for product development in these growing markets. To serve these needs, professionals have to be abreast of the needs of this new and growing sector and they must understand this diverse global consumer. This chapter focuses on Asian ethnic skin, which is a new category as defined elsewhere in this book and known as EP V-VII in the EP Global Skin Classification Scale.

By 2014, skin care will increase its already-sizeable lead in the beauty market to reach $91 billion (*Euromonitor International*). This increase is driven primarily by expansion of opportunities in the Asian market. Even in USA the Asian population grew faster than any other major race group between 2000 and 2010, increasing by 43% (U.S. Census Bureau).

By 2050, the U.S. population projections are that 51% of Americans will have skin of olive tones and dark-skinned racial backgrounds (Hispanics, Black, Asian, others) according to the PEW Research Center.

The most apparent difference in the skin of those from different ethnicities is, of course, the color, although there are also differences in skin thickness, vascularity, and predispositions to certain skin conditions and diseases. Pigmentation disorders are a primary concern for Asian ethnic skin as well as a tendency for acne for those with normal to oily skin.

The ingredients and methodology applied in creating effective corrective cosmeceuticals for this segment of the population must take these ethnic skin differences into account. Multiple symptoms and conditions, such as hyperpigmentation with oily skin, can then be treated with today's sophisticated formulations.

Market research shows that consumers are streamlining the number of products they buy and focusing on products that are targeted to correct more than one condition. It is therefore important for industry professionals to focus on development of "necessity products" in these skin care ranges.

TABLE OF CONTENTS

INTRODUCTION:

In modern-day India, a woman's worth is all too often determined by the color of her skin. In India, beauty lies not only in the eyes of the beholder but in societal pressure to be fair-skinned. Arranged marriages are still popular and mothers seek fair-skinned brides for their sons; in fact everyone seeks such brides/grooms. Being dark is undesirable and affects the marriage process; a darker-complexionrf girl, even with beautiful features, is not considered beautiful. Billboards all over India promote fairness, and ads on TV promote fairness with success and beauty.

Culturally this applies to Indians living in foreign countries as well: fair is considered beautiful. My personal experience in the west has been that Asians want lighter complexions and Caucasians want to be darker and tanned. It's like wanting what is not real. I feel we should all be happy with the complexion we are born with and not let societal or cultural pressure tell you otherwise. Taking care of your skin and bringing it back to optimum health by using good products is a necessity and no longer a luxury.

3.2.3.1 DEFINING THE ASIAN ETHNIC MARKET:

Pale skin has always been the ideal for women in Asian cultures for a long time. It has nothing at all to do with wanting to be more "white" in the racial or cultural sense. Up until the 1920s pale, unblemished skin for women was the ideal in western cultures as well. Browned skin was undesirable, since it was considered a trait of only the poor who endured hard labor outdoors. Well-off women used to apply all kinds of products to their skin to whiten them, and both Chinese and Japanese cultures have proverbs that imply "a white skin hides other flaws." Those sayings have existed for ages.

All across Asia, fair skin is highly prized. In dark-skinned South Asia, a fair complexion is considered the epitome of beauty while in already pale-skinned North and East Asia, pearly translucent white skin is a sign of affluence and glamour. In Asia, many people associate dark and tanned skin with menial work in the fields under the hot sun, and a pale complexion with a higher social standing and cultural refinement. Since the 1970s, Asia has been the fastest-growing sector in the global skin-lightening market. Asia is a lucrative market with high-growth potential because of a rising middle-class with increasing disposable income and centuries-old entrenched cultural impressions of beauty.

India's domestic cosmetics industry is expected to grow to US$3.6 billion by 2014, according to the Associated Chambers of Commerce and Industry of India. The skin-lightening cream market alone was worth US$432 million in 2010 and growing at 18% annually.

In Japan the cosmetics industry is growing at 17% a year and is expected to continue that rapid pace for a few more years at the very least, largely because of the hundreds of millions of emerging middle-class women who are spending their money on cosmetics. (1)

In China, where the skin care market is worth more than 35 billion yuan (US$5.5 billion), whitening products comprise a whopping 71% of the market. Elsewhere in Asia, a survey by the London-based market research firm Synovate found that four out of ten women in Hong Kong, Malaysia, the Philippines, South Korea, and Taiwan use a skin-whitening cream.

The cosmetics industry has also started to target men, selling them the same idea that a fairer complexion would make them more attractive. While skin-lightening products for women have been available for decades, products for men have only appeared in recent years, a trend that is rapidly growing. (2)

Japan dominates the global skin lighteners market with the lion's share, as stated in the new market research report from Global Industry Analysts, Inc. (GIA). The market for skin lighteners in Asia-Pacific is projected to cross the $2 billion mark by 2012, driven by the fast-growing markets of China and India. Apart from Asia, Western countries such as the United States and the United Kingdom are emerging as potential markets for skin-whitening products. The growing proportion of ethnic groups—Asians, Hispanics, and African Americans—in these regions is a major contributor to the enhanced demand for skin lighteners.

In Asia, skin-whitening products are very popular. The West seems to believe that these products are made because Asians want to become more Western, which isn't true. Fair skin has been a staple in beauty for Asian cultures for centuries; even old paintings in Asian cultures portray women as fair with flawless complexions.

Western society's obsession with skin tanning is well recognized, but we're often less aware of the aggressive pursuit of fair skin by those with darker skin. In communities where light skin is associated with success, prestige, and envy, women commonly turn to skin-lightening products to achieve and maintain their desired complexion.

In India, the appeal of fair skin is deeply rooted in the nation's culture and the caste system. Higher caste members traditionally had lighter skin and were less likely to be involved in manual work. Many years later, the ruling colonials had fair skin. And in the last century, film, TV, and advertisements have been saturated with images of attractive western actresses with fair skin. Skin-lightening creams are reportedly the most popular product on the Indian skin care market, with around 60% of Indian women using the products daily.

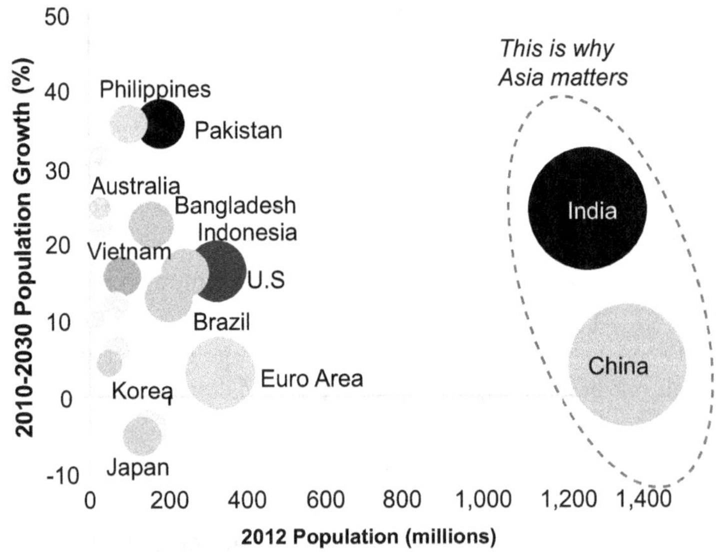

Data as at May 11, 2011. Source: United Nations World Population Prospects, Haver. Size of bubble indicates 2012 population.

Global diversity continues to grow throughout the world as Asian ethnicity remains a constant that makes up the majority of the world's population. The need for an assortment of products that are relevant to the specific multicultural market continues to drive research and technology in the skin care industry. Although Asian ethnic skin care products exist, the market struggles to find skin care products that are optimal in addressing their particular needs. It's important for brands to connect with ethnic consumers and address specific concerns to a wide array of skin types. Women and men of color around the world experience very distinctive issues related to their skin types, and the amount of pigment varies significantly between many ethnic groups. As noted in the EP Global Skin Classification Scale, each region/race has its unique skin color, characteristics, and related skin conditions.

A. Mediterranean/Asian I (EP Global Skin Classification V)

Afghanistan, Albania, Algeria, Armenia, Azerbaijan, Bahrain, Iraq, Iran, Israel, Jordan, Kazakhstan, Kuwait, Kyrgyzstan, Lebanon, Oman, Palestine, Qatar, Saudi Arabia, Syria, Tajikistan, Turkmenistan, UAE, Uzbekistan, Yemen

B. Asian II (EP Global Skin Classification VI)

Brunei Darussalam, Cambodia, China, Hong Kong, Indonesia, Japan, Korea, Laos, Macao, Malaysia, Mongolia, Philippines, Singapore, Taiwan, Thailand, East Timor, Vietnam

In Asia, a lighter skin color is associated with beauty and aristocracy. Asians have skin properties that set them apart from Caucasians. They have more yellow undertones, and skin color ranges from fair to dark. Sometimes Asian skin types can be deceiving and not appear to have a high content of melanin, which is why taking each person's ethnicity into account is crucial. Asian skin does in fact contain more pheomelanin pigments, which determines the yellow undertone skin color. Despite how Asians of different regions seem to sport different skin colors (Japanese are the fairest, with little redness in their skin; Indians are the darkest, with more skin redness), all actually have yellow undertones. Some might be stronger than others, like Asians of Malay origins (e.g., many Malaysians and Filipinos) have the most yellow "tones." Why yellow? It has to do with pheomelanin: high level of this type of melanin in the skin results in yellow undertones.

C. Asian III (EP Global Skin Classification VII)

Bangladesh, Bhutan, India, Maldives, Myanmar (Ex-Burma), Nepal, Pakistan, Sri-Lanka, Tibet

South Asians have a different skin type when compared to the Caucasians and require a different skin care schedule. Cosmetics used by Caucasians do not suit all Asian skin types. Asian skin is usually brownish, and skin tone varies according to the region of origin. Excessive melanin contributes to the brown color and also excessive melanin in the skin weaves a protection against skin cancer. In spite of excessive melanin content, South Asians are prone to pigmentation, age spots, freckles, etc. due to severe climatic conditions. Aging does not show up as wrinkles in South-Asians but rather as hyper pigmentation, dark spots, uneven skin tones, freckles, etc.

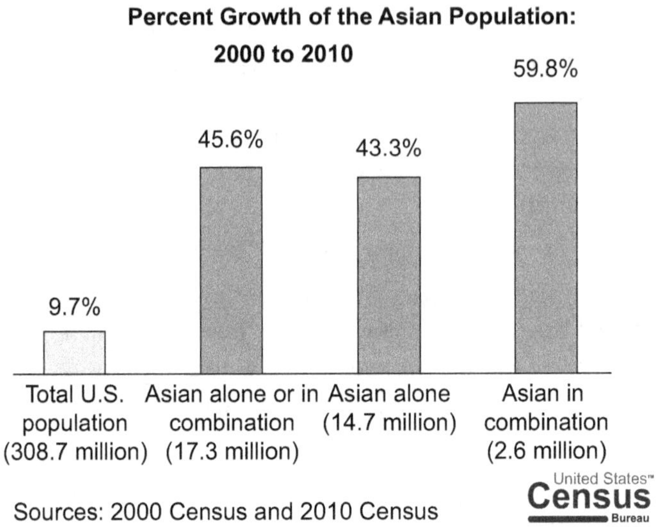

3.2.3.2 DIFFERENCES BETWEEN CONTENT LEVELS OF MELANIN IN THE SKIN

Differences between skin colors are determined by the amount of melanin produced by the melanocytes. Melanin comes in two different forms: pheomelanin, which gives the skin more red to yellow pigments, and eumelanin, which gives the skin dark brown to black pigment. The relative proportions of these two types of melanin determine the skin color. For example, lighter skin types produce a lesser amount of melanin whereas darker skin types produce more melanin. Also, some Asian skin types might appear to be fairer with strong yellow undertones; therefore their skin contains higher levels of the pheomelanin pigment. No matter the amount of melanin produced, we all have the same number of melanocytes in our skin, which are the cells that produce melanin (pigment). In darker skin types the melanocytes are more sensitive to irritation and react more aggressively to injuries. An example of injury can be as simple as extracting a blackhead and applying too much pressure on the skin, which results in trauma to the skin where a dark spot is formed, also known as post-inflammatory hyperpigmentation. This is a common problem associated with those who contain more melanin in their skin. Hyperpigmentation occurs more often in those with darker skin, which can be a result from burns, inflammation, scraps, cuts, or even a pimple. Those who suffer with acne, eczema, and ingrown hairs will also result in uneven skin tone and hyperpigmented spots.

Another key point of difference in those with darker skin is the sebaceous glands that produce oil/sebum. These glands tend to produce higher levels of oil, which results in excessive oil production and ultimately results in overdrying the skin. A huge benefit for those with higher melanin content or more color in their skin is that they will tend to see signs of aging later on in life. Melanin acts as a protector for our skin and helps to ward off the UV rays of the sun by absorbing them, and keeping them from penetrating the skin. Whenever the skin detects excess solar radiation it produces more melanin and more melanin means darker skin, hence, the suntan. This not to say that people of color do not get wrinkles; it just means that aging takes place differently and the propensity for irritation and hyperpigmentation is magnified for their skin type. Therefore a greater knowledge is required for product choice and professional treatment options. Most commonly Caucasian women tend to seek out skin care products for anti-aging properties and moisturizing, whereas women with more color look for products to correct and prevent uneven skin tone and blemishes.

3.2.3.3 COMMON SKIN CONDITIONS FOR ETHNIC SKIN AND TREATMENT METHODS

With social media and companies paying attention to wanting to help the consumer solve a skin care problem, I feel that the time has come in the industry where companies can collaborate to help educate consumers on how important prevention is and making lifestyle changes to support this. For example, if someone in their 30s wants to lighten their skin, it is mandatory that daily use of a SFP30 is also part of the regime. Direct sun avoidance during peak times is essential, and if not, a precaution such as a hat or additional protection measure should be taken.

With a collaborated campaign that is more educational, the message will reach out to consumers and change will happen. Social media plays a big role in that it can assist with getting the right message out to consumers, making it more fun and easier to grasp. In most Asian countries TV and media still play a big role in the lives of the masses, so some form of education via this method may also be very effective. Along with more education will come better preventative steps which will essential be the most successful approach to reduce dark spots.

Prevention is a key to successfully reducing the risk of hyperpigmentation in the future. A good skin care regimen followed a.m. and p.m. will help provide preventative results. A preventative regimen must include some type of mechanical or chemical exfoliation three times a week, a melanin-suppression formula, and sunscreen. The first step is to exfoliate the skin so that the dead skin cells are removed and to reveal brighter skin tone. Exfoliation will help increase the cellular turnover, so results are seen more quickly from the skin-brightening product. The second step is to use a skin-brightening product twice a day after cleansing the skin. There are a variety of skin-lightening products on the market, so the best thing to look for is the product containing the most amount of skin-lightening active ingredients. Some formulas contain hydroquinone and others do not. There are many alternatives in the market to address different skin types and pigment disorders. Refer to the list of skin-lightening actives. The last step will be to protect the skin from the harmful UV rays. Sun is the number one precursor to pigment formation. Protecting the skin with a broad-spectrum SPF of 30 will provide the best protection from UV-A and UV-B rays. If exposed to the sun for a long period of time reapply sunscreen every two hours for adequate protection. Below are common skin conditions and different causes and treatments.

Melasma (also known as chloasma or "pregnancy mask") is a common skin condition. It causes brown to gray patches of discoloration, very common in women during the reproductive years. Melasma is dark, irregular, well-demarcated hyperpigmented macules/patches commonly found on the upper cheek, nose, upper lip, and forehead. It can also appear on parts of the body that get excessive sun exposure such as forearms and neck and décolleté area.

Causes of Melasma: Hormonal changes in the body, genetics, and overexposure to sun. History of excessive or intermittent sun exposure. Pregnancy, birth control pills, HRT, other medications (diuretics, antibiotics, heart disease, diabetic, hypertension meds). Products or treatments that irritate the skin may cause an increase in melanin production and accelerate melasma symptoms.

People with olive or darker skin, like Hispanic, Asian, and Middle Eastern individuals, have higher incidences of melasma. People with a genetic predisposition or known family history of melasma are at an increased risk of developing melasma. Important prevention methods for these individuals include sun avoidance and application of extra sunblock to avoid stimulating pigment production.

An estimated 6 million women are living in the U.S. with melasma and 45–50 million women worldwide live with melasma; over 90% of all cases are women. Prevention is primarily aimed at facial sun protection and sun avoidance. Treatment requires regular UVA & UVB sunblock SPF 30 application and skin-lightening, -whitening and -brightening creams. (3)

Treatments for Melasma:

Microdermabrasion: utilizes vacuum suction and an abrasive material like fine diamond chips or aluminum oxide crystals to exfoliate the top layers of the skin. The vacuum pressure is adjusted depending on the sensitivity and tolerance of the skin. Typical microdermabrasion sessions can last anywhere from a few minutes to one hour. Minimal to no recovery time is needed after microdermabrasion. Microdermabrasion techniques can improve melasma, but dramatic results are not generally seen or expected after one or two treatments. Multiple treatments in combination with sunscreen and other creams yield best results.

Chemical peels: Many types and strengths of chemical peels are available for different skin types. The type of peel should be tailored for each individual and selected by a physician.

TCA: TCA peels are excellent and safe in the hands of an experienced dermatologist. This is a good option, particularly if you have severe melasma.

AHA +combinations: In treating melasma, 30–70% glycolic acid peels are very common. Various combination peels, including a mix of glycolic acid, kojic acid, lactic acid, etc., can be used to treat melasma. Usually six sittings at a gap of ten days produce good results.

Ultrasonic: Treatments with whitening jelly can be used in conjunction with chemical peels or MDA to further enhance results.

IPL treatments with pigmentation filter or currently Fractional Laser Treatments are being used to reduce pigmentation. Usually three to four treatments are needed at a gap of 15–20 days.

Although melasma tends to be a chronic disorder with periodic ups and downs, the prognosis for most cases is good. Just as melasma develops slowly, clearance also tends to be slow. The gradual disappearance of dark spots is based on establishing the right treatment combination for each individual skin type. Melasma that does not successfully respond to treatment is because sun exposure is not avoided.

Peri-Orbital Hypermelanosis (Undereye dark circles): This is a very common disorder among the Asian population, especially the Indian population. Undereye circles, which are dark pigments around the peri-orbital area, may be hereditary, or due to stress or eye strain. Also, those suffering from allergies seem to have dark circles. Smoking, drinking a lot of alcohol, coffee, soda, or caffeine beverages will usually make dark circles worse. Diet also plays a role and not having a healthy diet can affect it as well. A lack of sleep is a big culprit, so pulling all-nighters—whether for school or fun—can also contribute to dark circles around the eyes.

Treatments of Peri-Orbital Hypermelanosis: Once the cause has been identified there are several available solutions for treatment of this common disorder. Using a good eye cream that has ingredients specifically targeted to this delicate area, twice a day, will help prevent moisture loss, hydrate the area, and assist the delicate skin in absorbing the moisture and active ingredients, while stimulating the blood supply. Also wearing sunglasses can help prevent further pigmentation when exposed to the sun.

Photomelanosis: This is increased pigmentation due to sun exposure; it is also known as sun damage or photo-damage. The pigmentation occurs on exposed skin, commonly on the face, neck, and back. The pigmentation may be patchy or a diffused darkening of the exposed skin.

Hyperpigmentation: Hyperpigmentation is the production of excess melanin causing dark spots on the skin. Age spots, liver spots, freckles, sun spots, and pregnancy mask are all types of hyperpigmentation.

Causes of Hyperpigmentation: Common causes of skin hyperpigmentation are excessive sun exposure, hormonal changes, heredity, acne, and irritations from skin treatments and products. Hyperpigmentation may also be caused by inflammation, or by other skin injuries, including those related to acne vulgaris. In situations where hyperpigmentation is caused by acne or some other cause of skin inflammation, it is known as PIH, or post-inflammatory hyperpigmentation. People with darker Asian, Mediterranean, or African skin tones are also more prone to hyperpigmentation, especially if they have excess sun exposure.

Many forms of hyperpigmentation are caused by an excess production of melanin. Hyperpigmentation can be diffuse or focal, affecting such areas as the face and the back of the hands. Melanin is produced by melanocytes at the lower layer of the epidermis. Melanin is a class of pigment responsible for producing color in the body in places such as the eyes, skin, and hair. As the body ages, melanocyte distribution becomes less diffuse and its regulation less controlled by the body. UV light stimulates melanocyte activity, and where concentrations of the cells are denser than surrounding areas, hyperpigmentation is affected. It can also be caused by using skin-lightening lotions. (4)

Post-Inflammatory Hyperpigmentation: a very common condition for those with more color in their skin. Many types of trauma, inflammation, medications, cosmetics containing alcohol or fragrance, and skin conditions including: acne, eczema, contact dermatitis. Systemic disease such as Addison disease, liver disease, pregnancy, and pituitary tumors can also cause hyperpigmentation.

Acne Vulgaris: one of the biggest challenges to women with brown skin who seek clear, glowing complexions. In addition to the acne, women with brown skin must also face hyperpigmentation—skin darkening in spots or patches—which occurs in response to the acne outbreak.

Acne Rosacea: not one of the skin problems typically associated with skin of color. A main feature of rosacea is redness or erythema of the face. But rosacea does occur in people of color, including African Americans, Latinos, and Asians, and is often undiagnosed or misdiagnosed.

Eczema: one of the more common skin problems for individuals with brown skin, including those of Asian, Latino, and African descent. It is felt to be the second-most-common skin disease in African Americans. Although it is unknown if the incidence of eczema is increased in Latinos, one study found a significantly higher percent of Mexican American adolescents with eczema than white and African American adolescents.

Keloids: Abnormal healing of the skin occurs frequently in individuals with brown skin. When skin is injured, it may heal with one of several types of scars (keloids): normal (level with the surrounding skin), atrophic (depressed), hypertrophic (slightly raised), and keloidal (large and raised).

Seborrheic Dermatitis: often referred to as dandruff, is a common problem for many women with brown skin. Areas of involvement are the hairline and scalp, as well as the eyebrows, the area between the nose and corners of the mouth (nasolabial folds) and the ears.

Skin Cancer: People with brown skin often have a false sense of security when it comes to skin cancer. While individuals with increased skin pigmentation have added protection against the UV rays of the sun, it is dangerous to assume that darker skin exempts one from this serious skin problem.

Hypopigmentation: Areas of the skin that have lost their pigment completely when there are no longer functioning melanocytes in that area to create pigment, leaving white spots or patches on the skin. Hypopigmentation can result from overbleaching, or extensive trauma from UV light, lasers, or heat. Examples of hypopigmentation include:

Vitiligo: Vitiligo causes smooth, white patches on the skin. In some people, these patches can appear all over the body. It is an autoimmune disorder in which the pigment-producing cells are damaged. There is no cure for vitiligo, but there are several treatments, including cosmetic cover-ups, corticosteroid creams, or ultraviolet light treatments.

Albinism: Albinism is a rare inherited disorder caused by the absence of an enzyme that produces melanin. This results in a complete lack of pigmentation in skin, hair, or eyes. Albinos have an abnormal gene that restricts the body from producing melanin. There is no cure for albinism. People with albinism should use a sunscreen at all times because they are much more likely to get sun damage and skin cancer. This disorder can occur in any race, but is most common among whites.

Pigmentation loss as a result of skin damage: If you've had a skin infection, blisters, burns, or other trauma to your skin, you may have a loss of pigmentation in the affected area. The good news with this type of pigment loss is that it's frequently not permanent, but it may take a long time to repigment. Cosmetics can be used to cover the area, while the body regenerates the pigment. (5)

3.2.3.4 TIPS TO ACHIEVE HEALTHY, BEAUTIFUL SKIN

- Mandatory daily use of broad-spectrum UVA & UVB Sunblock – SPF30+
- Wash skin daily with mild nonsurfactant cleanser, use a clean towel to pat dry, do *not* rub the face harshly, or share towels with others. The face should be washed twice, both morning and evening.
- Drink water—an average adult typically needs 10–12 eight-ounce glasses a day. I prefer to drink room-temperature or hot water with a slice of lemon.
- Use quality skin care products that hydrate and repair the skin, and avoid products that clog your pores.
- Use lightweight facial makeup foundation or powders; this will allow the skin to breathe and prevent further breakouts. Personally I feel the less used the better; if you take care of your skin you will have a natural radiance.
- The skin is a very sensitive organ and given the level of abuse it goes through, is remarkably resilient. However, this resilience decreases as we age, and opens the door for bacteria, viruses, microbes, parasites, etc. that invade the skin. In climates such as Asia where it is hot and polluted, especially in the cities, environmental damage also plays a role in the aging process.
- If you have a tendency to break out, seek professional help to treat it and go for the root cause of the blemish, rather than using makeup to cover skin blemishes and trauma. This can save you permanent damage with scars and or ice-pick marks.
- Avoid skin trauma like tattoos, body piercing, etc. These abuses can age the skin, and expose it to bacteria and other viruses.
- When you notice skin discomfort, dryness, itchiness, reddening, discoloration, blemishes, lesions, bruising, tags, moles, bumps, warts, corns, calluses, or other skin trauma, seek professional help, as some conditions may get worse over time if not treated.
- Diet plays a crucial part in skin health, so eat wisely. Your diet should contain plenty of green leafy vegetables. Eat seasonal fruits and add nuts to your diet; if you have health issues it is wise to seek a nutritionist, or dietician, to establish a healthy diet to suit your unique skin and bodily needs.
- Make regular monthly visits with a skin care professional to help maintain healthy skin. Having topical treatments such as Lactic Peels, chemical peels, microdermabrasion, and laser therapy specific for Asian skin.
- Treat yourself to regular spa treatments; having a regular full-body massage is not only relaxing but good for you too. A deep massage is good to maintain healthy skin, since the kneading breaks up old fat deposits and releases toxins. The sauna and steam bath are recommended to help keep

skin moist, supple, healthy, and toned. Drink water to hydrate before and after your sessions.

- Minimize exposure to tanning machines, lamps, beds, etc. The tanning process is actually a form of skin abuse, and can result in premature aging of the skin and promote hyperpigmentation.
- Always use high-quality and well-made skin care products. Using a daily program that consists of cleanser, exfoliator, moisturizer, and SPF 30 is highly recommended. The reward is to enjoy clear, healthy, blemish-free, radiant, glowing, beautiful skin for many years.
- Avoid cheaply made skin creams with a lot of chemicals. Products that are highly fragranced, with artificial colors, binders, emulsifiers, etc., can cause some people to develop allergies, leading to rashes and pigmentation issues.
- In order to maintain healthy skin and overall health, a total avoidance of alcohol, tobacco, and illegal drugs is advisable. These are all toxic to the body and after many years of such abuse, the skin can become wrinkled, saggy, dry, and itchy, and can lose its suppleness. Reducing or eliminating caffeine, sugar, and soft drinks will also benefit the skin and overall health.

REFERENCES:

1. Japan Ref: Jeff D. Opdyke, the Sovereign Investor, Jan 2013.
2. Asian Scientist (Sep. 18, 2012).
3. Freedberg, Irwin M., et al. Fitzpatrick's Dermatology in General Medicine. 4th ed. Vol. 1. New York: McGraw-Hill, 1993.
4. "Hyperpigmentation". Dermatalogic Disease Database. American Osteopathic College of Dermatology. Retrieved 2006-03-08. Hyperpigmentation (Age Spots) Hyperpigmentation, Chloasma & Melasma, KAVI.
5. WebMD Sources:

   Merck Manual Home Health Handbook: "Overview of Skin Pigment."

   American Osteopathic College of Dermatology: "Hyperpigmentation."

   American Academy of Dermatology: "Melasma."

   National Institute of Arthritis and Musculoskeletal and Skin Diseases: "Healthy Skin Matters."

COMPROMISED SKIN IN THE ELDERLY

Authors
R. Randall Wickett, Ph.D., Martha Tate, Ph.D.

Randall Wickett, Ph.D.
Emeritus Professor
Pharmaceutics and Cosmetic Science
Univ. Cincinnati College of Pharmacy
3225 Eden Ave
Cincinnati, Oh 42567

Martha Tate, Ph.D.
Research and Engineering
Kimberly-Clark Corporation
1400 Holcomb Bridge Road
Roswell, GA 30076

ABSTRACT

This chapter provides a thorough look at the structure and chemistry of the skin. It draws upon, and consolidates, the enormous body of literature on the subject and brings it together to form a solid foundation for the reader's understanding of skin aging as well as describing treatments of aging skin with selected effective "cosmeceuticals." We live in a culture that values a youthful appearance at a time when the population is aging rapidly in developed countries. According to the United States census there were ~57 million Americans age 60 and older in 2010, nearly a 25% increase in the ten years since the 2000 census. As people live longer, populations in Western Europe and Japan are also aging.

It is well known that the appearance of the skin can have dramatic effects on the overall impression of age. Both wrinkles (1, 2) and inhomogeneity of skin color (3–6) contribute significantly to the apparent age of individuals. The combination of the effect of skin appearance on apparent age and an aging population with the desire to look youthful has, not surprisingly, led to enormous interest in products that might make skin appear more youthful.

Skin aging is often broken into two categories referred to as intrinsic aging and extrinsic aging (7–9). *Intrinsic aging is the unavoidable effect of time.* It occurs on all body sites and is considered to be independent of lifestyle. Extrinsic aging results from lifestyle choices. The main factor is photo-aging brought about by exposure to ultraviolet (UV) light from the sun (7, 10–12). While sun exposure is considered the main extrinsic factor leading to skin damage, it is becoming increasingly clear that exposure to cigarette smoke can lead to significant skin compromise both in smokers(13–21) and in nonsmoking spouses of smokers (22).

This chapter reviews the consequences of both intrinsic and extrinsic skin aging. Mechanisms underlying photo-aging will be discussed, as will attempts to improve aging skin and at least partially reverse the effects of time and extrinsic insults.

TABLE OF CONTENTS

3.2.4.1 STRUCTURE OF THE SKIN

We begin with a brief review of skin structure to facilitate our discussion of skin aging. This subject is discussed in more detail in other chapters to this book. Discussion of the structure of skin will naturally refer to its various layers (23, 24) or strata. The skin's multiple layers work together to perform its multiple functions. Figure 1 is a hematoxyln and eosin (H&E) stained image of a cross-section of human skin.

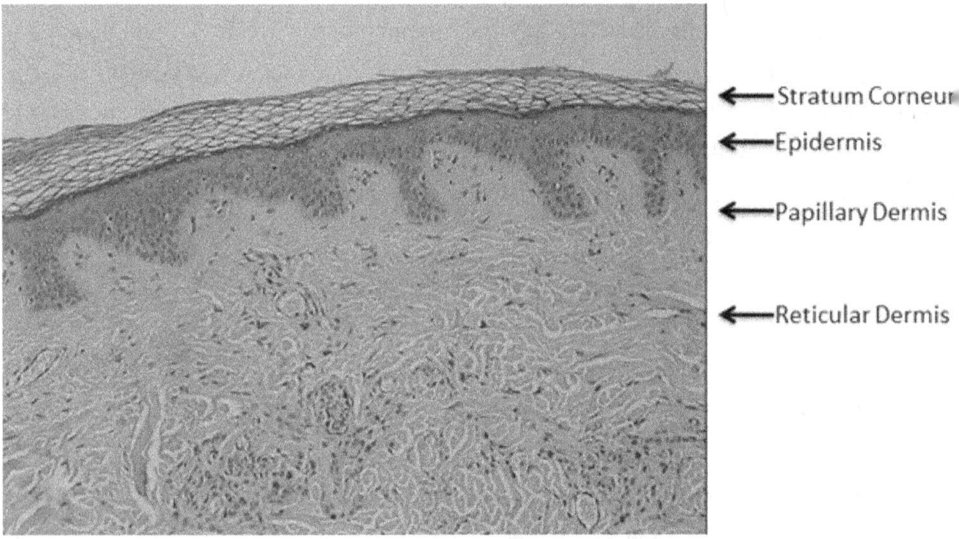

Figure 1 (H&E stained cross section of human skin labeled to show the various layers. The "basket weave" appearance of the *stratum corneum* is an artifact of processing. http://en.wikipedia.org/wiki/Epidermis_(skin) public domain image)

The epidermis and dermis are fundamentally different types of tissue. The epidermis overlays the papillary dermis and is composed of cells. The main type of cell of the epidermis is the **keratinocyte**. Keratinocytes are found from the basal layer to the granular layer where they are transformed into the corneocytes of the *stratum corneum* (SC). Keratinocytes make many proteins including keratins, the main structural proteins of the SC (25). Two other important cells in the epidermis are melanocytes and Langerhans cells.

The **dermis** has two layers, papillary and reticular. The hypodermis or subcutaneous tissue is sometimes considered part of the dermis but will not be considered in this review. The dermis is a fibrous tissue composed primarily of collagen, elastin, and proteoglycans, which form the dermal matrix. The papillary dermis is named for the dermal papilla protruding into the epidermis (Figure 1). The fibroblasts, which make the proteins and proteoglycans of the dermis, are found in the dermal matrix (24).

The main structural protein of the dermis is collagen. Collagen has a unique amino acid sequence. Every third amino acid is glycine, which does not have a side chain. This allows collagen to form a compact triple-helix with three collagen chains winding around each other as if in a braid. Each triple helix is about 300 nm long and 1.5 nm in diameter (26). Collagen is synthesized in fibroblasts as pro-collagen and exported from the cell into the dermal matrix where it is processed by proteolytic enzymes, which remove sections from both ends of pro-collagen to form 300-nm filaments. These filaments then aggregate in the extracellular space to form collagen fibers.

The matrix in the papillary dermis is loosely packed with fibers compared to the tightly packed reticular dermis (24). The papillary dermis contains type III collagen, which is found at relatively low levels in the reticular dermis where type I collagen predominates (27–29). Oxytalan fibers are thin (10–12nm) elastic fibers found perpendicular to the dermal-epidermal junction in the papillary dermis (30, 31). Elaunin fibers are also found in the papillary dermis parallel to the plane of the skin (30).

Elastin provides elasticity to skin (32). In elastin, four protein chains are bound together through the desmosine cross-link. Elastin has an amino acid residue called allysine, made from lysine by the enzyme lysyl oxidase. The desmosine cross-link is formed between three allylisine chains and one lysine chain. Amorphous elastin fibers surrounded by fibrillin microfibrils are found predominately in the reticular dermis (33, 34) (Figure 2).

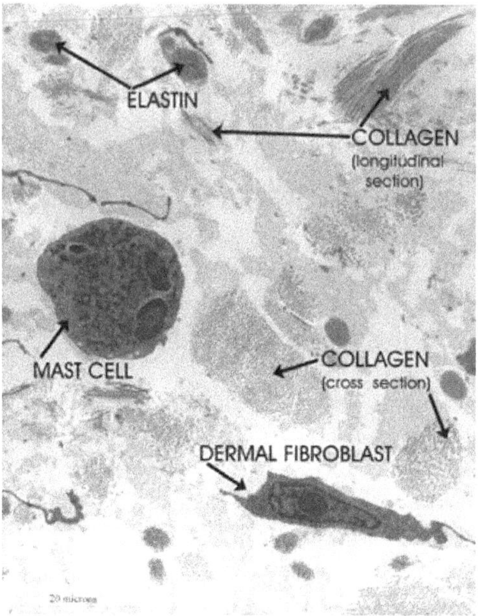

Figure 2: Electron micrograph of the reticular dermis showing collagen, elastin, a fibroblast, and a mast cell. (© Raymond Boissy, used with permission)

Glycosaminoglycans or GAGS bind water in the dermal matrix (35) keeping the dermis hydrated. Hyaluronic acid (HA), a major component of GAGS, is a very high molecular weight. GAGs such as chondroitin sulfate and keratan sulfate bind to core proteins to form proteoglycans. Proteins called link proteins bind proteoglycans to HA in a noncovalent proteoglycan complex that is very hygroscopic.

Figure 2 is an electron micrograph of the reticular dermis showing collagen and elastin fibers as well as a fibroblast and a mast cell. Mast cells contain histamine granules and release histamine in response to heat or irritants. The reticular dermis is much more densely packed with fibers than the papillary dermis.

The dermal matrix is significantly affected by both intrinsic and extrinsic aging as will be discussed below.

Skin barrier function resides primarily in the epidermis and barrier may be considered "*la raison d'être*" of the epidermis (36). Layers of the epidermis are shown schematically in Figure 3.

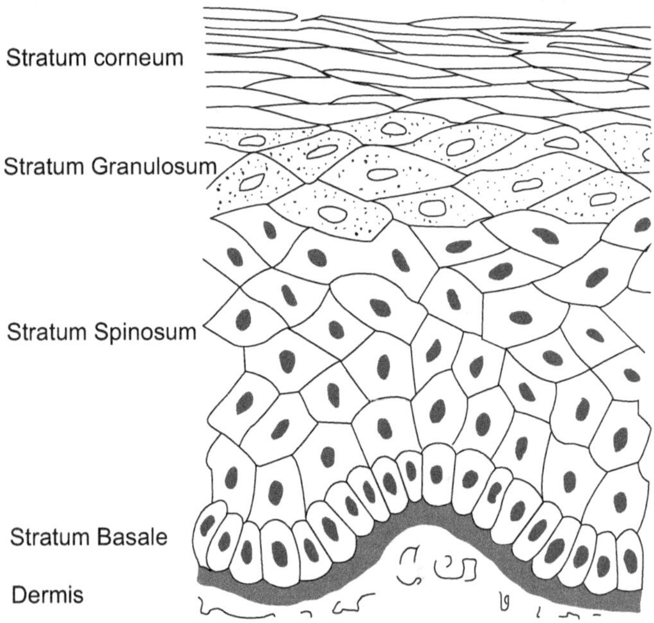

Figure 3: Diagram showing layers of the epidermis (illustration by Robin M. Wickett)

The epidermal barrier defends the body from water loss to the environment, absorption of noxious chemicals from the environment, and microbial infection. These defensive functions depend critically on the top layer, the *stratum corneum* (SC), and are thought to be integrated with SC formation and homeostasis (37, 38).

For 30 years the most common model used to organize thinking about the SC barrier has been the "bricks and mortar" model proposed by Elias (39). This model is based on the fact that corneocytes are surrounded by the extracellular lipids of the SC. Thus the corneocytes are modeled as bricks and the lipids as mortar. The model has proven useful for representing the phenomena associated with describing ingredient skin penetration. Moderately hydrophobic molecules are thought to penetrate the SC by diffusing through the lipid mortar, winding their way around the corneocytes bricks (40). Harding has described an updated version of the bricks-and-mortar model that includes the presence of the desmosomes that hold SC cells together prior to desquamation and the role of natural moisturizing factor in SC function (41). This model is illustrated in Figure 4.

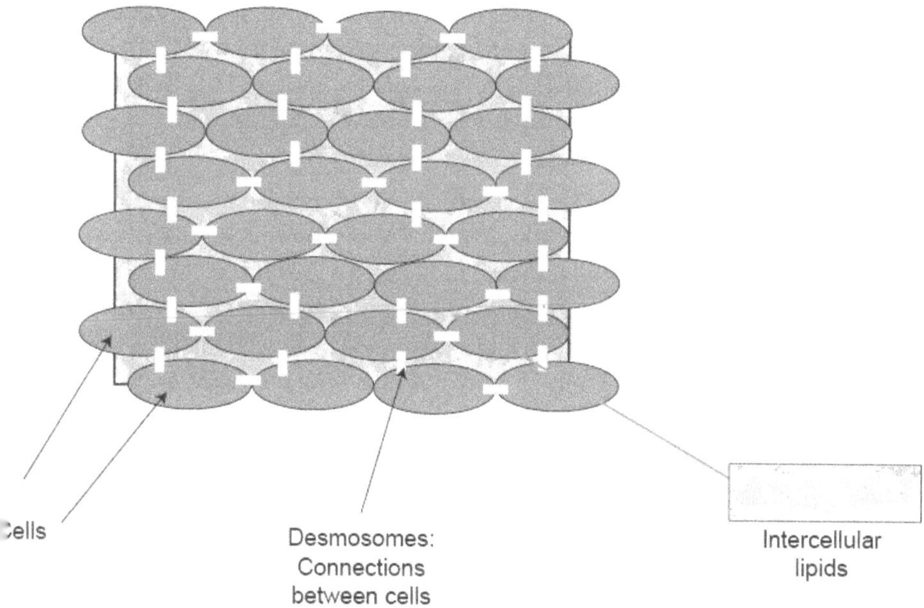

Figure 4: Schematic of the "bricks and mortar" model for human *stratum corneum* illustrating the corneocyte "bricks," the intercellular lipid "mortar," and the desmosomes connecting the corneocytes. (M.O. Visscher, used with permission)

The "bricks and mortar" of the SC barrier are formed in the *stratum granulosum* (SG) (Figure 4) where keratinocytes are transformed to form the corneocytes "bricks" and lipids are released into the intercellular space to form the "mortar." The SG is named for the two types of granules that appear in the cells, keratohyalin granules (24) that are composed of protein and lamellar bodies that primarily contain lipids (42, 43).

A complex process occurs in the SG: the nucleus is digested, the cytoplasm disappears, and lipids are released into the intercellular space to form the mortar (39, 44, 45). The keratin intermediate filaments aggregate to form microfibrils (46, 47) inside the corneocytes (48, 49). aided by filaggrin from the keratohyalin granules.

Filaggrin is an acronym for filament-aggregating protein (50–53). Filaggrin contains a high level of positively charged amino acids, allowing it to interact with the negatively charged epidermal keratins (54). Filaggrin is then modified to come off the microfibrils, through conversion of the positively charged amino acid arginine to uncharged citruline by the enzyme peptidyl arginine deminase (PAD) (55, 56). After release from the microfibrils filaggrin is digested by proteolytic enzymes to produce the amino acid components of the natural moisturizing factor (NMF) of the *stratum corneum* (57–62).

NMF consists of lactate, amino acids from filaggrin breakdown, and pyrollidone carboxylic acid (PCA) formed from the amino acid glutamine (63–65). These natural moisturizers are important to maintain proper hydration of the SC allowing it to be flexible and to desquamate properly (57, 66–69). Digestion of filaggrin to NMF is thought to happen in the mid-*stratum corneum* (70).

In the *stratum granulosum* (SG) the keratinocyte cell membrane is replaced by the corneocyte cell envelope, a very tough structure made of cross-linked protein with lipids covalently attached to its surface (71–75). The resulting corneocytes or squames (the bricks) are flat cells that tend to be in the shape of either a hexagon or pentagon. Corneocyte size and distribution have been investigated by several authors. A single corneocyte is about 25 μm on a side, with a surface area ranging from about 550 to 1300 μm^2 depending on age and body site (76–79), and a thickness of about 0.5–1.0 μm (80, 81). Rougier et al. (79) reported corneocyte surface area on most body sites investigated to range from 900 to 1100 μm^2 but to be as low as 500 μm^2 on the forehead. A negative correlation was found between corneocyte size and the penetration of benzoic acid through skin *in vivo*. The *stratum corneum* is 12–16 cell layers thick on most body sites, but it can vary from as little as nine cell layers on the forehead or eyelids to as much as 25 on the dorsum of the hand and 50 or more on the palms or the soles of the feet (82, 83).

The lipids that are released into the intercellular space as the SC forms are glucosyl ceramides, cholesterol, cholesterol esters, and long-chain fatty acids. In the intercellular space the glucosyl ceramides are converted to ceramides (84, 85). SC ceramides are polar lipids, but much less hydrophilic than the phospholipids of the original cell membrane. Figure 5 shows the structure of some of the main SC ceramides with both the original and new nomenclature that is used for them. Phospholipids from the keratinocytes of the viable layers are broken down by phospholipases (86–88) in the lower *stratum corneum*. After this extracellular processing, SC lipids spontaneously organize into multiple layers between the SC cells (89). This layered structure is critical to the barrier function of the skin.

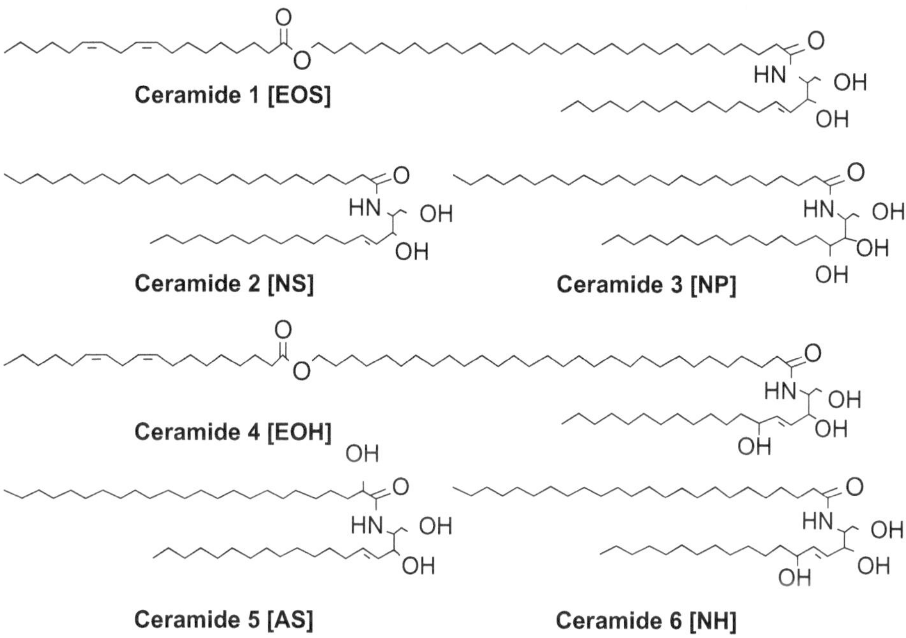

Figure 5: Key ceramides of the SC barrier.

3.2.4.2 SKIN AGING: CHANGES IN THE EPIDERMIS AND *STRATUM CORNEUM*

A general trend for corneocytes to increase in surface area with age has been reported by several groups (77, 79, 90-93). The reported increase in surface area between young adults and adults over 55 ranges from 8 to 14% depending on body site and method of measurement. Figure 6 shows corneocyte size data from two different age groups reported by Grove et al. (91, 93).

Note the extreme variability in the data from the older age group compared to the narrower distribution in the younger group. The average size of corneocytes is increased in the older age group but there is considerable overlap between the two data sets.

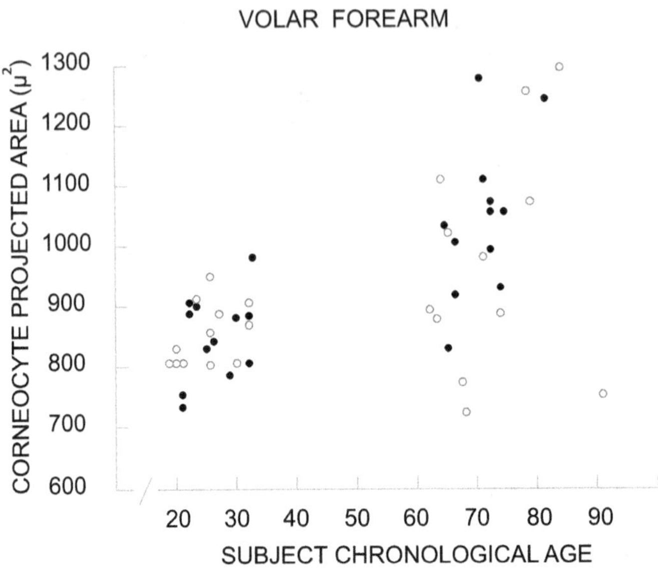

Figure 6: Projected corneocyte surface area for two age ranges for men (•) and women (○). Reprinted from Grove et al. (93) with permission of the Society of Cosmetic Chemists.

While the "bricks" of the SC may increase in size with age, the "mortar" content is apparently decreasing. Imokawa et al. reported a gradual decrease in total SC ceramides with age (94). Rogers et al. reported progressive reductions in fatty acids, ceramides and cholesterol with age in subjects ranging in age from 21–60 years on the hands, legs, and face (95). The reduction in ceramide I (EOS) linolate was especially noteworthy.

SC barrier function is affected by both intrinsic and extrinsic aging (96), but it is relatively robust to both and changes are not always in the direction that one might expect. The most common and best-validated method for determining SC barrier function *in vivo* is by measurement of the passive diffusion of water through the skin by measuring the rate water evaporates from the surface of dry nonsweating skin. This parameter is known as trans-epidermal water loss (TEWL) (97–99).

Several groups have studied the effects of age on SC barrier function by measuring TEWL. Results have varied. Roskos and Guy (100) reported no correlation between baseline TEWL on the ventral forearm and age for subjects ranging in age from 20 to 90 years, and Marks et al. (101) did not see a significant correlation to age on the forearm with a similar age range, but a trend to *lower* TEWL was observed for subjects above 55. Rougier et al. found no significant change in TEWL on the upper outer arm in subjects ranging in age from 20 to 80 years (79).

Kligman (102) reported that TEWL on both the forearm and lower legs averaged slightly *lower* for a group of individuals aged 66–81 compared to a 19–26 year old cohort. Leveque et al. (77) reported TEWL from the arm to be approximately constant from 25 to 65 years of age but to decline slightly between ages 65 and 75.

Wilhelm et al. (103) compared TEWL data from a young group (26.7±2.8 years) and an older group (70.5±13.8 years) on several body sites. TEWL was significantly *lower* from the older age group on all sites except the palm. Saijo et al. (104) measured TEWL from the dorsum of the hand and the dorsum of foot on children from one to five years of age, young adults from 21 to 34 years of age, and older adults ranging from 63 to 78 years of age. Aged individuals had the lowest TEWL values on both body sites. There was no difference in TEWL from the dorsum of the hand between children and young adults. Ghadially et al. (105) reported average TEWL of 4.43±0.16 g/(m^2-hr) for a group of six individuals over 80 compared to 6.41±0.93 g/(m^2-hr) for a group of 21 subjects under 30.

Schwindt et al. (106) found significantly lower TEWL on the backs of subjects averaging 69.8 years of age compared to subjects averaging 27.7 years old. In a recent study Luebberding et al. reported TEWL data from six different body sites on 150 women divided equally into five age groups, 18–29, 30–39, 40–49, 50–59, and 60–80 (107). No correlation was found between TEWL and age on the neck, forearm, or back of the hand. TEWL was negatively correlated to age on the forehead and cheek. Interestingly, TEWL on the décolleté area was positively correlated to age, ranging from 5.62 gm/m^2-hr on the youngest group to 7.86 gm/m^2-hr on the oldest, with a high level of statistical significance. In our review of the literature these data from the décolleté are the only ones to show a statistically significant increase in TEWL with age.

The SC barrier to penetration of compounds into the skin has also been evaluated as a function of age. Roskos et al. compared the penetration of six drugs of differing polarity into the skin of subjects 22–40 years of age and over 65 years old *in vivo* (108). Permeation rates for the two most hydrophobic drugs, testosterone and estradiol, were not significantly different between the two age groups but hydrocortisone, benzoic acid, acetylsalicylic acid, and caffeine all penetrated the skin of the older group at a significantly *lower* rate than into the younger. Rougier et al. also reported that benzoic acid penetrated older skin significantly more slowly than younger *in vivo* (79).

Analysis of all these results leads to the somewhat surprising conclusion that basal SC barrier function is relatively unaffected by age from childhood through late middle age and then may actually begin to increase slightly sometime after age 60. It is notable that this apparent improvement in baseline barrier function occurs in spite of the reduction in SC barrier lipids discussed above. Rogers et al. point out that while lipids decrease, the ratio of ceramides to other SC structural lipids remain approximately constant (95). It is also possible that skin permeation of some compounds through SC is slower because of the larger corneocytes. Rougier at al. found a negative correlation between corneocyte size and the skin permeation rate of benzoic acid *in vivo* (79).

Most studies indicate that the reactivity of skin to irritant may actually decrease with age, or at least is not more marked with age as one might expect. Bettley and Donoghue reported fewer reactions to patch testing with soap in subjects 50 and older compared to subjects 10–49 years of age (109). Grove et al. reported lower skin reactivity to a variety of irritants including dimethyl sulfoxide, ethyl nicotinate, and lactic acid (93, 110) in older subjects. Maibach and coworkers (106, 111) and Robinson (112) observed lower reactivity of older skin to sodium lauryl sulfate (SLS). Robinson also reported that reaction to another strong irritant, octanoic acid, was significantly lower in subjects more than 55 years old while reactions to the weaker irritants acetic acid and decanol were only directionally reduced with age (112). Bowman et al. performed a ten-day cumulative irritation test comparing 26 subjects age 18–45 with 26 subjects age 65–80 using 11 products of widely varying irritancy (113). They found no statistically significant differences in response between the age groups, but the response was directionally less in the older age group for all the compounds that produced significant irritation.

While the static barrier function of the epidermis does not seem to diminish with age, recovery of barrier function after disruption has been found to be significantly slower in older skin. Ghadially et al. disrupted SC by either tape stripping or acetone treatment to the point that TEWL was increased to the range of 20–30 g/m^2-hr (105). Recovery of the barrier was quantified by measuring TEWL over the next several days. After acetone treatment young skin (under age 30) recovered its barrier function by 50% at 24 hours, while older skin (over 80) had only recovered 15% at 24 hours. Younger subjects took about four days to recover to 90% of their original SC barrier to TEWL while older skin required seven days to reach this level of recovery regardless of the type of insult (tape or acetone). The slower recovery of barrier function may be related to slower rates of epidermal renewal in older skin.

It is well known that corneocytes are continually shed into the environment and are being continually replaced by cells generated in the SG (see above). The SC "turnover time" is most frequently measured by staining the SC with the fluorescent dye, dansyl chloride, and monitoring the rate of dye disappearance with a UV light. When all of the fluorescence has disappeared, the SC has turned over completely (114). Grove and coworkers reported that SC turnover time is increased in elderly skin (76, 93). The turnover time for SC on the volar forearm increased from 19.8 ± 1.4 days in cohort under 35 years old to 28.1 ± 2.7 days in an over 60 age group. Similar changes were seen on the inner arm. These results confirmed the positive correlation between age and the time to turn over the SC reported by Roberts and Marks (115).

Grove found the number of SC cell layers was approximately constant between age groups, indicating that the increased SC turnover time results from decreased epidermal cell proliferation rates with age. Marks reported a small but statistically significant decline with age in the number of epidermal cells in the DNA synthesis phase (116). Engelke et al. investigated differences between young normal skin, young dry skin, aged normal skin, and aged dry skin (117) using an antibody that stains the nuclei of proliferating cells (Ki-S3) (118). Antibody staining indicated a significant reduction in epidermal proliferation rate in aged "normal skin" compared to young normal skin. A slower rate of epidermal cell proliferation is consistent with the increased time to repair a disrupted SC barrier as reported by Ghadially (105). Grove also reported that small chemically induced blisters healed more slowly in subjects between 65 and 70 years of age than in subjects 18–25 years of age (119).

The greater tendency of older subjects to develop dry skin is well known (120–122). Elderly dry skin seems to be especially prone to itching (120, 123–126), which can sometimes be severe. Dry skin in the elderly tends to develop some distinctive patterns, especially on the legs. Figure 7 below shows dry skin that developed on the legs of three elderly subjects who lived in the desert Southwest. These pictures were taken after one week of washing twice daily with a standard soap and no use of moisturizers. Notice the distinct pattern of lines on some of the subjects.

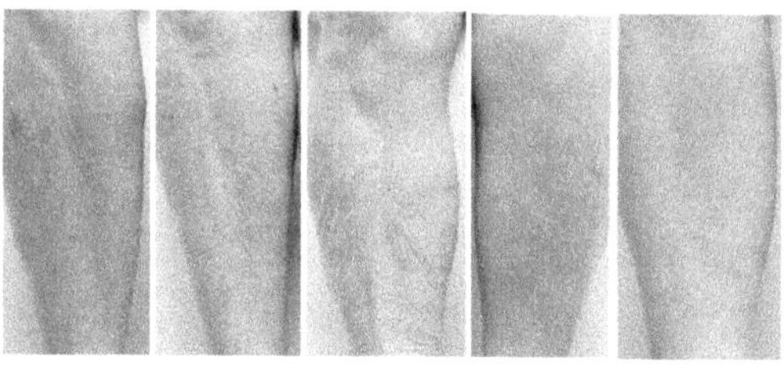

Figure 7: Dry skin on the lower legs of elderly subjects (70–90 y.o.) after washing twice daily with a standard soap and avoidance of moisturizer use.

This pattern of lines frequently develops in elderly subjects but occurs rarely if at all in younger subjects (R.R. Wickett, personal observations). Treatment with an effective moisturizer reduces or eliminates the pattern in some subjects but not in others. In Figure 8 below we see that moisturizer treatment of the right legs has nearly eliminated the pattern in the subject on the left but had little effect on the subject on the right.

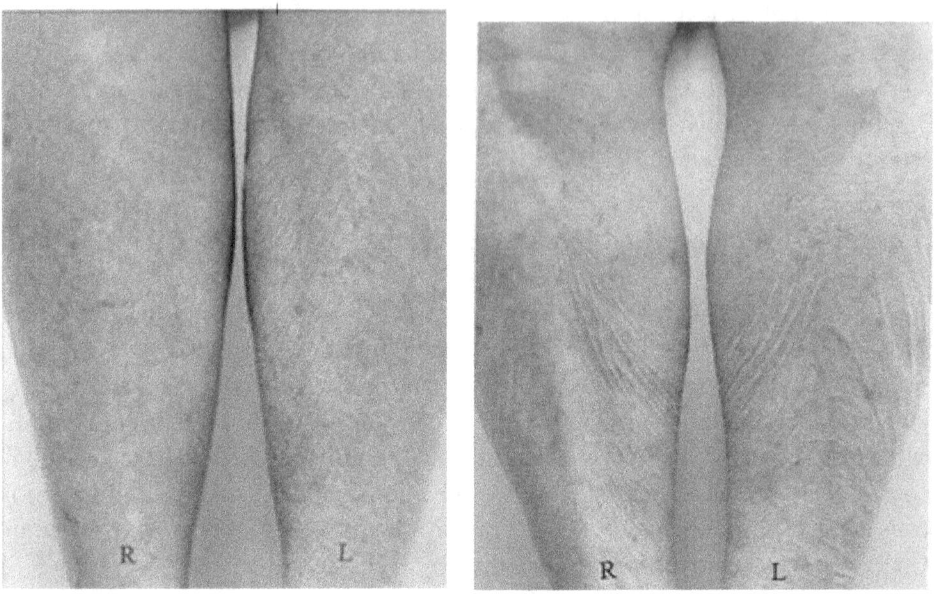

Figure 8: Dry skin resulting from soap use on the legs two elderly subjects. After one week of washing with soap and no moisturizer use the right leg of each subject was treated with an effective moisturizing lotion for two weeks while soap treatment continued on both legs.

It is not entirely clear why the elderly are so much more prone to developing dry skin. One possibility is reduction of levels of NMF (see above) in elderly skin. It has been shown that NMF levels are lower in dry skin (62). Data on the effect of age on NMF levels do not present a consistent picture. One of the key moisturizing components of NMF is the very hydrophilic molecule pyrollidone carboxylic acid (PCA) (56, 57) (see above). Harding et al. reported lower levels of PCA in elderly subjects and the difference was more marked deeper in the *stratum corneum* (70). Horii et al. reported a general decrease in free amino acids with increasing levels of dry skin in elderly subjects (127).

On the other hand, Jacobson et al. found that some SC amino acids decreased with age while others increased, but no difference was seen in total NMF free amino acids (FAA) normalized to protein content between young and old subjects (128). Takahashi and Tezuka (129) reported that NMF FAA actually increased in older subjects. However, both of these groups sampled the *stratum corneum* by scraping skin flakes from the surface rather than tape stripping to sample from lower levels of the SC as Harding et al. did. Further, as Tagami (96) has pointed out, Takahashi and Tezuka reported their results as FAA/corneocyte. Thus the higher levels of NMF FAA they report could be due to the presence of larger corneocytes in older skin (77, 78, 93) as discussed above.

Lactate is a component of the NMF that may be derived either from sweat (130, 131) or through anaerobic metabolism in the upper epidermis (132). Nakagawa et al. investigated the correlation between NMF components and SC stiffness, pH and hydration in summer and winter with healthy subjects (67). The only components that correlated significantly to SC stiffness and hydration were lactate and potassium. One might expect that the slower metabolism of aging skin reflected by the lower SC turnover rate might lead to lower levels of lactate in the SC. However, Prahl and coworkers reported that keratinocytes from aging skin produce higher levels of lactate *ex vivo* (133). It is well established that sweating rates decrease with age (134), which might lead to lower levels of lactate and thus stiffer, less well-hydrated SC.

Another factor in skin aging may be the reduction of sebum production that occurs with age (135). Fluhr et al. have presented data from studies of asebic mice, indicating that glycerol derived from the hydrolysis of sebum contributes to skin hydration (136). Sebum production declines dramatically in women at menopause but does not really decline much in men before age 80 (135), so this seems unlikely to be the whole story either. It seems likely that the tendency for elderly subjects to develop dry skin has multiple contributing factors including lower PCA levels, the slower rate of SC renewal, lower levels of lactic acid due to reduced sweating, possibly reduced glycerol due to reduced sebum production, and other factors that have yet to be discovered.

There are been relatively few studies specifically comparing the effects of intrinsic and extrinsic aging on the SC. Tagami's group studied the dorsum of the hands of Japanese golfers who only wore a golfing glove on one hand (96, 137). Roughness of the skin surface was measured from silicon replicas. Interestingly, there was a significant negative correlation between the difference in roughness between exposed and covered hands and a golfer's handicap. Better golfers (lower handicap) had larger increases in roughness on their exposed hand. Hydration as measured by higher-frequency conductance was lower for the exposed site indicating a drier skin surface, but there was no difference in barrier function as measured by TEWL.

3.2.4.3 AGING AND THE DERMIS

Both intrinsic aging and photo-aging affect the dermis far more dramatically than the epidermis. The papillary dermis is strongly affected by both intrinsic aging and chronic sun exposure. Figure 9 shows the effect of aging on abdominal skin of 18- and 76-year-old females. At the time these micrographs were published (1955) the abdominal skin of women received very little sun exposure, so the changes represent the effect of intrinsic aging.

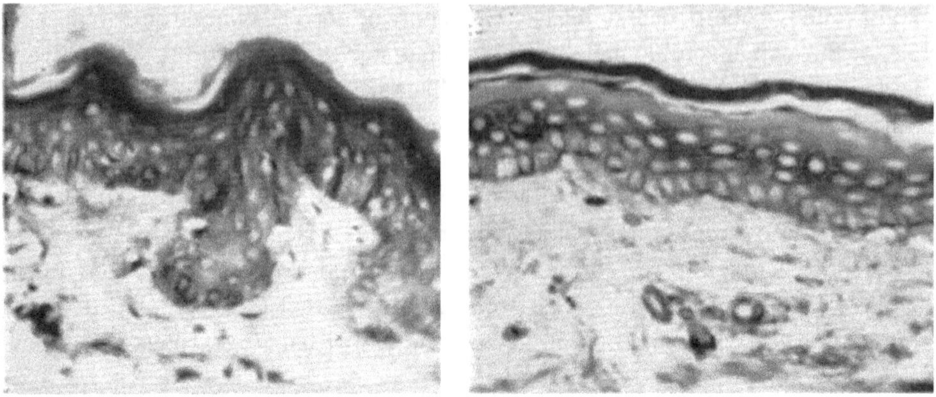

Figure 9: Abdominal skin from an 18-year-old female (left) and a 76-year-old female (right). Note the flattening of the dermal-epidermal junction as the papillary dermis diminishes with age.- (modified from Andrew [138] with permission of the Society of Cosmetic Chemists).

This flattening of the papillary dermis makes the skin less resistant to shearing stress, and the skin of elderly people is more easily ulcerated than that of younger people.

The thickness of the skin varies with age and changes depend on body site. In general, skin thickness increases for the first two decades of life. After this initial period, skin thickness may be fairly constant until about age 60. De Rigal et al. reported ultrasound results showing that skin thickness on both the ventral and dorsal forearm decreased significantly with age, but only after age 60 (139). Gniadecka and Jemec, however, reported a gradual decline in skin thickness on the forearms and ankles starting at about age 20 (140). Skin on the forehead and buttocks was found to increase in thickness with age. Takema et al. also found skin thickness to decrease with age on the forearms and increase on the forehead, corners of the eyes, and the cheeks (141). They interpreted this increased thickness as the result of sun exposure on the face.

3.2.4.4 THE DERMATOGLYPHIC PATTERN OF THE SKIN

Young skin shows a complex pattern of shallow lines on the surface. This dermatoglyphic pattern is altered on aging and a pattern with fewer but deeper lines that become more oriented emerges (93). Natural lines of tension in the skin called Langer's lines may influence the directional orientation. Hassan Zahouani and coworkers have studied these line patterns in detail (142–144). Figure 10 shows typical patterns from subject in various age ranges, pseudo-colored to indicate topography.

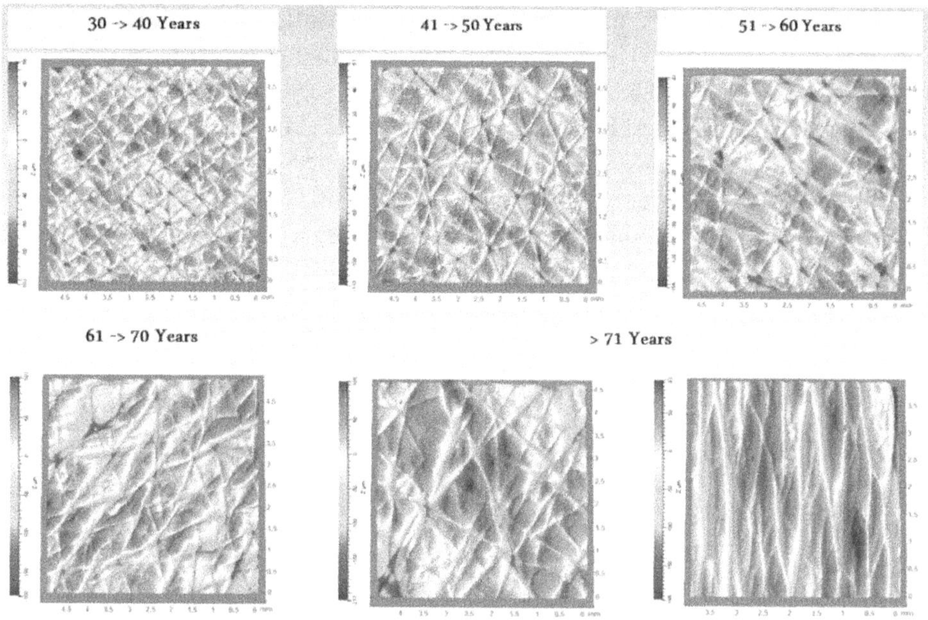

Figure 10: Changes with age in the dermatoglyphic pattern of human skin. Figure courtesy of Hassan Zahouani, used with permission.

A highly aligned dermatogyphic pattern can also be seen on the legs of some of the subjects in Figure 8 above.

In addition to the flattened dermal-epidermal junction (Figure 9) and changes in the dermatoglyphic pattern, intrinsically aged skin has diminished collagen synthesis leading to reduced levels of collagen in the dermis (145–147). El-Domyati et al. reported that there is gradual loss of the transverse elaunin fiber network and shortening and eventual reduction of the oxytalin fibers, which were nearly gone by the ninth decade of life in sun-protected skin. Underlying elastic fibers in the mid to deep reticular dermis of sun-protected skin remained relatively unchanged in amount with age (146). Focal loss of elastin and clumping of elastin fiber bundles has been observed in sun-protected elderly skin in some individuals (148).

3.2.4.5 AGING AND MECHANICAL PROPERTIES OF SKIN

Skin is a viscoelastic material. Measurement of mechanical properties of skin *in vivo* is complicated by its complex, layered nature (Part 1). It is difficult to deform the SC without producing significant deformations in the underlying layers, and of course it is impossible to deform the dermis without deforming the SC. The general principle is that smaller deformations (minimum strain) will help to localize the response to the SC, and larger deformation will reflect more on the properties of the underlying layers (149).

The most commonly used instrument for measuring skin elasticity is the Cutometer® (150–152). The Cutometer uses negative pressure to pull the skin vertically into the opening of the probe (151, 152). Negative pressures can be controlled between 20 and 500 mbar. The height the skin raises into the probe is determined by an optical system. Probes with diameters of 2, 4, 6, and 8 mm are available. In the most widely used mode, deformation is measured while vacuum is applied quickly, held constant for a defined period of time, and then released (Figure 11).

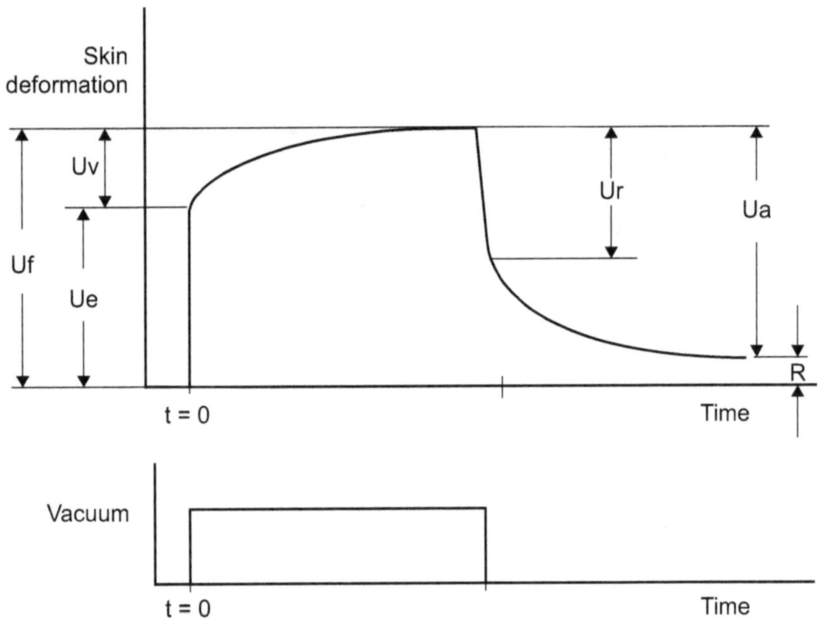

Figure 11: Schematic of Response of Skin to Cutometer

Table 1 defines parameters that can be obtained from the Cutometer curve.

TABLE 1 Cutometer Parameters from Figure 11

Ue	Elastic deformation of the skin due to the application of stress (vacuum)
Uv	Viscoelastic creep occurring after the elastic deformation
Uf	Total extensibility of the skin during stress application
Ur	Elastic recovery due to stress removal
Ua	Total recovery at the end of the stress-off period
R	Amount of deformation not recovered by the end of the stress-off period
Ua/Uf	Overall elasticity of the skin, including creep and creep recovery
Ur/Ue	Pure elasticity ignoring viscoelastic creep
Uv/Ue	Ratio of viscoelastic to elastic extension, called the viscoelastic ratio
Ur/Uf	Ratio of elastic recovery to total deformation

Cua, et al. (153) used the Cutometer® to evaluate age and body site differences in the viscoelastic properties of skin in a study with 33 subjects, 17 of them elderly averaging about 75 years, and 16 young subjects averaging about 28 years. Measurements were performed on 11 body sites. Generally, Uv/Ue increased while Ur/Uf decreased with age, but differences were not significant for all body sites.

Smalls et al. (154, 155) investigated the effects of age, body site and skin thickness on mechanical properties of skin with the Cutometer® using the 6-mm probe in a 30-subject study. Uf on the shoulder measured by the Cutometer® was negatively correlated to age with $r = -0.78$ and $p<0.001$. Results are shown in Figure 12.

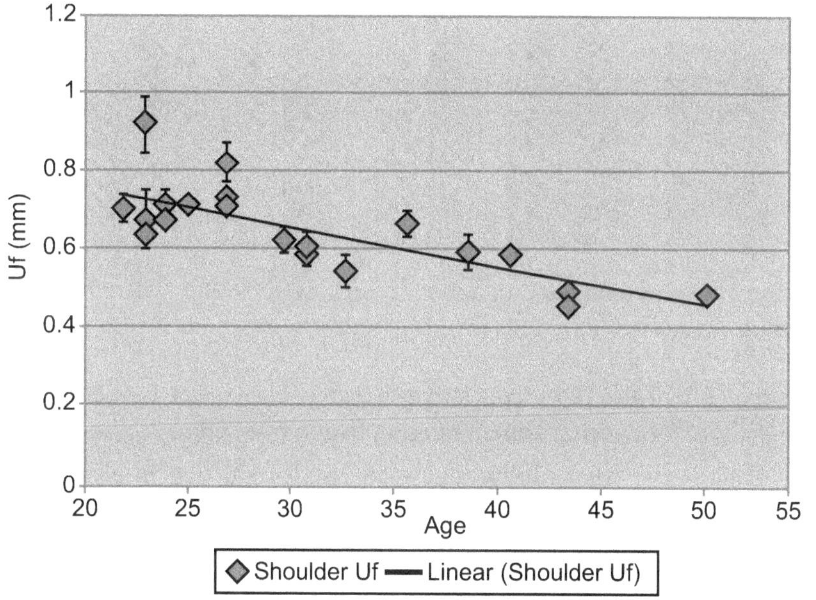

Figure 12: Uf on the shoulder versus age. Slope = –0.78, Reprinted from (155) with permission.

Ur and Ur/Uf also showed significant negative correlations with age.

Krueger et al. (156) investigated the effect of age and body site on Cutometer parameters with a panel of 120 women divided evenly into four age groups as follows.

Group	Age Range
I	20–29
II	30–39
III	40–49
IV	50–65

All of the viscoelastic parameters in Table 1 were measured. The mean correlation of Uf with age was –0.56. The parameter that had the strongest correlation with age was Ur/Uf, the ratio of immediate recovery to total deformation ($R^2 = 0.656$). Figure 13 shows their Ur/Uf results for each age group and body site.

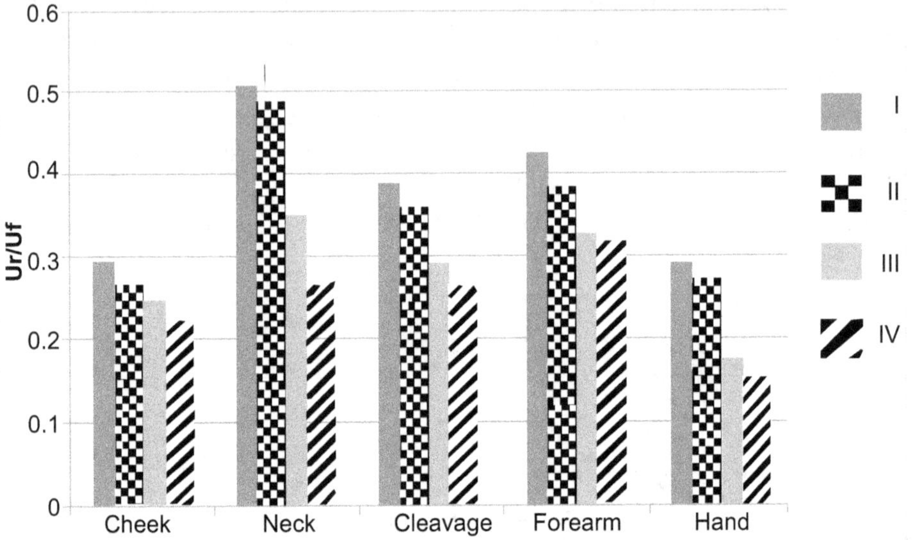

Figure 13: Ur/Uf as a function of age for five body sites. Data taken from Krueger et al. (156).

Ryu et al. (157) also reported a strong negative correlation between Ur/Uf and age in a study of 96 Korean women ranging in age from 20 to 75 years.

The reduction in extensibility and even larger reduction in elastic recovery with age is consistent with studies showing changes in the elastic fiber network of skin with aging and photo-aging (146, 158–161). Ezure et al. (162) reported that Ur/Uf decreased as "sagging" scores increased on the cheeks of Japanese women. Warrier et al. found significantly lower elastic recovery (Ur) on the cheeks of Caucasian women compared to age-matched African American women (163) and attributed the difference to less photo-damage on the face of African American women because of sun protection by melanin. Other studies have also shown that Ur/Uf is negatively correlated with age (141, 164). Increases in Ur/Uf by product treatment could possibly be used to substantiate anti-aging effects on skin elasticity.

On the other hand, dynamic indentation experiments performed by Boyer et al. indicate that the skin becomes more extensible with age (165). The authors attribute this difference to the fact that the indentation experiments were made without a "guard ring." The Cutometer deforms a small, well-defined area, determining the rheological properties of the skin, while dynamic indentation experiments deform a wider area and are proposed to be more reflective of the natural tension in the skin. Further discussion on the measurement and evaluation of skin elasticity and its relation to wrinkles and skin topology are extensively discussed in this book in the section on skin testing.

3.2.4.6 TELANGIECTASIA

Telangiectasia is the presence of visible blood vessels on the surface of the skin. It can occur both in sun-exposed and -protected areas of the skin with age. On sun-protected areas telangiectasia may develop because of thinning of the dermis.

Figure 14: Visible blood vessels (telangiectasia) on the outer thigh of a 64-year-old male (nonsmoker).

Chronic sun exposure may lead to the development of telangiectasia (166, 167). Yano and coworkers have shown that acute sun exposure induces blood-vessel growth both by up-regulation of vascular endothelial growth factor (VEGF) and down-regulation of an important endogenous inhibitor of blood-vessel growth, thrombospondin (TSP-1) (168, 169). Up-regulation of VEGF and down-regulation of TSP-1 was seen in epidermal keratinocytes, endothelial cells, and dermal fibroblasts after UV-B exposure equivalent to two times the minimal erythema dose. Not surprisingly, new blood-vessel growth was also observed (169). The correlation between sun exposure and telangiectasia seems to be stronger in men than in women (21). Current smoking has also been reported to be strongly associated with the presence of telangiectasia (170).

3.2.4.7 PHOTO-AGING MECHANISMS

The major factor in extrinsic aging of the skin is chronic sun exposure. It is well known that the majority of negative changes in skin's appearance, especially on the face, are primarily due to photo-aging (171). Ultraviolet radiation affects skin cells through two mechanisms. The first is direct damage to DNA by UV-induced formation of DNA lesions, primarily pyrimidine dimers (7, 12, 172–174). DNA may also be damaged by reactive oxygen species (ROS) generated under the influence of UV exposure (175, 176). The ability to repair DNA damage through the Nucleotide Excision Repair system has been reported to decline with age (177), perhaps contributing to further compromise of sun-exposed elderly skin. Telomeres are especially sensitive to UV damage (178) and telomere shortening may significantly affect photo-aging (172, 179, 180).

The second major factor in extrinsic aging is damage mediated by ROS, which in addition to damaging DNA, can cause skin changes either by direct action on cell surface receptors or by inducing the generation of cytokines (12, 173, 181–183). Figure 15 illustrates the effect of ROS-induced cytokine release on keratinocytes and fibroblasts.

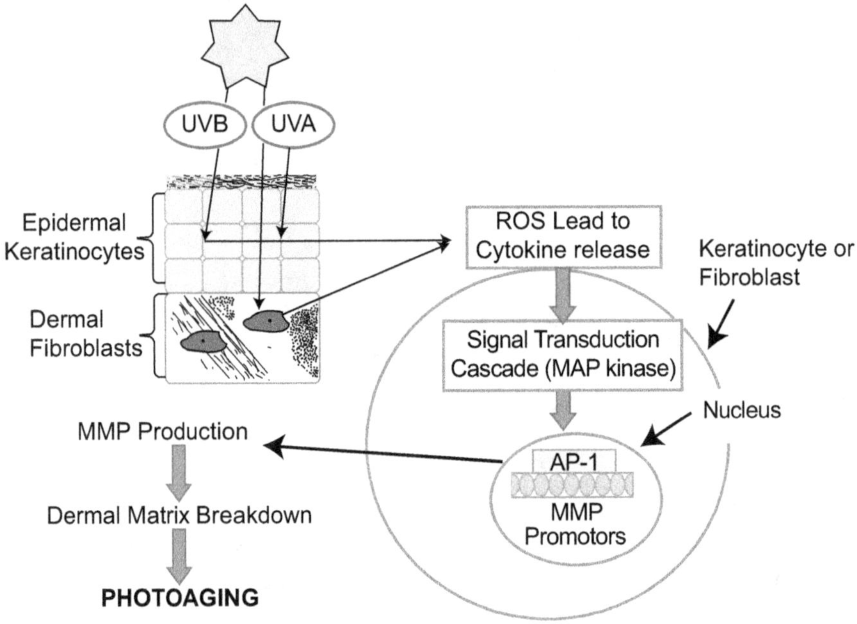

Figure 15: UV radiation affects keratinocytes and fibroblasts through similar mechanisms. Reactive Oxygen Species (ROS) generated by UV exposure lead to cytokine production that stimulates the Mitogen-Activated Protein kinase pathway. MAP kinases are generated that cause the production of the transcription factor AP-1 and promotion of the synthesis of Matrix Metalo Proteinases (MMP) that break down collagen in the dermal matrix.

In both cases the Mitogen-Activated Protein kinase pathway is activated (181). This pathway involves a complex cascade of protein kinases (enzymes that catalyze the phosphorylation of other enzymes) that leads to the formation of the transcription factor AP-1 (184, 185). AP-1 has two important effects that contribute to photo-aging. It promotes the transcription of messenger RNA for the production of collagenase and other matrix metalloproteinases that break down the dermal matrix, and it reduces the sensitivity of fibroblasts to transforming growth factor beta (TGF-β), reducing collagen production (173).

The hallmarks of photo-aging in histology are seen in Figure 16. Both type I and type III collagen are reduced (146, 186, 187) except in the thin band right below the epidermis called the Grenz zone. The SC and epidermis may be slightly thickened, though not all authors agree on this point. The major characteristic difference between photo-aging and intrinsic aging is the presence of elastosis (146–148, 188). There is actually a large accumulation of elastic fibers in the dermis of severely photo-aged skin, but these fibers are dystrophic, with large accumulations of condensates including lysozyme and amyloid P protein (189), which protect the deranged elastin from digestion by elastase (190). The fibers that result from actinic elastosis provide little or no elasticity to the skin.

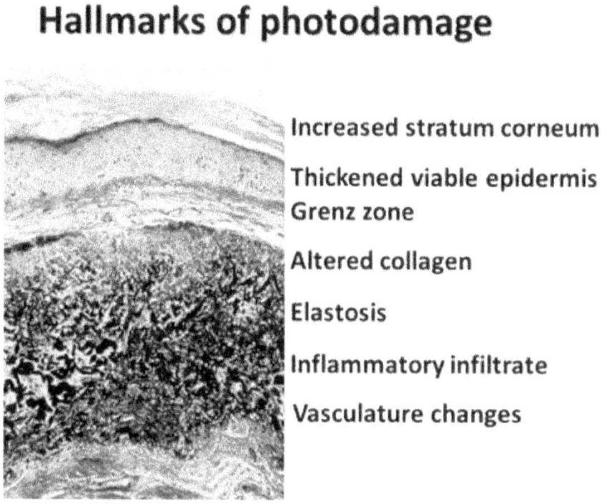

Figure 16: Hallmarks of photo-damage as seen in histology. From Robert Lavker, MD. Skin aging and photo-aging: Presented to Congress of the International Society for Bioengineering and the Skin, Orlando, FL. October 28, 2004, reprinted with permission.

As solar damage progresses, inflammatory cells migrate into the dermis. The vasculature changes that may result in telangiectasia have been discussed above.

3.2.4.8 PHOTO-AGING AND APPEARANCE

The visual signs of photo-damage are well known and include wrinkles around the eyes and mouth, hyperpigmentation (age spots), telangiectasia, and deep furrows in the skin in exposed body sites (158, 191–193). Figure 17 shows classic signs of photo-aging on some well-known faces.

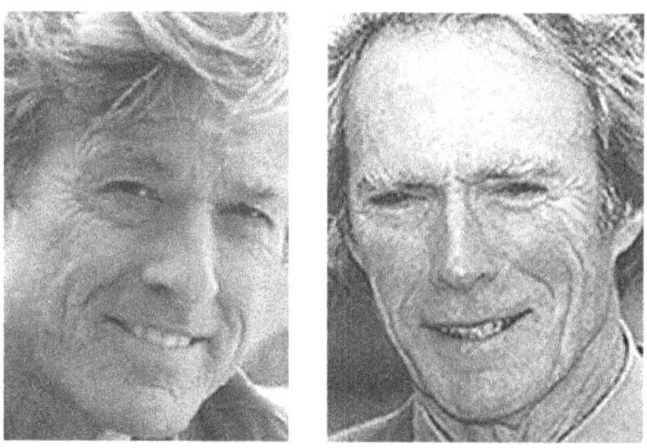

Figure 17: Classic signs of photo-aging (public domain publicity stills taken from www.skinema.com)

Both subjects have extensive wrinkling in the around the eyes in the peri-orbital or so-called crow's-foot area and around the mouth. The subject on the right spent much time filming in the sun while wearing a cowboy hat. Notice that the skin on the forehead looks better than the skin lower on the face.

Corcuff et al. analyzed wrinkling in the peri-orbital area on 81 subjects ranging in age from six to 76 years (194) using image analysis of silicone replicas. Results are reprinted in Figure 18.

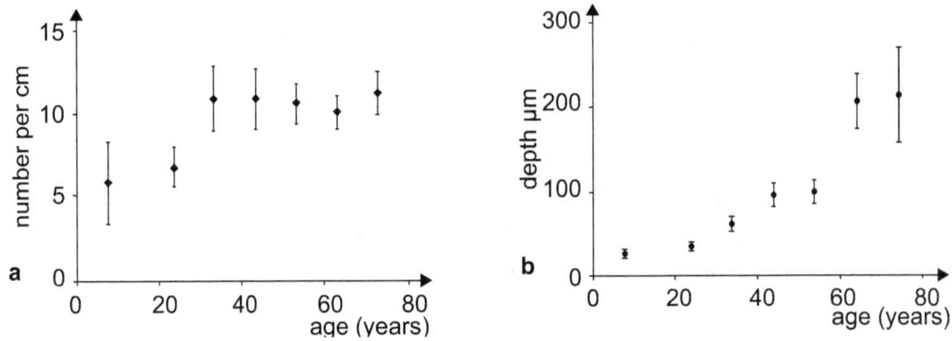

Figure 18: Evolution of "crow's-foot" wrinkles with age. Number of wrinkles per $cm^2 \pm$ S.E. b. means depth of wrinkles ($\mu m \pm$ S.E.). Reprinted from (194) with permission of the Society of Cosmetic Chemists.

Interestingly, the number of wrinkles peaked at about age 35, but mean wrinkle depth increased by eightfold between age 35 and 65.

Sun-induced changes can occur at an early age if sun exposure is sufficiently extreme. Corcuff, de Rigal, and Leveque did a very interesting study on riders in the 1985 Tour de France (195). Professional cyclists spend many hours in the sun and wear tight-fitting short-sleeved shirts while training, providing a sharp divide between exposed and sun-protected areas of skin. Even though the average age of the riders was 25 years, there were dramatic differences between protected and exposed skin. The line pattern on the exposed skin sites of these young cyclists resembled that seen in the >71-year age group in Figure 10. The average furrow depth in the exposed sites was 42 ± 1.5 mm on the exposed sites compared to 29.5 ± 1.0 mm on protected sites.

3.2.4.9 COMPROMISED ELDERLY SKIN TREATMENTS

a. Sunscreens—an ounce of prevention

Since sun exposure plays such an important role in compromising skin, it seems obvious that sunscreen use is a good strategy to prevent damage. However, this is difficult to prove in humans. Long-term studies are required, and it is not ethical to give people a "placebo" sunscreen.

The most convincing study on sunscreen use and photo-aging that has been published to date was done as part of the Nambour Skin Cancer Prevention Trial, a randomized, community-based trial in Nambour, Australia (196, 197). In this study, conducted from 1992 to 1996, some subjects were required to apply an SPF 15+ sunscreen daily while others only used sunscreens at their discretion. The photo-aging trial was conducted on a subset comprised of 903 subjects who were under 55 years of age to emphasize the effect of photo-aging compared to intrinsic aging (198). Dietary supplementation with β-carotene was also investigated. Photo-aging was measured by using a validated method based on grading silicone replicas from the backs of the hands on a scale ranging from 1 (no damage) to 6 (deep horizontal lines and loss of vertical lines) (199, 200). Reported sun exposure was similar between the daily and discretionary sunscreen groups. Participants with initial grades of three or four showed reduced skin aging in the daily sunscreen group compared to discretionary use and significantly reduced skin aging after 4.5 years in the study, compared to those who only used sunscreens at their discretion. Results with the group given oral supplementation with β-carotene were not different from placebo.

The study described above showed that regular sunscreen use can have a significant effect on the rate of photo-aging. When we consider that modern sunscreens tend to be higher SPF and broader spectrum compared to those used in the early 1990s, it seems logical that they could provide an even better protective effect, but the data indicate that very regular use is likely to be required, rather than just casual application when one goes out for prolonged exposure.

b. All-Trans Retinoic Acid (Tretinoin): The Gold Standard

Tretinoin is the only drug approved by the United States Food and Drug Administration for the treatment of wrinkles. It was first reported to have positive effects on photo-aged skin by Albert Kligman and colleagues (201) in 1986. During the 1990s, tretinoin was investigated in double-blind, vehicle-controlled clinical studies (202–204). Olsen et al. performed a 320-subject multicenter study comparing 0.05%, 0.01%, and 0.001% tretinoin to vehicle on the face (205). After 24 weeks of treatment, 0.05% tretinoin produced statistically significant improvements in grades for overall severity of photo-damage, mottled hyperpigmentation, fine wrinkling, and skin roughness compared to vehicle. Other studies showed that tretinoin was very effective for treating "liver spots" associated with photo-damage (206) and hyperpigmented spots in Asian subjects (207). Grove and coworkers used image analysis of silicone replicas to demonstrate that 0.05% tretinoin consistently improved skin topography more than vehicle (208).

c. Cosmeceutical Treatments for Aging Skin

Tretinoin is a pharmaceutical product and an approved drug. Cosmetic treatments designed to improve aged skin are often referred to as "Cosmeceuticals." While Albert Kligman, MD, is often said to have coined this term in the 1980s, it actually predates that time. The first published use of the term we are aware of is by Raymond Reed, published in the *Journal of the Society of Cosmetic Chemists* in January 1962 (209). However, Reed's definition is so broad as to include simple moisturizers and other ingredients that probably wouldn't be considered "cosmeceuticals" today. Certainly Kligman popularized the term and played a significant role in the development of its current usage to refer to cosmetic ingredients that have activities that provide skin effects such as anti-aging (210). It is also important to keep in mind what the FDA says about "cosmeceuticals (211)"

The FD&C Act does not recognize any such category as "cosmeceuticals." A product can be a drug, a cosmetic, or a combination of both, but the term "cosmeceutical" has no meaning under the law.

Perhaps this is why, even today, the exact definition of cosmeceutical is not totally clear (212, 213). A significant literature exists on cosmeceuticals, even though the FDA says the term has no legal meaning and there are many reviews on the subject (212, 214–227). We will now briefly review a few of the many "cosmeceutical" actives.

d. Vitamin A and "Cosmeceutical" Derivatives

Retinol and retinol esters are popular ingredients in skin care products designed to treat the signs of skin aging. Retinol produces some changes in skin that are similar to tretinoin (228). It is much less effective but also less irritating (228, 229). Pierard-Franchimont et al. showed that retinol treatment can produce improvements in the mechanical properties and topography of skin (230). Retinol still has the potential for skin irritation and can be unstable. This has led to investigation of retinol derivatives such as acetate, proprionate, and palmitate esters (216, 231). These esters are presumably metabolized to retinol and the free acid in the skin as has been demonstrated with retinyl palmitate (232). Bissett presented data showing that 0.15% retinol and 0.3% retinyl propionate can have positive effects on both wrinkling and hyperpigmentation after 12 weeks of treatment (216). Retinol has also been reported to improve intrinsically aged skin (233).

e. Niacinamide

Niacinamide, also known as nicotinamide, is the amide of nicotinic acid (vitamin B_3). In the cell it is incorporated in nicotinamide adenine dinucleotide and nicotinamide adenine dinucleotide phosphate, which are vital to energy metabolism. Topical application of niacinamide has been shown to have many positive effects on the skin, including improving barrier function (234–237), reducing the appearance of fine lines and wrinkles (234, 238), and improving hyperpigmentation (239, 240). The improvement in skin pigmentation is apparently through a reversible effect on the transfer of melanosomes from melanocytes to keratinocytes (240, 241).

f. Alpha and Beta Hydroxy Acids

As pointed out above, the turnover rate of the SC decreases with age. Lactic acid had been well known as a moisturizer for many years (242–244), but the observation that lactic and glycolic acid increase the rate of SC turnover (245, 246) led to great interest in their application as potential anti-aging treatments. Stiller et al. published a double-blind placebo-controlled study comparing 8% lactic and 8% glycol acids to vehicle on signs of photo-aging on both the face and forearm (247). Both lactic acid and glycol acid were significantly better than vehicle in improving global photo-aging scores, and the two hydroxy acids were not different from each other. The so-called beta hydroxy acid products are based on salicylic acid, usually at about 2% concentration. This topic is described in great depth elsewhere in this book under the Ingredient section.

g. Antioxidants

Since reactive oxygen species play such an important role in photo-aging, it is not surprising that antioxidants have been a major focus of cosmetic research. Vitamins E and C are probably the most studied for their potential to protect the skin from photo-aging and treat its symptoms (216, 248–259). Raschke reported that 3% ascorbate had a significant effect on reduction of facial wrinkles compared to vehicle, but only when delivered from an "optimized formulation" (256). Antioxidants from plant sources are also under study. Green tea polyphenols have been the most studied ingredients in this regard. While studies in murine skin have shown promise (260, 261), human skin clinical trials of both topical (262) and oral (263) green tea treatment have failed to show visible benefits on skin aging. Histological evaluation after topical treatment for eight weeks did show significantly improved elastic tissue compared to placebo (262).

h. Other actives

A wide variety of other ingredients that can potentially improve the condition of compromised elderly skin are under investigation or have been investigated. They include peptides (221, 264, 265), topical application of estrogen cream (266) (a pharmaceutical not a cosmeceutical), anti-glycation compounds (267), and a variety of botanical ingredients (268).

CONCLUSIONS

As we age, our skin undergoes obvious changes. Some changes occur even on body sites not exposed to the sun or other insults. This intrinsic aging results from the unavoidable effects of the passage of time. Some of our daily activities not only accelerate the aging of skin but also alter its consequences, thereby leading to extrinsic aging. The most important contributor to extrinsic aging is exposure to the sun, though exposure to cigarette smoke may also contribute. Sun-exposed skin ages more rapidly than unexposed skin and differences in histology appear. For example, in chronically sun-exposed skin collagen decreases but elastin increases, though it is often highly dystrophic, while in intrinsic aging both collagen and elastin decrease.

This chapter has reviewed the effects of both intrinsic and extrinsic aging on the skin. Perhaps because of its vital function, the *stratum corneum* barrier is relatively unaffected by age, though barrier repair and wound healing may be slowed. The tendency of the Aged to develop dry skin is clear, and this may contribute to the appearance of fine lines and wrinkles. Changes in the dermis result in changes in the dermatoglyphic pattern of the skin and deeper wrinkles. Chronic sun exposure has profound effects on skin, leading to solar elastosis and the development of deep wrinkles and "age spots."

We have also reviewed prevention and treatment of skin damage. Skin damage from the sun may be reduced or even prevented by frequent use of sunscreens. Tretinoin is the only FDA-approved drug for the treatment of wrinkles. Studies over the past three decades have shown the effect of tretinoin on photo-damage, hyperpigmentation, wrinkles, and skin roughness.

Many cosmetic ingredients and products are alleged to provide effective treatment for the appearance of aged skin. The literature on some of the most common of these treatments was reviewed. Retinol derivatives, antioxidants, and niacinamide are among the treatments reviewed. While there is ample evidence that some "cosmeceutical" treatments may be effective for treatment of the signs and symptoms of skin aging, manufacturers must be careful that claims about product efficacy are restricted to those appropriate for cosmetics based on existing regulatory statutes in the U.S. and elsewhere.

REFERENCES

(1) Fink B, Matts PJ. The effects of skin colour distribution and topography cues on the perception of female facial age and health. J Eur Acad Dermatol Venereol 2008;22:493–8.

(2) Mark LS, Pittenger JB, Hines H, Carelio C, Shaw RE, Todd JT. Wrinkling and head shape as coordinated sources of age level information. Perception and Psychopysics 1980;27:117–24.

(3) Fink B, Matts PJ, Roder S, Johnson R, Burquest M. Differences in visual perception of age and attractiveness of female facial and body skin. Int J Cosmet Sci 2011;33:126–31.

(4) Fink B, Bunse L, Matts PJ, D'Emiliano D. Visible skin colouration predicts perception of male facial age, health and attractiveness. Int J Cosmet Sci 2012;34:307–10.

(5) Fink B, Matts PJ, D'Emiliano D, Bunse L, Weege B, Roder S. Colour homogeneity and visual perception of age, health and attractiveness of male facial skin. J Eur Acad Dermatol Venereol 2012;26:1486–92.

(6) Matts PJ, Fink B, Grammer K, Burquest M. Color homogeneity and visual perception of age, health, and attractiveness of female facial skin. J Am Acad Dermatol 2007;57:977–84.

(7) Gilchrest BA. Skin aging and photoaging. Dermatol Nurs 1990;2:79–82.

(8) Kohl E, Steinbauer J, Landthaler M, Szeimies RM. Skin ageing. J Eur Acad Dermatol Venereol 2011;25:873–84.

(9) Puizina-Ivic N. Skin aging. Acta Dermatovenerol Alp Panonica Adriat 2008;17:47–54.

(10) Berneburg M, Plettenberg H, Krutmann J. Photoaging of human skin. Photodermatol Photoimmunol Photomed 2000;16:239–44.

(11) Fisher GJ. The pathophysiology of photoaging of the skin. Cutis 2005;75:5–8.

(12) Gilchrest BA. Photoaging. J Invest Dermatol 2013;133:E2–E6.

(13) Chung JH, Lee SH, Youn CS, Park BJ, Kim KH, Park KC, et al. Cutaneous photodamage in Koreans: influence of sex, sun exposure, smoking, and skin color. Arch Dermatol 2001;137:1043–51.

(14) Kadunce DP, Burr R, Gress R, Kanner R, Lyon JL, Zone JJ. Cigarette smoking: risk factor for premature facial wrinkling. Ann Intern Med 1991;114:840–4.

(15) Koh JS, Kang H, Choi SW, Kim HO. Cigarette smoking associated with premature facial wrinkling: image analysis of facial skin replicas. Int J Dermatol 2002;41:21–7.

(16) Martires KJ, Fu P, Polster AM, Cooper KD, Baron ED. Factors that affect skin aging: a cohort-based survey on twins. Arch Dermatol 2009;145:1375–9.

(17) Morita A. Tobacco smoke causes premature skin aging. J Dermatol Sci 2007;48:169–75.

(18) Ortiz A, Grando SA. Smoking and the skin. Int J Dermatol 2012;51:250–62.

(19) Petitjean A, Mac-Mary S, Sainthillier JM, Muret P, Closs B, Humbert P. Effects of cigarette smoking on the skin of women. Journal of Dermatological Science 2006;42:259–61.

(20) Yin L, Morita A, Tsuji T. Skin premature aging induced by tobacco smoking: the objective evidence of skin replica analysis. J Dermatol Sci 2001;27 Suppl 1:S26–S31.

(21) Kennedy C, Bastiaens MT, Bajdik CD, Willemze R, Westendorp RG, Bouwes Bavinck JN. Effect of smoking and sun on the aging skin. J Invest Dermatol 2003;120:548–54.

(22) Muizzuddin N, Marenus K, Vallon P, Maes D. Effect of cigarette smoke on skin. J Soc Cosmet Chem 1997;48:235–42.

(23) Draelos ZD, Pugliese PT. Physiology of the Skin. 3rd ed. Carol Stream Il.: Allured Books; 2011.

(24) Odland G F. Structure of the Skin. In: Goldsmith LA, editor. Physiology, Biochemistry and Molecular Biology of the Skin. Second Edition ed. New York: Oxford University Press; 1991. p. 3–62.

(25) Steinert PM. Structure, Function and Dynamics of Keratin Intermediate Filamaments. J Invest Dermatol 1993;100:729–34.

(26) Wenstrup, R.J., Murad S, Pinnell S. Collagen. In: Goldsmith LA, editor. Physiology, Biochemistry and Molecular Biology of the Skin. Second Edition ed. New York: Oxford University Press; 1991. p. 481–508.

(27) Meigel WN, Gay S, Weber L. Dermal architecture and collagen type distribution. Arch Dermatol Res 1977;259:1–10.

(28) Epstein EH, Jr., Munderloh NH. Human skin collagen. Presence of type I and type III at all levels of the dermis. J Biol Chem 1978;253:1336–7.

(29) Weber L, Kirsch E, Muller P, Krieg T. Collagen type distribution and macromolecular organization of connective tissue in different layers of human skin. J Invest Dermatol 1984;82:156–60.

(30) Cotta-Pereira G, Guerra RF, Bittencourt-Sampaio S. Oxytalan, elaunin, and elastic fibers in the human skin. J Invest Dermatol 1976;66:143–8.

(31) HASEGAWA J. "Oxytalan" fibers of the dermal-epidermal junction. Arch Dermatol 1960;82:250–2.

(32) Bauer EA, Goldberg GL, Eisen AZ, Welgus HG. Elastic Fibers of the Connective Tissue. In: Goldsmith LA, editor. Physiology,

Biochemistry and Molecular Biology of the Skin. Second Edition ed. New York: Oxford University Press; 1991. p. 530–57.

(33) Kielty CM, Sherratt MJ, Shuttleworth CA. Elastic fibres. J Cell Sci 2002;115:2817–28.

(34) Baldwin AK, Simpson A, Steer R, Cain SA, Kielty CM. Elastic fibres in health and disease. Expert Rev Mol Med 2013;15:e8.

(35) Goetinck PF, Winterbottom N. Proteglycans: Modular Macromolecules of the Extracellular Matrix. In: Goldsmith LA, editor. Physiology, Biochemistry and Molecular Biology of the Skin. Second Edition ed. New York: Oxford University Press; 1991. p. 558–75.

(36) Madison KC. Barrier function of the skin: "la raison d'etre" of the epidermis. J Invest Dermatol 2003;121:231–41.

(37) Elias PM, Choi EH. Interactions among stratum corneum defensive functions. Exp Dermatol 2005;14:719–26.

(38) Elias PM. Stratum corneum defensive functions: an integrated view. J Invest Dermatol 2005;125:183–200.

(39) Elias PM. Epidermal lipids, barrier function, and desquamation. J Invest Dermatol 1983;80 Suppl:44s–9s.

(40) Talreja P, Kleene N, Pickens W, Wang T, Kasting G. Visualization of the lipid barrier and measurement of lipid pathlength in human stratum corneum. AAPS PharmSci JID - 100897065 2001;3:E13.

(41) Harding CR. The stratum corneum: structure and function in health and disease. Dermatol Ther 2004;17 Suppl 1:6–15.

(42) Oashi M, Sawada Y, Makita R. Odland body and intercellular substances. Acta Derm Venereol Suppl (Stockh) 1973;73:47–54.

(43) ODLAND GF. A submicroscopic granular component in human epidermis. J Invest Dermatol 1960;34:11–5.

(44) Elias PM, Grayson MA, Lampe MA, Williams ML, Brown BE. The Intercorneocyte Space. In: Marks R, Plewig G, editors. Stratum Corneum.New York: Springer-Verlag; 1983. p. 53–67.

(45) Elias PM, Menon GK. Structural and lipid biochemical correlates of the epidermal permeability barrier. Adv Lipid Res 1991;24:1–26.

(46) Dale BA, Resing KA, Lonsdale-Eccles JD. Filaggrin: a keratin filament associated protein. Ann N Y Acad Sci 1985;455:330–42.

(47) Steinert PM, North AC, Parry DA. Structural features of keratin intermediate filaments. J Invest Dermatol 1994;103:19S–24S.

(48) Norlen L, Emilson A, Forslind B. Stratum corneum swelling. Biophysical and computer assisted quantitative assessments. Arch Dermatol Res 1997;289:506–13.

(49) Robbins CR, Fernee K. Some observations on the swelling of behavior of human epidermal membrane. J Soc Cosmet Chem 1983;34:21–34.

(50) Dale BA, Holbrook KA, Kimball JR, Hoff M, Sun TT. Expression of epidermal keratins and filaggrin during human fetal skin development. J Cell Biol 1985;101:1257–69.

(51) Dale BA. Filaggrin, the matrix protein of keratin. Am J Dermatopathol 1985;7:65–8.

(52) Dale BA, Resing KA, Lonsdale-Eccles JD. Filaggrin: a keratin filament associated protein. Ann N Y Acad Sci 1985;455:330–42.

(53) Lynley AM, Dale BA. The characterization of human epidermal filaggrin. A histidine-rich, keratin filament-aggregating protein. Biochim Biophys Acta 1983;744:28–35.

(54) Dale BA, Presland RB, Lewis SP, Underwood RA, Fleckman P. Transient expression of epidermal filaggrin in cultured cells causes collapse of intermediate filament networks with alteration of cell shape and nuclear integrity. J Invest Dermatol 1997;108:179–87.

(55) Nachat R, Mechin MC, Takahara H, Chavanas S, Charveron M, Serre G, et al. Peptidylarginine deiminase isoforms 1–3 are expressed in the epidermis and involved in the deimination of K1 and filaggrin. J Invest Dermatol 2005;124:384–93.

(56) Rawlings AV, Matts PJ. Stratum corneum moisturization at the molecular level: an update in relation to the dry skin cycle. J Invest Dermatol 2005;124:1099–110.

(57) Rawlings AV, Scott IR, Harding CR, Bowser PA. Stratum corneum moisturization at the molecular level. J Invest Dermatol 1994;103:731–41.

(58) Scott IR, Harding CR, Barrett JG. Histidine-rich protein of the keratohyalin granules. Source of the free amino acids, urocanic acid and pyrrolidone carboxylic acid in the stratum corneum. Biochim Biophys Acta 1982;719:110–7.

(59) Scott IR, Harding CR. Filaggrin breakdown to water binding compounds during development of the rat stratum corneum is controlled by the water activity of the environment. Dev Biol 1986;115:84–92.

(60) Hoste E, Kemperman P, Devos M, Denecker G, Kezic S, Yau N, et al. Caspase-14 is required for filaggrin degradation to natural moisturizing factors in the skin. J Invest Dermatol 2011;131:2233–41.

(61) Kamata Y, Taniguchi A, Yamamoto M, Nomura J, Ishihara K, Takahara H, et al. Neutral cysteine protease bleomycin hydrolase is essential for the breakdown of deiminated filaggrin into amino acids. J Biol Chem 2009;284:12829–36.

(62) Harding CR, Aho S, Bosko CA. Filaggrin - revisited. Int J Cosmet Sci 2013.

(63) Cler EJ, Fourtanier A. L'acide purrolidone caboxylique(PCA) et la peau. Int J Cosmet Sci 1981;3:101.

(64) Marty JP. [NMF and cosmetology of cutaneous hydration]. Ann Dermatol Venereol 2002;129:131–6.

(65) SPIER HW, PASCHER G. [Analytical and functional physiology of the skin surface.]. Hautarzt 1956;7:55–60.

(66) Jokura Y, Ishikawa S, Tokuda H, Imokawa G. Molecular analysis of elastic properties of the stratum corneum by solid-state 13C-nuclear magnetic resonance spectroscopy. J Invest Dermatol 1995;104:806–12.

(67) Nakagawa N, Sakai S, Matsumoto M, Yamada K, Nagano M, Yuki T, et al. Relationship between NMF (lactate and potassium) content and the physical properties of the stratum corneum in healthy subjects. J Invest Dermatol 2004;122:755–63.

(68) Robinson MH, Wickett RR. Biochemical and bioengineering analysis of the skin's natural moisturizing factors. J Cosmet Sci 2004;55:211–2.

(69) Yamamura T, Tezuka T. The water-holding capacity of the stratum corneum measured by 1H-NMR. J Invest Dermatol 1989;93:160–4.

(70) Harding CR, Watkinson A, Rawlings AV, Scott IR. Dry skin, moisturization and corneodesmolysis. Int J Cosmet Sci 2000;22:21–52.

(71) Nemes Z, Steinert PM. Bricks and mortar of the epidermal barrier. Exp Mol Med 1999;31:5–19.

(72) Yoneda K, McBride OW, Korge BP, Kim IG, Steinert PM. The cornified cell envelope: loricrin and transglutaminases. J Dermatol 1992;19:761–4.

(73) Candi E, Schmidt R, Melino G. The cornified envelope: a model of cell death in the skin. Nat Rev Mol Cell Biol 2005;6:328–40.

(74) Kalinin A, Marekov LN, Steinert PM. Assembly of the epidermal cornified cell envelope. J Cell Sci 2001;114:3069–70.

(75) Marekov LN, Steinert PM. Ceramides Are Bound to Structural Proteins of the Human Foreskin Epidermal Cornified Cell Envelope. J Biol Chem 1998;273:17763–70.

(76) Grove GL, Kligman AM. Age-associated changes in human epidermal cell renewal. J Gerontol 1983;38:137–42.

(77) Leveque JL, Corcuff P, de RJ, Agache P. In vivo studies of the evolution of physical properties of the human skin with age. Int J Dermatol 1984;23:322–9.

(78) Marks R, Barton SP. The significance of the size and shape of corneocytes. In: Marks R, Plewig G, editors. Stratum Corneum.New York: Springer-Verlag; 1983. p. 161–70.

(79) Rougier A, Lotte C, Corcuff P, Maibach HI. Relationship between skin permeability and corneocyte size according to anatomic site, age and sex in man. J Soc Cosmet Chem 1988;39:15–26.

(80) Mark R, Barton SP. The significance of the size and shape of corneocytes. In: Marks R, Plewig G, editors. Stratum Corneum.New York: Springer-Verlag; 1983. p. 161–70.

(81) Plewig G, Scheuber E, Reuter B, Waidelich W. Thickness of Corneoctyes. In: Marks R, Plewig G, editors. Stratum Corneum.New York: Springer-Verlag; 1983. p. 171–4.

(82) Holbrook KA, ODLAND GF. The fine structure of developing human epidermis: light, scanning, and transmission electron microscopy of the periderm. J Invest Dermatol 1975;65:16–38.

(83) Ya-Xian Z, Suetake T, Tagami H. Number of cell layers of the stratum corneum in normal skin - relationship to the anatomical location on the body, age, sex and physical parameters. Arch Dermatol Res 1999;291:555–9.

(84) Holleran WM, Takagi Y, Menon GK, Jackson SM, Lee JM, Feingold KR, et al. Permeability barrier requirements regulate epidermal beta-glucocerebrosidase. J Lipid Res 1994;35:905–12.

(85) Holleran WM, Takagi Y, Menon GK, Legler G, Feingold KR, Elias PM. Processing of epidermal glucosylceramides is required for optimal mammalian cutaneous permeability barrier function. J Clin Invest 1993;91:1656–64.

(86) Fluhr JW, Kao J, Jain M, Ahn SK, Feingold KR, Elias PM. Generation of free fatty acids from phospholipids regulates stratum corneum acidification and integrity. J Invest Dermatol JID - 0426720 2001;117:44–51.

(87) Mao-Qiang M, Feingold KR, Jain M, Elias PM. Extracellular processing of phospholipids is required for permeability barrier homeostasis. J Lipid Res 1995;36:1925–35.

(88) Mao-Qiang M, Jain M, Feingold KR, Elias PM. Secretory phospholipase A2 activity is required for permeability barrier homeostasis. J Invest Dermatol 1996;106:57–63.

(89) Swartzendruber DC, Wertz PW, Kitko DJ, Madison KC, Downing DT. Molecular models of the intercellular lipid lamellae in mammalian stratum corneum. J Invest Dermatol 1989;92:251–7.

(90) Marks R. Measurement of biological ageing in human epidermis. Br J Dermatol 1981;104:627–33.

(91) Grove GL. Exfoliative cytological procedures as a nonintrusive method for dermatogerontological studies. J Invest Dermatol 1979;73:67–9.

(92) Plewig G. Regional differences of cell sizes in the human stratum corneum. II. Effects of sex and age. J Invest Dermatol 1970;54:19–23.

(93) Grove GL, Lavker RM, Hoelzle E, Kligman AM. Use of non-intrusive tests to monitor age associated changes in human skin. J Soc Cosmet Chem 1981;32:15–26.

(94) Imokawa G, Abe A, Jin K, Higaki Y, Kawashima M, Hidano A. Decreased level of ceramides in stratum corneum of atopic dermatitis: an etiologic factor in atopic dry skin? J Invest Dermatol 1991;96:523–6.

(95) Rogers J, Harding C, Mayo A, Banks J, Rawlings A. Stratum corneum lipids: the effect of ageing and the seasons. Arch Dermatol Res 1996;288:765–70.

(96) Tagami H. Functional characteristics of the stratum corneum in photoaged skin in comparison with those found in intrinsic aging. Arch Dermatol Res 2008;300 Suppl 1:S1–S6.

(97) Fluhr JW, Feingold KR, Elias PM. Transepidermal water loss reflects permeability barrier status: validation in human and rodent in vivo and ex vivo models. Exp Dermatol 2006;15:483–92.

(98) Nilsson GE. Measurement of water exchange through the skin. Med Biol Eng Comput 1977;15:209–18.

(99) Berardesca E, Maibach HI. Transepidermal water loss and skin surface hydration in the non invasive assessment of stratum corneum function. Derm Beruf Umwelt 1990;38:50–3.

(100) Roskos KV, Guy RH. Assessment of skin barrier function using transepidermal water loss: effect of age. Pharm Res 1989;6:949–53.

(101) Marks R, Lawson A, Nicholls S. Age-Related Changes in Stratum Corneum, Structure and Function. In: Marks R, Plewig G, editors. Stratum Corneum. New. York: Springer-Verlag; 1983. p. 175–80.

(102) Kligman AM. Perspectives and problems in cutaneous gerontology. J Invest Dermatol 1979;73:39–46.

(103) Wilhelm KP, Cua AB, Maibach HI. Skin aging. Effect on transepidermal water loss, stratum corneum hydration, skin surface pH, and casual sebum content. Arch Dermatol 1991;127:1806–9.

(104) Saijo S, Hashimoto-Kumasaka K, Takahashi M, Tagami H. Functional Changes of the Stratum Corneum Associated with Aging and Photoaging. J Cosmet Sci 1991;42:379–83.

(105) Ghadially R, Brown BE, Sequeira-Martin SM, Feingold KR, Elias PM. The aged epidermal permeability barrier. Structural, functional, and lipid biochemical abnormalities in humans and a senescent murine model. J Clin Invest 1995;95:2281–90.

(106) Schwindt DA, Wilhelm KP, Miller DL, Maibach HI. Cumulative irritation in older and younger skin: a comparison. Acta Derm Venereol 1998;78:279–83.

(107) Luebberding S, Krueger N, Kerscher M. Age-related changes in skin barrier function - quantitative evaluation of 150 female subjects. Int J Cosmet Sci 2013;35:183–90.

(108) Roskos KV, Maibach HI, Guy RH. The effect of aging on percutaneous absorption in man. J Pharmacokinet Biopharm 1989;17:617–30.

(109) Bettley FR, Donghue E. The irritant effect of soap upon the normal skin. Br J Dermatol 1960;72:67–76.

(110) Grove GL. Age-Associated Chages in Integumental Reactivity. In: Leveque JL, Agache P, editors. Aging Skin.New York: Marcel Dekker; 1993. p. 227–38.

(111) Cua AB, Wilhelm KP, Maibach HI. Cutaneous sodium lauryl sulphate irritation potential: age and regional variability. Br J Dermatol 1990;123:607–13.

(112) Robinson MK. Population differences in acute skin irritation responses. Race, sex, age, sensitive skin and repeat subject comparisons. Contact Dermatitis 2002;46:86–93.

(113) Bowman JP, Kligman AM, Stoudemayer T, Nicholson J. Effects of age on human cumulative irritation responses. J Cosmet Sci 2005;56:213–8.

(114) Jansen LH, Hojyo-Tomoko MT, Kligman AM. Improved fluorescence technique for estimating stratum corneum turnover time. Br J Dermatol 1974;90:9–11.

(115) Roberts D, Marks R. The determination of regional and age variations in the rate of desquamation: a comparison of four techniques. J Invest Dermatol 1980;74:13–6.

(116) Marks R. Influence of Age on Stratum Corneum Cohesion, Desquamation and Epidermal Turnover. In: Leveque JL, Agache P, editors. Aging Skin.New York: Marcel Dekker; 1993. p. 217–26.

(117) Engelke M, Jensen JM, Ekanayake-Mudiyanselage S, Proksch E. Effects of xerosis and ageing on epidermal proliferation and differentiation. Br J Dermatol 1997;137:219–25.

(118) Kreipe H, Heidebrecht HJ, Hansen S, Rohlk W, Kubbies M, Wacker HH, et al. A new proliferation-associated nuclear antigen detectable in paraffin-embedded tissues by the monoclonal antibody Ki-S1. Am J Pathol 1993;142:3–9.

(119) Grove GL. Age-related differences in healing of superficial skin wounds in humans. Arch Dermatol Res 1982;272:381–5.

(120) Norman RA. Xerosis and pruritus in the elderly: recognition and management. Dermatol Ther 2003;16:254–9.

(121) Seyfarth F, Schliemann S, Antonov D, Elsner P. Dry skin, barrier function, and irritant contact dermatitis in the elderly. Clin Dermatol 2011;29:31–6.

(122) White-Chu EF, Reddy M. Dry skin in the elderly: complexities of a common problem. Clin Dermatol 2011;29:37–42.

(123) Berger TG, Shive M, Harper GM. Pruritus in the older patient: a clinical review. JAMA 2013;310:2443–50.

(124) Norman RA. Xerosis and pruritus in elderly patients, Part 2. Ostomy Wound Manage 2006;52:18–20.

(125) Norman RA. Xerosis and pruritus in elderly patients, Part 1. Ostomy Wound Manage 2006;52:12–4.

(126) Patel T, Yosipovitch G. The management of chronic pruritus in the elderly. Skin Therapy Lett 2010;15:5–9.

(127) Horii I, Nakayama Y, Obata M, Tagami H. Stratum corneum hydration and amino acid content in xerotic skin. Br J Dermatol 1989;121:587–92.

(128) Jacobson TM, Yuksel KU, Geesin JC, Gordon JS, Lane AT, Gracy RW. Effects of aging and xerosis on the amino acid composition of human skin. J Invest Dermatol 1990;95:296–300.

(129) Takahashi M, Tezuka T. The content of free amino acids in the stratum corneum is increased in senile xerosis. Arch Dermatol Res 2004;295:448–52.

(130) +àStrand I. Lactate Content in Sweat. Acta Physiologica Scandinavica 1963;58:359–67.

(131) Patterson MJ, Galloway SD, Nimmo MA. Variations in regional sweat composition in normal human males. Exp Physiol 2000;85:869–75.

(132) Ronquist G, Andersson A, Bendsoe N, Falck B. Human epidermal energy metabolism is functionally anaerobic. Exp Dermatol 2003;12:572–9.

(133) Prahl S, Kueper T, Biernoth T, Wohrmann Y, Munster A, Furstenau M, et al. Aging skin is functionally anaerobic: importance of coenzyme Q10 for anti aging skin care. Biofactors 2008;32:245–55.

(134) Fenske NA, Lober CW. Structural and functional changes of normal aging skin. J Am Acad Dermatol 1986;15:571–85.

(135) Pochi PE, Strauss JS, Downing DT. Age-related changes in sebaceous gland activity. J Invest Dermatol 1979;73:108–11.

(136) Fluhr JW, Mao-Qiang M, Brown BE, Wertz PW, Crumrine D, Sundberg JP, et al. Glycerol regulates stratum corneum hydration in sebaceous gland deficient (asebia) mice. J Invest Dermatol 2003;120:728–37.

(137) Kikuchi-Numagami K, Suetake T, Yanai M, Takahashi M, Tanaka M, Tagami H. Functional and morphological studies of photodamaged skin on the hands of middle-aged Japanese golfers. Eur J Dermatol 2000;10:277–81.

(138) Andrew W. The Anatomy and Histology of Aging Skin. J Soc Cosmet Chem 1955;6:299–313.

(139) de Rigal J, Escoffier C, Querleux B, Faivre B, Agache P, Leveque JL. Assessment of aging of the human skin by in vivo ultrasonic imaging. J Invest Dermatol 1989;93:621–5.

(140) Gniadecka M, Jemec GB. Quantitative evaluation of chronological ageing and photoageing in vivo: studies on skin echogenicity and thickness. Br J Dermatol 1998;139:815–21.

(141) Takema Y, Yorimoto Y, Kawai M, Imokawa G. Age-related changes in the elastic properties and thickness of human facial skin. Br J Dermatol 1994;131:641–8.

(142) Guinot C, Latreille J, Mauger E, Ambroisine L, Gardinier S, Zahouani H, et al. Reference ranges of skin micro-relief according to age in French Caucasian and Japanese women. Skin Res Technol 2006;12:268–78.

(143) Pailler-Mattei C, Debret R, Vargiolu R, Sommer P, Zahouani H. In vivo skin biophysical behaviour and surface topography as a function of ageing. J Mech Behav Biomed Mater 2013;28:474–83.

(144) Zahouani H, Vargiolu R. Skin Line Morphology: Trees and Branches. In: Agache P, Humbert P, editors. Measuring the Skin.Berlin: Springer-Verlag; 2004. p. 40–59.

(145) Chung JH, Seo JY, Choi HR, Lee MK, Youn CS, Rhie G, et al. Modulation of skin collagen metabolism in aged and photoaged human skin in vivo. J Invest Dermatol 2001;117:1218–24.

(146) El Domyati M, Attia S, Saleh F, Brown D, Birk DE, Gasparro F, et al. Intrinsic aging vs. photoaging: a comparative histopathological, immunohistochemical, and ultrastructural study of skin. Exp Dermatol 2002;11:398–405.

(147) Uitto J, Fazio MJ, Olsen DR. Molecular mechanisms of cutaneous aging. Age-associated connective tissue alterations in the dermis. J Am Acad Dermatol 1989;21:614–22.

(148) Braverman IM, Fonferko E. Studies in cutaneous aging: I. The elastic fiber network. J Invest Dermatol 1982;78:434–43.

(149) Wickett RR. Stretching the Skin Surface: Skin Elasticity. Cosmetics and Toiletries 2001;116:47–54.

(150) Barel AO, Courage W, Clarys P. Suction method for measurement of skin mechanical properties: The Cutometer. In: Serup J, Jemec GBE, editors. Handbook of Non-invasive methods and the Skin.Ann Arbor: CRC Press; 1995. p. 335–40.

(151) Berndt U, Elsner P. Hardware and Measuring Principle: The Cutometer. In: Elsner P, Berardesca E, Wilhelm KP, Maibach HI, editors. Bioengineering of the Skin Skin Biomechanics. 1st ed. Boca Raton: CRC Press; 2001. p. 91–7.

(152) Barel AO, Lambrecht R, Clarys P. Mechanical Function of the Skin:State of the Art. In: Elsner P, Barel AO, Berardesca E, Gabard B, Serup J, editors. Skin Bioengineering Techniques and Applications in Dermatology and Cosmetology.Basel: Karger; 1998. p. 69–83.

(153) Cua AB, Wilhelm KP, Maibach HI. Elastic properties of human skin: relation to age, sex, and anatomical region. Arch Dermatol Res 1990;282:283–8.

(154) Smalls LK, Wickett R R, Visscher M. Effect of Dermal Thickness, Tissue Composition, and Body Site on Skin Biomechanical Properties. Skin Research and Technology 2006;12:43–9.

(155) Small LK. Development of quantitative models for the investigation of gynoid lipodistrophy (cellulite) [Docteral Dissertation] University of Cincinnati; 2005.

(156) Krueger N, Luebberding S, Oltmer M, Streker M, Kerscher M. Age-related changes in skin mechanical properties: a quantitative evaluation of 120 female subjects. Skin Res Technol 2011;17:141–8.

(157) Ryu HS, Joo YH, Kim SO, Park KC, Youn SW. Influence of age and regional differences on skin elasticity as measured by the Cutometer. Skin Res Technol 2008;14:354–8.

(158) Chung JH. Photoaging in Asians. Photodermatol Photoimmunol Photomed 2003;19:109–21.

(159) Balin AK, Pratt L A. Physiological consequences of human skin aging. Cutis 1989;43:431–6.

(160) Bouissou H, Pieraggi M, Julian M, Savit T. The elastic tissue of the skin: a comparison of spontaneous and actinic (solar) aging. 1988. Int J Dermatol 1988;27:327–35.

(161) Fazio MJ, Olsen DR, Uitto J. Skin aging: lessons from cutis laxa and elastoderma. Cutis 1989;43:437–44.

(162) Ezure T, Hosoi J, Amano S, Tsuchiya T. Sagging of the cheek is related to skin elasticity, fat mass and mimetic muscle function. Skin Res Technol 2009;15:299–305.

(163) Warrier AG, Kligman AM, Harper RA, Bowman J, Wickett RR. A comparison of black and white skin using noninvasive methods. J Soc Cosmet Chem 1996;47:229–40.

(164) Boyer G, Laquieze L, Le BA, Laquieze S, Zahouani H. Dynamic indentation on human skin in vivo: ageing effects. Skin Res Technol 2009;15:55–67.

(165) Boyer G, Pailler MC, Molimard J, Pericoi M, Laquieze S, Zahouani H. Non contact method for in vivo assessment of skin mechanical properties for assessing effect of ageing. Med Eng Phys 2012;34:172–8.

(166) Wlaschek M, Tantcheva-Poor I, Naderi L, Ma W, Schneider LA, Razi-Wolf Z, et al. Solar UV irradiation and dermal photoaging. J Photochem Photobiol B 2001;63:41–51.

(167) Toyoda M, Nakamura M, Luo Y, Morohashi M. Ultrastructural characterization of microvasculature in photoaging. J Dermatol Sci 2001;27 Suppl 1:S32–S41.

(168) Yano K, Kajiya K, Ishiwata M, Hong YK, Miyakawa T, Detmar M. Ultraviolet B-induced skin angiogenesis is associated with a switch in the balance of vascular endothelial growth factor and thrombospondin-1 expression. J Invest Dermatol 2004;122:201–8.

(169) Yano K, Kadoya K, Kajiya K, Hong YK, Detmar M. Ultraviolet B irradiation of human skin induces an angiogenic switch that is mediated by upregulation of vascular endothelial growth factor and by down-regulation of thrombospondin-1. Br J Dermatol 2005;152:115–21.

(170) Green AC, Hughes MC, McBride P, Fourtanier A. Factors associated with premature skin aging (photoaging) before the age of 55: a population-based study. Dermatology 2011;222:74–80.

(171) Gilchrest BA. Skin aging and photoaging: an overview. J Am Acad Dermatol 1989;21:610–3.

(172) Gilchrest BA, Eller MS, Yaar M. Telomere-mediated effects on melanogenesis and skin aging. J Investig Dermatol Symp Proc 2009;14:25–31.

(173) Yaar M, Gilchrest BA. Photoageing: mechanism, prevention and therapy. Br J Dermatol 2007;157:874–87.

(174) Tewari A, Grage MM, Harrison GI, Sarkany R, Young AR. UVA1 is skin deep: molecular and clinical implications. Photochem Photobiol Sci 2013;12:95–103.

(175) Aust AE, Eveleigh JF. Mechanisms of DNA oxidation. Proc Soc Exp Biol Med 1999;222:246–52.

(176) Rai P. Oxidation in the nucleotide pool, the DNA damage response and cellular senescence: Defective bricks build a defective house. Mut Res -Genetic Toxicology and Environmental Mutagenesis 2010;703:71–81.

(177) Takahashi Y, Moriwaki S, Sugiyama Y, Endo Y, Yamazaki K, Mori T, et al. Decreased gene expression responsible for post-ultraviolet DNA repair synthesis in aging: a possible mechanism of age-related reduction in DNA repair capacity. J Invest Dermatol 2005;124:435–42.

(178) Rochette PJ, Brash DE. Human telomeres are hypersensitive to UV-induced DNA Damage and refractory to repair. PLoS Genet 2010;6:e1000926.

(179) Buckingham EM, Klingelhutz AJ. The role of telomeres in the ageing of human skin. Exp Dermatol 2011;20:297–302.

(180) Kosmadaki MG, Gilchrest BA. The role of telomeres in skin aging/photoaging. Micron 2004;35:155–9.

(181) Fisher GJ, Kang S, Varani J, Bata-Csorgo Z, Wan Y, Datta S, et al. Mechanisms of photoaging and chronological skin aging. Arch Dermatol 2002;138:1462–70.

(182) Kondo S. The roles of cytokines in photoaging. J Dermatol Sci 2000;23 Suppl 1:S30–S36.

(183) Rittie L, Fisher GJ. UV-light-induced signal cascades and skin aging. Ageing Res Rev 2002;1:705–20.

(184) Bode AM, Dong Z. Mitogen-activated protein kinase activation in UV-induced signal transduction. Sci STKE 2003;2003:RE2.

(185) Geilen CC, Wieprecht M, Orfanos CE. The mitogen-activated protein kinases system (MAP kinase cascade): its role in skin signal transduction. A review. J Dermatol Sci 1996;12:255–62.

(186) Talwar HS, Griffiths CE, Fisher GJ, Hamilton TA, Voorhees JJ. Reduced type I and type III procollagens in photodamaged adult human skin. J Invest Dermatol 1995;105:285–90.

(187) Bernstein EF, Chen YQ, Kopp JB, Fisher L, Brown DB, Hahn PJ, et al. Long-term sun exposure alters the collagen of the papillary dermis. Comparison of sun-protected and photoaged skin by northern analysis, immunohistochemical staining, and confocal laser scanning microscopy. J Am Acad Dermatol 1996;34:209–18.

(188) Lavker RM. Structural alterations in exposed and unexposed aged skin. J Invest Dermatol 1979;73:59–66.

(189) Suwabe H, Serizawa A, Kajiwara H, Ohkido M, Tsutsumi Y. Degenerative processes of elastic fibers in sun-protected and sun-exposed skin: immunoelectron microscopic observation of elastin, fibrillin-1, amyloid P component, lysozyme and alpha1-antitrypsin. Pathol Int 1999;49:391–402.

(190) Park PW, Biedermann K, Mecham L, Bissett DL, Mecham RP. Lysozyme binds to elastin and protects elastin from elastase-mediated degradation. J Invest Dermatol 1996;106:1075–80.

(191) Akazaki S, Nakagawa H, Kazama H, Osanai O, Kawai M, Takema Y, et al. Age-related changes in skin wrinkles assessed by a novel three-dimensional morphometric analysis. Br J Dermatol 2002;147:689–95.

(192) Flament F, Bazin R, Laquieze S, Rubert V, Simonpietri E, Piot B. Effect of the sun on visible clinical signs of aging in Caucasian skin. Clin Cosmet Investig Dermatol 2013;6:221–32.

(193) Scharffetter-Kochanek K, Brenneisen P, Wenk J, Herrmann G, Ma W, Kuhr L, et al. Photoaging of the skin from phenotype to mechanisms. Exp Gerontol 2000;35:307–16.

(194) Corcuff P, Leveque JL, Grove GL, Kligman AM. The impact of aging on the microrelief of peri-orbital and leg skin. J Soc Cosmet Chem 1987;38:145–52.

(195) Corcuff P, Francois AM, Leveque JL, Porte G. Microrelief changes in chronically sun-exposed human skin. Photodermatol 1988;5:92–5.

(196) Darlington S, Williams G, Neale R, Frost C, Green A. A randomized controlled trial to assess sunscreen application and beta carotene supplementation in the prevention of solar keratoses. Arch Dermatol 2003;139:451–5.

(197) Green A, Battistutta D, Hart V, Leslie D, Marks G, Williams G, et al. The Nambour Skin Cancer and Actinic Eye Disease Prevention Trial: design and baseline characteristics of participants. Control Clin Trials 1994;15:512–22.

(198) Hughes MC, Williams GM, Baker P, Green AC. Sunscreen and prevention of skin aging: a randomized trial. Ann Intern Med 2013;158:781–90.

(199) Battistutta D, Pandeya N, Strutton GM, Fourtanier A, Tison S, Green AC. Skin surface topography grading is a valid measure of skin photoaging. Photodermatol Photoimmunol Photomed 2006;22:39–45.

(200) Hughes MC, Strutton GM, Fourtanier A, Green AC. Validation of skin surface microtopography as a measure of skin photoaging in a subtropical population aged 40 and over. Photodermatol Photoimmunol Photomed 2012;28:153–8.

(201) Kligman AM, Grove GL, Hirose R, Leyden JJ. Topical tretinoin for photoaged skin. J Am Acad Dermatol 1986;15:836–59.

(202) Olsen EA, Katz HI, Levine N, Nigra TP, Pochi PE, Savin RC, et al. Tretinoin emollient cream for photodamaged skin: results of 48-week, multicenter, double-blind studies. J Am Acad Dermatol 1997;37:217–26.

(203) Weiss JS, Ellis CN, Headington JT, Tincoff T, Hamilton TA, Voorhees JJ. Topical tretinoin improves photoaged skin. A double-blind vehicle-controlled study. JAMA 1988;259:527–32.

(204) Weinstein GD, Nigra TP, Pochi PE, Savin RC, Allan A, Benik K, et al. Topical tretinoin for treatment of photodamaged skin. A multicenter study. Arch Dermatol 1991;127:659–65.

(205) Olsen EA, Katz HI, Levine N, Shupack J, Billys MM, Prawer S, et al. Tretinoin emollient cream: a new therapy for photodamaged skin. J Am Acad Dermatol 1992;26:215–24.

(206) Rafal ES, Griffiths CE, Ditre CM, Finkel LJ, Hamilton TA, Ellis CN, et al. Topical tretinoin (retinoic acid) treatment for liver spots associated with photodamage. N Engl J Med 1992;326:368–74.

(207) Griffiths CE, Goldfarb MT, Finkel LJ, Roulia V, Bonawitz M, Hamilton TA, et al. Topical tretinoin (retinoic acid) treatment of hyperpigmented lesions associated with photoaging in Chinese and Japanese patients: a vehicle-controlled trial. J Am Acad Dermatol 1994;30:76–84.

(208) Grove GL, Grove MJ, Leyden JJ, Lufrano L, Schwab B, Perry BH, et al. Skin replica analysis of photodamaged skin after therapy with tretinoin emollient cream. J Am Acad Dermatol 1991;25:231–7.

(209) Reed RE. The definition of cosmecuticals. J Soc Cosmet Chem 1962;13:99–102.

(210) Kligman AM. Why Cosmeceuticals. Cosm & Toil 1993;108:37–8.

(211) FDA Office of Cosmetics and Colors. What about "cosmeceuticals"? 4-30-2012. FDA.Gov, United States Food and Drug Adminstration Office of Cosmetics and Colors.

REF TYPE: ONLINE SOURCE

(212) Draelos ZD. The cosmeceutical realm. Clin Dermatol 2008;26:627–32.

(213) Draelos ZD. Cosmeceuticals: undefined, unclassified, and unregulated. Clin Dermatol 2009;27:431–4.

(214) Babamiri K, Nassab R. Cosmeceuticals: the evidence behind the retinoids. Aesthet Surg J 2010;30:74–7.

(215) Bergstrom KG. Beyond tretinoin: cosmeceuticals for aging skin. J Drugs Dermatol 2009;8:674–7.

(216) Bissett DL. Common cosmeceuticals. Clin Dermatol 2009;27:435–45.

(217) Bruce S. Cosmeceuticals for the attenuation of extrinsic and intrinsic dermal aging. J Drugs Dermatol 2008;7:s17–s22.

(218) Green BA, Yu RJ, Van Scott EJ. Clinical and cosmeceutical uses of hydroxyacids. Clin Dermatol 2009;27:495–501.

(219) Griffiths TW. Cosmeceuticals: coming of age. Br J Dermatol 2010;162:469–70.

(220) Hexsel D, Soirefmann M. Cosmeceuticals for cellulite. Semin Cutan Med Surg 2011;30:167–70.

(221) Lupo MP. Cosmeceutical peptides. Dermatol Surg 2005;31:832–6.

(222) Malerich S, Berson D. Next generation cosmeceuticals: the latest in peptides, growth factors, cytokines, and stem cells. Dermatol Clin 2014;32:13–21.

(223) Millikan LE. Cosmetology, cosmetics, cosmeceuticals: definitions and regulations. Clin Dermatol 2001;19:371–4.

(224) Morganti P. Cosmeceuticals. Clin Dermatol 2008;26:317.

(225) Rupani R, Gilbert E. Cosmeceutical and nutraceutical horizons. J Drugs Dermatol 2011;10:24–5.

(226) Sorg O, Antille C, Kaya G, Saurat JH. Retinoids in cosmeceuticals. Dermatol Ther 2006;19:289–96.

(227) Thornfeldt C. Cosmeceuticals containing herbs: fact, fiction, and future. Dermatol Surg 2005;31:873–80.

(228) Kang S, Duell EA, Fisher GJ, Datta SC, Wang ZQ, Reddy AP, et al. Application of retinol to human skin in vivo induces epidermal hyperplasia and cellular retinoid binding proteins characteristic of retinoic acid but without measurable retinoic acid levels or irritation. J Invest Dermatol 1995;105:549–56.

(229) Fluhr JW, Vienne MP, Lauze C, Dupuy P, Gehring W, Gloor M. Tolerance profile of retinol, retinaldehyde and retinoic acid under maximized and long-term clinical conditions. Dermatology 1999;199 Suppl 1:57–60.

(230) Pierard-Franchimont C, Castelli D, Cromphaut IV, Bertin C, Ries G, Cauwenbergh G, et al. Tensile properties and contours of aging facial skin. A controlled double-blind comparative study of the effects of retinol, melibiose-lactose and their association. Skin Research and Technology 1998;4:237–43.

(231) Mukherjee S, Date A, Patravale V, Korting HC, Roeder A, Weindl G. Retinoids in the treatment of skin aging: an overview of clinical efficacy and safety. Clin Interv Aging 2006;1:327–48.

(232) Boehnlein J, Sakr A, Lichtin JL, Bronaugh RL. Characterization of esterase and alcohol dehydrogenase activity in skin. Metabolism of retinly palmitate to retinol (Vitamin A) during absorption. Pharmaceutical Research 1994;11:1155–9.

(233) Kafi R, Kwak HS, Schumacher WE, Cho S, Hanft VN, Hamilton TA, et al. Improvement of naturally aged skin with vitamin A (retinol). Arch Dermatol 2007;143:606–12.

(234) Bissett DL, Oblong JE, Saud A, Berg CA, Trejo AV, Biedermann KA. Topical niacinamide provides skin aging appearance benefits while enhancing barrier function. JOURNAL OF CLINICAL DERMATOLOGY-NANJING- 2003;32:S9.

(235) Bissett D. Topical niacinamide and barrier enhancement. Cutis 2002;70:8–12.

(236) Draelos ZD, Ertel K, Berge C. Niacinamide-containing facial moisturizer improves skin barrier and benefits subjects with rosacea. Cutis 2005;76:135–41.

(237) Christman JC, Fix DK, Lucus SC, Watson D, Desmier E, Wilkerson RJ, et al. Two randomized, controlled, comparative studies of the stratum corneum integrity benefits of two cosmetic niacinamide/glycerin body moisturizers vs. conventional body moisturizers. J Drugs Dermatol 2012;11:22–9.

(238) Bissett DL, Oblong JE, Berge CA. Niacinamide: A B vitamin that improves aging facial skin appearance. Dermatol Surg 2005;31:860–5.

(239) Bissett DL, Miyamoto K, Sun P, Li J, Berge CA. Topical niacinamide reduces yellowing, wrinkling, red blothiness, and hyperpigmented spots in aging facial skin. Int J Cosmet Sci 2004;26:231–8.

(240) Hakozaki T, Minwalla L, Zhuang J, Chhoa M, Matsubara A, Miyamoto K, et al. The effect of niacinamide on reducing cutaneous pigmentation and suppression of melanosome transfer. Br J Dermatol 2002;147:20–31.

(241) Greatens A, Hakozaki T, Koshoffer A, Epstein H, Schwemberger S, Babcock G, et al. Effective inhibition of melanosome transfer to keratinocytes by lectins and niacinamide is reversible. Exp Dermatol 2005;14:498–508.

(242) Middleton JD. Development of a skin cream designed to reduce dry and flaky skin. J Soc Cosmet Chem 1974;25:519–34.

(243) Rogers RS, Callen J, Wehr R, Krochmal L. Comparative efficacy of 12% ammonium lactate lotion and 5% lactic acid lotion in the treatment of moderate to severe xerosis. J Am Acad Dermatol 1989;21:714–6.

(244) Takahashi M, Machida Y, Tsuda Y. The influence of hydroxy acids on the rheological properties of stratum corneum. J Soc Cosmet Chem 1985;36:177–87.

(245) Smith WP. Hydroxy acids and skin aging. Cosmetics and Toiletries 1994;109:41–8.

(246) Thueson DO, Chan EK, Oechsli LM, Hahn GS. The roles of pH and concentration in lactic acid-induced stimulation of epidermal turnover. Dermatol Surg 1998;24:641–5.

(247) Stiller MJ, Bartolone J, Stern R, Smith S, Kollias N, Gillies R, et al. Topical 8% glycolic acid and 8% L-lactic acid creams for the treatment of photodamaged skin. A double-blind vehicle-controlled clinical trial. Arch Dermatol 1996;132:631–6.

(248) Burke KE. Interaction of vitamins C and E as better cosmeceuticals. Dermatol Ther 2007;20:314–21.

(249) Colven RM, Pinnell SR. Topical vitamin C in aging. Clin Dermatol 1996;14:227–34.

(250) Fitzpatrick RE, Rostan EF. Double-blind, half-face study comparing topical vitamin C and vehicle for rejuvenation of photodamage. Dermatol Surg 2002;28:231–6.

(251) Fryer MJ. Evidence for the photoprotective effects of vitamin E. Photochem Photobiol 1993;58:304–12.

(252) Fuchs J, Kern H. Modulation of UV-light-induced skin inflammation by D-alpha-tocopherol and L-ascorbic acid: a clinical study using solar simulated radiation. Free Radic Biol Med 1998;25:1006–12.

(253) Jurkiewicz BA, Bissett DL, Buettner GR. Effect of topically applied tocopherol on ultraviolet radiation- mediated free radical damage in skin. J Invest Dermatol 1995;104:484–8.

(254) Krol ES, Kramer-Stickland KA, Liebler DC. Photoprotective actions of topically applied vitamin E. Drug Metab Rev 2000;32:413–20.

(255) Lopez-Torres M, Thiele JJ, Shindo Y, Han D, Packer L. Topical application of alpha-tocopherol modulates the antioxidant network and diminishes ultraviolet-induced oxidative damage in murine skin. Br J Dermatol 1998;138:207–15.

(256) Raschke T, Koop U, Dusing HJ, Filbry A, Sauermann K, Jaspers S, et al. Topical activity of ascorbic acid: from in vitro optimization to in vivo efficacy. Skin Pharmacol Physiol 2004;17:200–6.

(257) Thiele JJ, Hsieh SN, Ekanayake-Mudiyanselage S. Vitamin E: critical review of its current use in cosmetic and clinical dermatology. Dermatol Surg 2005;31:805–13.

(258) Wolf R, Wolf D, Ruocco V. Vitamin E: the radical protector. J Eur Acad Dermatol Venereol 1998;10:103–17.

(259) Zahouani H, Rougier A, Creidi P, Richard A, Humbert P. Interest of a 5% vitamin C w/o emulsion in the treatment of skin aging: effects on skin relief. Eur J Dermatol 2002;12:XXIII–XXXVI.

(260) Vayalil PK, Elmets CA, Katiyar SK. Treatment of green tea polyphenols in hydrophilic cream prevents UVB-induced oxidation of lipids and proteins, depletion of antioxidant enzymes and phosphorylation of MAPK proteins in SKH-1 hairless mouse skin. Carcinogenesis 2003;24:927–36.

(261) Vayalil PK, Mittal A, Hara Y, Elmets CA, Katiyar SK. Green tea polyphenols prevent ultraviolet light-induced oxidative damage and matrix metalloproteinases expression in mouse skin. J Invest Dermatol 2004;122:1480–7.

(262) Chiu AE, Chan JL, Kern DG, Kohler S, Rehmus WE, Kimball AB. Double-blinded, placebo-controlled trial of green tea extracts in the clinical and histologic appearance of photoaging skin. Dermatol Surg 2005;31:855–60.

(263) Janjua R, Munoz C, Gorell E, Rehmus W, Egbert B, Kern D, et al. A two-year, double-blind, randomized placebo-controlled trial of oral green tea polyphenols on the long-term clinical and histologic appearance of photoaging skin. Dermatol Surg 2009;35:1057–65.

(264) Lintner K, Peschard O. Biologically active peptides: from a laboratory bench curiosity to a functional skin care product. Int J Cosmet Sci 2000;22:207–18.

(265) Robinson LR, Fitzgerald NC, Doughty DG, Dawes NC, Berge CA, Bissett DL. Topical palmitoyl pentapeptide provides improvement in photoaged human facial skin. Int J Cosmet Sci 2005;27:155–60.

(266) Creidi P, Faivre B, Agache P, Richard E, Haudiquet V, Sauvanet JP. Effect of a conjugated oestrogen (Premarin) cream on ageing facial skin. A comparative study with a placebo cream. Maturitas 1994;19:211–23.

(267) Farris PK. Innovative cosmeceuticals: sirtuin activators and anti-glycation compounds. Semin Cutan Med Surg 2011;30:163–6.

(268) Baumann L. Botanical ingredients in cosmeceuticals. J Drugs Dermatol 2007;6:1084–8.

PART 11

TESTING, CHARACTERIZATION AND PERFORMANCE CLAIMS

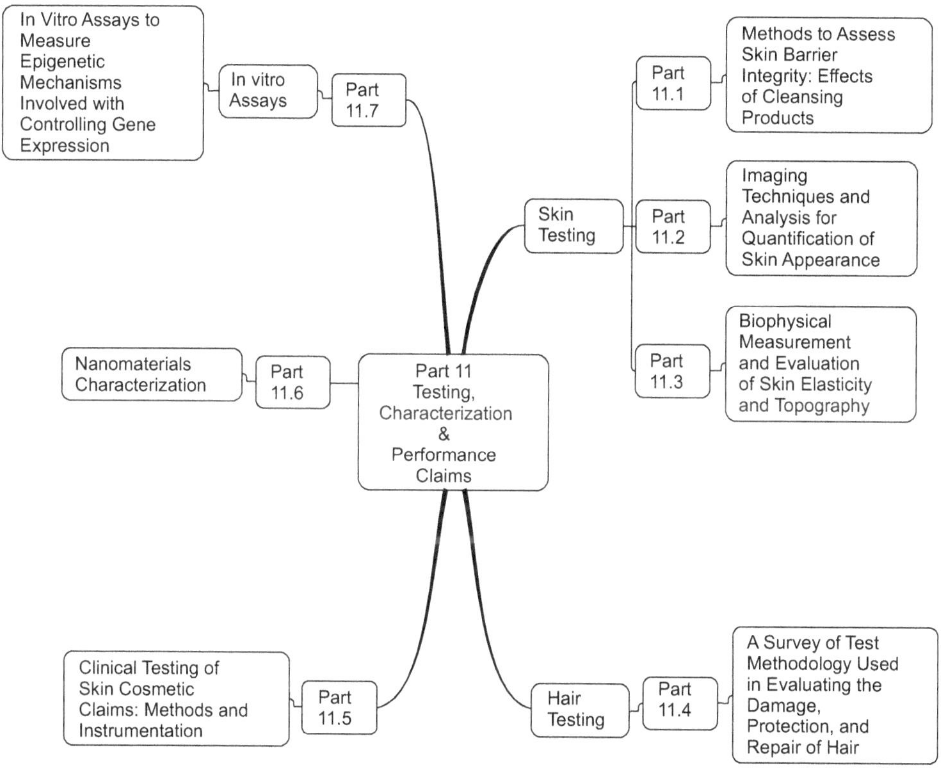

PART 11.1

METHODS TO ASSESS SKIN BARRIER INTEGRITY: EFFECTS OF CLEANSING PRODUCTS

Guojin Lu, Roger L. McMullen, and David J. Moore
Ashland Specialty Ingredients

ABSTRACT

Protecting skin barrier integrity is vital to maintaining the health of human skin. While providing skin hygiene, surfactant-containing cleansing formulations can damage the skin and reduce its natural defensive barrier function. Such formulations can also cause dry, flaky, or itchy skin as a result of irritation due to surfactant absorption and penetration. Several mechanisms have been proposed to describe the interaction of surfactants with the *stratum corneum* (SC). These include protein denaturation, natural moisturizing factor (NMF) removal, selective SC lipid removal, and disruption of SC lipid organization leading to increased permeability through the SC.

In this chapter, we discuss the effects of cleansing stresses (e.g., surfactants, pH, and cleansing product temperature) on skin barrier integrity. We also describe some practical methods that can be used for evaluating the extent of skin barrier damage induced by cleansing formulations, as well as the advantages and disadvantages of each measurement technique.

TABLE OF CONTENTS

11.1.1 INTRODUCTION

a. Skin structure and functions

In addition to being the largest organ of the human body, the skin is the interface between the organism and the external environment and protects the body from external insults. In the design of skin care products or formulations, the ultimate consumer experience, as well as skin health and appearance, are determined by formulation ingredients and their material properties. The physical and chemical activity of these ingredients and their interactions with each other influence both skin/*stratum corneum* (SC) structure and their biochemistry. In order for the cosmetic scientist to improve skin condition or reduce the skin damage caused by cleansing products, an understanding of skin structure and function is essential. This is especially true concerning the basic physiology of the outer epidermal layer, SC.

There have been many articles that reviewed skin structure and functions in detail, which is however not the primary focus of this chapter[1–3]. Briefly speaking, skin is a complex multilayered organ consisting of three components. Looking from the outside towards the inside, these components are the viable epidermis, the dermis, and hypodermis. Major skin functions include: i. the protective and defensive barrier (its vital function) to prevent uncontrolled water loss and to protect the body from a variety of environmental insults (e.g., abrasion, microorganism invasion, UV or other radiation damage, exogenous chemical agents such as surfactants and solvents, and other daily insults); ii. thermo-regulation function through blood flow and sweating to maintain normal body temperature; iii. immune system function; iv. sensory function via the nervous system; and v. psychological function for skin visual appearance and social acceptance.

In practice, it is generally accepted that topical skin care is primarily concerned with protecting the skin barrier[4]. A widely employed analogy for the SC organization is a brick-mortar (corneocyte-lipid) model[5]. Overwhelming evidence indicates that SC lipid composition and organization governs skin permeability and plays a critical physiological role in regulating water loss/uptake through the skin. In healthy skin, lipids are typically in a lamellar bi-layer crystalline state. The organization of the SC lipid membranes is very complex and is comprised of three major components: free fatty acids (FFA), ceramides (CER), and cholesterol (CHO). Together they form the highly ordered lipid phase of the SC.

The SC lipid matrix, and also the mixed SC lipid model systems that have been widely used to study the SC, do not exist as homogenous or uniformly mixed single phases, but rather form separate domains (and bi-layer phases) in the SC lipid membranes[6–8]. Although the exact ratio of the phases has not been determined experimentally, fluid (liquid crystalline) and solid phases (both hexagonal and orthorhombic) of lipids do coexist, which is a crucial requirement for the barrier properties and flexibility of the SC lipid layers.

b. Cleansing and commonly used surfactant systems in cleansing formulations

As part of their daily routine, consumers frequently use surfactant-containing cleansing products such as soap bars, detergents, as well as liquid hand soaps, body washes, cleansing lotions, liquid face washes, (hand) dish wash, etc. These surfactant-based preparations are efficacious cleansing systems that help remove unwanted materials such as dirt, oil, sweat, debris, pathogenic microorganisms, and other excess body and cutaneous serums from different substrates (skin, hair, fabrics, dishes, etc.). Cleansing efficacy is very important for hygiene and is achieved by means of surfactant properties such as solubilization/emulsification of grease in liquids, and dispersion or suspension of solids in liquids. These properties arise from the ability of surfactants to concentrate at the interface, leading to a reduction in interfacial tension. Because of their characteristics, surfactants are among the most important cosmetic ingredients.

Surfactants are amphiphilic (two-part) molecules that are composed of a hydrophobic portion (tail group, almost always a hydrocarbon structure) and a hydrophilic portion (head group). When the solution concentration of a surfactant reaches its critical micelle concentration (CMC), surfactant molecules tend to form association structures of dynamic aggregates such as micelles. These micelles are typically spherical in nature with the hydrophobic portion facing inwards. As a result of this structure, they can dissolve oils easily by incorporating oil within the inner portion of the micelles and by associating their hydrocarbon tail with the oil surface, thereby causing the solubilized oil to lift up from the surface of the substrate. Depending on the composition or charge of the surfactant molecule (head group), surfactants can be classified as anionic, cationic, nonionic, and amphoteric or zwitterionic (the charge of the head groups changes with pH) surfactants.

For most skin-cleansing formulations, anionic surfactants with hydrocarbon chains of various length especially those with C12 chain length are typically used as primary surfactants (e.g., sodium lauryl sulfate [SLS] or sodium laureth sulfate [SLES]) due to their desirable detergency, foaming, and lather features. Amphoteric surfactants, such as betaines, are normally used as co-surfactants in liquid cleansers that are milder with respect to the skin barrier. Nonionic and cationic surfactants are less frequently used in skin-cleansing systems. With regard to the extent of harshness, the following order is well known: anionic surfactants (highest) > amphoteric surfactants > nonionic surfactants. Among the anionic surfactants, besides soap surfactants that are originated from animal or plant sources (e.g., SDS [or SLS], ALS, or SLES), synthetic detergents (syndets) are also frequently used as they are milder surfactants. For a surfactant with given chain length, the larger the head group size, the lower its tendency to cause skin damage due to steric hindrance. Other factors that affect harshness of a surfactant include its critical micelle concentration (CMC) and micelle size.

c. Skin damages by cleansing products

Due to personal cleansing activities, human skin is constantly exposed to surfactants, which are well known to compromise the essential barrier function of healthy skin. Skin barrier damage can be accompanied by after-wash skin tightness, dryness, scaly skin, or even erythema, irritation, and itch due to surfactant absorption and penetration into the skin. These surfactant-induced, undesirable visible manifestations of skin and uncomfortable skin feeling are greater when the ambient temperature and humidity levels are relatively low in the winter environment. These undesirable side effects are also interrelated.

In addition to adverse effects, the alteration of skin barrier function by surfactants can be managed to enhance the penetration of topically applied materials, such as transdermally delivered drugs. In the case of surfactant use, a careful balance has to be maintained between maximum drug penetration enhancement and minimum skin irritant response, since any surfactant that has the capability to reduce the cutaneous barrier function for certain drugs could also enhance the permeation of other ingredients, including any excipients used as well as the surfactants themselves.

To understand the interactions of surfactants with the skin and their effect on skin barrier integrity—especially with the outer SC—it is essential to develop qualitative and quantitative measurement methods (both *in vitro* and *in vivo*) to predict, evaluate, and demonstrate the effect of different surfactant chemistries, formulation ingredients, and cleansing conditions.

In this chapter, we discuss surfactant-skin interaction mechanisms and the effects of cleansing stresses (e.g., surfactants, pH, and cleansing product temperature) on skin-barrier integrity. We also describe some practical methods for evaluating the extent of skin-barrier damage induced by cleansing formulations as well as the advantages and disadvantages of each measurement technique. We conclude with a discussion of employing these methods to assess the benefits provided by harshness-reducing technologies applicable in skin-cleansing formulations.

11.1.2 PHYSICOCHEMICAL INTERACTIONS BETWEEN SURFACTANTS AND SKIN

As a system having a heterogeneous surface as well as a bulk material phase, the skin is very complex and surfactants applied to its surface can interact with many different targets in the skin structure in multiple ways. Only a few skin components will be discussed in this chapter: the SC (including intercellular SC lipids and dead cells of protein-containing corneocytes), keratin, and living cells of the epidermis.

It is generally accepted that surfactant-SC interactions and disruption of skin-barrier properties occur when surfactants have penetrated into the skin barrier. Several mechanisms have been proposed regarding the subsequent interaction of surfactants with the SC and skin components. These include, but are not limited to: enzyme disruption, skin permeation and penetration, protein denaturation and dissolution, SC swelling that causes enhanced water penetration, and removal of natural moisturizing factor (NMF) from corneocytes[9–10]. Such insults lead to reduced water-holding capacity and dry skin, selective SC lipid extraction or removal, and disruption of SC lipid organization/structure. They can also lead to a change of lipid composition, which generates an increased permeability through the SC lipid bi-layers that are responsible for the SC barrier function[11–12]. The above phenomena may also trigger some biological responses from the skin, such as the scenario described in the "dry skin cycle" model by Rawlings[13]. If the cleansing stresses (e.g., surfactant concentration, application period, pH, temperature, etc.) are strong enough, or the skin is not rinsed sufficiently, surfactant residue left on the skin will continue to penetrate into the viable epidermis, and perhaps even into the dermis. This process will cause further disruption of living skin cell homeostasis, ultimately leading to an inflammatory response. It is worth noting that the above-mentioned mechanisms are not independent from each other but rather related in a cycle.

Most of the mechanisms described above also involve water loss, either directly or indirectly. In other words, surfactant-based cleansing products cause water loss and reduce the water-holding capability of the SC by disturbing the skin's normal mechanisms for regulating water content[14]. In fact, maintaining of optimal water content is a key factor (if not the most important one) for sustaining the practical function of the SC[15–16].

a. SC protein binding, denaturation, dissolution, and SC swelling

Surfactant interaction with skin proteins can adversely affect skin hydration and viscoelasicity. It is widely reported that surfactants can bind to skin keratin with high affinity[17–22]. This binding reduces the ability of skin protein to bind and retain water, thereby causing dry and tight skin. This binding could also lead to the development of repulsive forces, causing some protein denaturation (separation of the protein matrix, uncoiling of the filaments, and exposing more water-binding sites), SC conformation change, and transient swelling/hyperhydration. These events are often followed by water evaporation causing skin drying[17–18]. This effect is thought to saturate at about the CMC since protein binding and denaturation are associated with surfactant monomers, although this hypothesis remains controversial[11, 19–22].

In general, surfactants that bind more strongly to SC proteins have a higher potential to cause significant protein denaturation and severe skin-barrier damage. For anionic surfactants, the skin swells as water content increases with increase in charge—protein unfolding and dissolution may occur. An increase in water uptake only hydrates the skin temporarily, while eventually it will reduce the skin's water-holding capability due to surfactant adsorption onto protein hydration sites. After rinsing, as the water evaporates, the hydration level of the skin is lower than the preexposure level. As the result, the skin will be even drier than before cleansing due to additional water evaporation and SC swelling. For other surfactant systems, there is little change with increase/decrease in surfactant charge and therefore minimal SC swelling is observed. Indeed, SC swelling can be reduced by the addition of secondary surfactants (such as betaine) even though the total surfactant concentration is increased by mixing[23]. This phenomenon can be explained by the reduced binding of the harsher surfactant due to the competition between them for binding sites, and the lowering of the CMC by the addition of a surfactant with lower CMC. Another way to reduce SC swelling is to increase the size of the head or polar group of surfactant, which will provide an additional barrier in the form of steric hindrance.

Surfactant and even water adsorption on the SC may dissolve some components of the water-soluble natural moisturizing factor, leading to a reduction in their levels in skin[24]. NMF is a heterogeneous mixture of hygroscopic amino acids in the corneocytes and it is one of the major components responsible for water holding (other two major water-holding SC factors are intercellular lamellar lipid organization and corneodesmosome function)[25]. NMF adsorbs water from the atmosphere to provide sufficient hydration to help keep skin flexible and smooth, as well as to support a variety of enzymatic reactions in the dermis. It is very water soluble and can be very easily leached by water if the protecting lipid bi-layers surrounding the corneocytes get damaged, as for example, by surfactant exposure. Consequences of reduced NMF include reduced hydration of the SC, reduced activities of SC enzymes leading to reduced desmosome breakdown, increased stiffness of the SC leading to the possibility of cracking around joints, and erythema due to inflammation associated with an undesirable biochemical response.

b. SC lipid extraction and selective removal

SC lipids are the major barrier to permeability of the SC and play a critical role in skin functions ensuring cellular cohesion, skin-barrier properties, water-holding capability, and normal healthy-looking skin. Indeed, skin or SC with disordered lipid structure or abnormal composition would be more water permeable and more vulnerable to external attacks. Mainly due to the effect on the lipid layers, surfactant exposure would increase the ability of exogenous compounds to penetrate the skin and to increase water loss through the skin.

It is reported that lipid extraction is possible above the CMC, and cholesterol and free fatty acids (not ceramides) are generally removed[24, 26–29]. In one study, Loden concluded that lipid extraction/solubilization was caused by surfactant micelles and therefore is concentration dependent[30]. When the SDS concentration is relatively high, more surfactant molecules are available for skin binding and penetration and thereby "consume" the lipid matrix. This concept is used to explain the mechanism of damage to SC by surfactants at concentrations above their CMC[21, 31].

The solubilization and removal of SC lipid by a large amount of absorbed surfactant molecules has been reported in lipid films[32]. Lipid content in the skin SC is normally observed to decrease because of delipidization after cleansing with soap products[33]. In a study of recovery in SDS-treated skin by daily topical application of SC lipid fractions, Imokawa and colleagues strongly supported deficiency of intercellular lipids as an essential mechanism in surfactant-induced skin damage[27]. The concept of disruption of the lipid matrix (degreasing) is the dominant hypothesis for explaining the damage induced in SC lipid organization by surfactants. A few groups have challenged this idea of lipid extraction by conducting experiments suggesting that only very small amounts of lipids are removed from the SC by surfactants, even at high concentrations (above CMC), if the surfactant treatment time is not excessive (less than a few minutes)[28–29].

c. Disruption of SC lipid organization/structure and change of lipid composition

While extraction of SC lipids by surfactants remains controversial and may not be the critical factor affecting lipid barrier function, alterations in lipid phase behavior and organizational structure, and disruption of the integrity of the lipid bi-layer barrier have attracted more attention. Surfactant exposure can cause expansion of intercellular spaces of the lipid lamellar structure and surfactant molecules will intercalate into the lipid network[34]. It is also reported that anionic surfactants induce intercellular lipid structure disruption, disordering, and, possibly lipid fluidization[32, 35]. Changes in lipid organization will impact skin irritation and alter the penetration of irritant molecules in the SC. This process also includes affecting desmosomal cleavage between corneocytes[9].

Prolonged water and surfactant contact, although very different in their chemical nature, are both deleterious to the skin barrier since they disrupt SC lipid structure[24, 36]. In many situations human skin is exposed to both stresses, as for example during cleansing, as well as in many workplace environments. Lipid disruption not only leads to increased water loss through the skin, but also enhances penetration of other chemical substances including toxic and irritating compounds through the skin.

Long-term exposure to surfactants will also modify the lipid composition and cause phase transitions and changes in the overall phase behavior of the lipid bi-layer systems[37]. Lipid composition is of paramount importance for the SC organization and its barrier properties[38–40]. In fact, it is known that lipid composition in the SC is different between individuals, between anatomical skin sites, and a function of skin damage and diseases[41]. The alteration of the ratio of the three major lipid components may also cause phase separation of lipids at the surface of the *stratum corneum* and result in crystallization of the lipid matrix[42]. These phase changes in turn will affect the water-holding capability and barrier properties of the SC, causing dry skin and/or skin irritation[37, 43–44]. Evidence indicates that diminishing amount of ceramide and increasing levels of fatty acid (nearly doubled) are related to soap-induced winter xerosis[42].

Based on literature reports, SC lipid-surfactant interactions likely progress as follows: (1) initial water loss due to osmosis or surfactant-induced water swelling or hydration to open up the lipid structure; (2) surfactant penetration/insertion into the lipids that further alters lipid phase, structure, and even composition, leading to extra water uptake by the lipid layers; (3) after extended exposure to surfactant solutions for a long period, part of the lipid matrix is removed by dissolution and the lipid barrier function is further damaged, causing water loss and dry skin due to reduced water-holding capability; and (4) SC disruption by surfactants stimulates SC formation and this new formation typically proceeds too quickly, leading to abnormal architecture and inadequate barrier function thereby causing low hydration and abnormal desquamation (scaly appearance).

d. pH effect

Another factor that can aggravate the deleterious effects of surfatcant-skin interactions is the pH of the cleansing formulation. It is well known that pH plays a very significant role in the alteration of skin intergrity by surfactants. The effect of pH on SC barrier function and skin permeability to drug molecules has been the subject of many studies[9, 45–51]. The results of these studies demonstrate that the enviromental pH to which skin is exposed has a significant impact on SC lipid composition and organization. Further it impacts SC cohesion, protein swelling, and skin irritation. Indeed, a predictable relationship between the solution pH and skin irratancy has been demonstrated, although it has been reported that the influence of pH on the chemistry of surfactant-based washing compositions is more important than that of the direct contribution of pH on the SC[52].

Since the pH of a healthy SC is acidic (generally around pH 5), the attaction and penetration of basic surfactant solutions is more favorable. Under basic pH conditions anionic surfactants bind primarily by hydrophobic functional groups to hydrophobic sites on the skin to minimize the repulsion of negative charges, thus leading to swelling of the SC in the presence of more alkaline surfactants[35]. The effect of surfactant pH on SC was further demonstrated to negatively influence the barrier repair mechanism by the daily use of soap-based cleansers with greater pH[53].

Soap-based cleansers are alkaline in nature (pH 10, e.g., for regular soap bars) while milder synthetic detergents (syndets, such as Dove bar) are mostly neutral (pH ~7 for Dove soap bar). The fact that detergents with higher pH are less mild is not surprising since there is more binding to keratin by anionic surfactants[52]. It has been reported that alkaline pH alone, in the absence of surfactants, induces an increase of SC swelling and irreversible lipid phase changes in SC[9, 45, 54].

11.1.3 APPROACHES AND METHODS TO ASSESS THE EFFECTS OF CLEANSING STRESSES ON SKIN-BARRIER INTEGRITY

Requirements from consumers have stimulated the development of milder cleansing products, which makes it difficult to differentiate minor variations between products. Exaggerated and more progressive application tests (i.e., "accelerated" testing), where test conditions are modified to be harsher (e.g., more concentrated, elevated temperature, longer exposure period, etc.), are usually conducted to enhance the skin reactions.

For clinical tests utilizing human subjects, the procedures are regulated by ethical recommendations and test guidelines to ensure safety and standardization. More details may be found in a published series of testing procedures and guidelines by the European Group for Efficacy Measurements on Cosmetics and Other Topical Products (EEMCO) for tests related to different skin properties, such as dry skin and xerosis[55–56], skin hydration by electrical methods[57], TEWL in cosmetic sciences[58], skin surface pH[59], tensile functional properties[60], skin color[61], skin microcirculation[62], and skin topography[63].

While it is the most straightforward method to assess the harshness of skin-cleansing products, consumer perception and expert grading is not objective and, therefore, not always reproducible or reliable[35, 64]. As a result, a large number of subjects are required and different consumer habits and practices have to be considered. It is also difficult to distinguish the small differences between relatively mild cleansing products using such methods. These problems make it difficult, expensive, and time consuming to directly compare skin-cleansing products solely by consumer perception tests. Consequently, various exaggerated methods and approaches have been developed for formulation screening and product development, leaving consumer testing as a tool mostly used for claim substantiation of final products.

Noninvasive biophysical and bioengineering methods offer insights into the different aspects of skin structure and functions. These methods are primarily based on sophisticated scientific instrumentations and have been used to measure skin characteristics following environmental exposure (e.g., UV exposure) and cosmetic treatment (e.g., surfactants, skin care products, etc.) as well as monitoring skin aging and diseases. They are sensitive, easy to use, fast, mostly portable, and not costly. They are practical approaches that can be used to monitor and assess topical treatments for *in vivo* human skin in real time and to obtain objective, quantitative, and reproducible information on skin conditions after surfactant challenge.

In the last several decades, various experimental approaches have been utilized to better serve different application needs. There are *in vivo* methods where human skin is subjected to various imaging and instrumental methods. Often tape stripping is applied to provide more in-depth information. Frequently *in vitro* approaches are employed. In these cases, full thickness human or porcine skin, isolated *stratum corneum*, or extracted lipids may be used. Porcine skin is commonly employed due to its physiological similarity to human skin. Other than real skin samples, some model materials have been recently developed to study surfactant interactions with skin, SC, lipid, or proteins. These include lipid models, protein models, synthetic membrane substrates (vitro skin, vitro corneum, episkin®, silicone membrane, etc.).

To model the interactions of surfactants with the skin and their effect on skin-barrier integrity, especially with a focus on the outer SC, it is essential to develop qualitative and quantitative measurement methods (both *in vitro* and *in vivo* approaches) to predict, evaluate, and demonstrate the effect of different surfactant chemistries, formulation ingredients, and cleansing conditions.

Because surfactants can interact with skin in a variety of ways, there are many properties of skin that can be characterized to assess cleanser mildness. Each single property cannot represent the comprehensive skin condition by itself. In the discussion below, the effects of surfactant-based cleansing products on the skin-barrier integrity will be discussed according to the following three categories: surfactant-skin/SC interactions, surfactant-lipid interactions, and surfactant-protein interactions.

a. Surfactant-skin/SC interactions

1. Sensory testing and substantiating instrumental methods

Sensory methods such as visual or tactile methods through consumer perception and expert grading after actual use are often used to evaluate various skin parameters and assess skin/SC damage by cleansing products, evaluating parameters such as after-wash dryness, roughness (scaling), tightness, erythema (redness), and irritation/itching or even pain. This approach is generally rapid and inexpensive but it is subjective and not quantitative. Skin damage has to be significant and visible, therefore it may not indicate subclinical skin damage.

With the assistance of modern image analysis techniques, skin surface texture, dryness, and roughness can be visualized by skin replicas (commonly silicone replicas). This replica methodology can be used to provide an imprint of the skin surface and the scanned images of the replicas can be quantitatively analyzed with image analysis.

Skin color change and erythema can be evaluated by expert grading. This can also be conducted by color measuring instruments based on the quantification of skin's optical and thermal properties. These portable instruments (such as

Erythema Meter from Dia-Stron, Minolta Chroma Meter, and DermaSpectrometer from Cortex) monitor skin reflection with different light or utilize the three-dimensional color coordinate system (L, a, and b) to measure skin redness[65–66]. Another way to characterize skin redness is by measuring blood flow and vascular status of skin (e.g., utilizing laser Doppler technology).

Based on measurements of redness or erythema, the harshness and irritancy of surfactant systems or cleansing formulations can be assessed by exaggerated exposure tests such as the soap chamber test or patch test, where the volar forearms of human volunteers are treated with surfactants and subsequently the condition of the skin barrier is determined. For example, the soap chamber test has been used to compare the beneficial effects of syndet bars over regular soap bars[67–68].

2. Microscope, video microscopy for skin surface topography

Optical or light microscopy is most commonly used to visualize the skin surface and study the effects of environmental and physiological (e.g., aging) factors on the appearance of the skin surface. With recent technological advancements, high-quality images with high resolution and large depth of field can be obtained and quantified.

Digitalized optical microscopes (e.g., Scopeman Video Microscope from Moritex and Visioscope from Courage & Khazaka) can collect images of the skin surface, allowing real-time visualization of skin condition and texture after image analysis[69]. The introduction of noninvasive confocal microscopy imaging (e.g., VivaScope from Lucid and Vectra 3D imaging systems from Canfield) and advanced image analysis software now provide specialized photographic 3-D skin surface images with high optical resolution and contrast to facilitate skin studies and enhanced understanding of skin at the cellular level.

Profilometry is another commonly used method to quantify skin surface topography such as skin scaling and roughness[70]. Skin surface changes induced by cleansing products and the benefits from cosmetic treatments can be visualized in three-dimensional images.

Compared to optical microscopy, scanning electron microscopy (SEM), transmission electron microscopy (TEM), and atomic force microscope (AFM) can provide microscopic images of the SC ultrastructure with greater resolution[24, 36, 42, 71–74].

3. Skin penetration/permeability by Franz cell and impedance measurements

Skin penetration and permeation by surfactants can be measured using Franz diffusion cells. In a typical experimental protocol, a skin sample is placed as a diffusion barrier between two components of a diffusion cell. The amount of surfactant that permeates through the SC membrane after a certain period of exposure can be measured by several techniques (e.g., HPLC)[75].

Skin's electrical impedance can be used to evaluate skin integrity and skin-barrier damage and recovery[12]. Skin-barrier perturbation due to exposure to different chemicals can be quantitatively expressed by measuring changes in skin impedance. When the skin barrier is perturbed, skin electrical impedance is expected to decrease since the transport rate of ions flowing across the skin is higher. It has been shown by different research groups, and for different applications, that skin impedance correlates well with skin permeability[12, 21, 76]. Thus, for example, Ghosh and Blankschtein[21] have reported a positive relationship between *in vitro* manitol transdermal permeability and *in vitro* skin electric current when exposing pig skin to sodium dodecyl sulfate solutions. In other studies of drug permeation across human skin, Karande et al.[12] demonstrated a correlation between skin permeability and skin impedance for different solutes in various formulations. They also showed the feasibility of using impedance as an alternative indicator for increased skin permeability induced by chemical penetration enhancers.

With relatively straightforward *in vitro* skin impedance studies and high-throughput or combinatorial technologies, it is possible to quantitatively examine *in situ* skin-barrier perturbation induced by surfactants, and other physical or chemical stresses including temperature, time of exposure, and pH. Previous reports have demonstrated that results from *in vitro* impedance measurements are consistent with *in vivo* findings in terms of ranking the extent of surfactant-induced skin-barrier damage[77]. Using this approach, one can simultaneously examine, screen, and rank many simple formulations and dramatically reduce the time and efforts needed for skin-related formulation improvements including product development and marketing.

In a recent study, *in vitro* skin electrical current (impedance) measurements were conducted in a Franz diffusion cell (Figure 1) to quantitatively monitor changes in skin-barrier integrity as a function of surfactant chemistry and concentration[54]. In addition, time of exposure, temperature, pH, and the addition of chemical constituents (such as glycerin) were also evaluated. One example is shown in Figure 2, where skin damage by SDS and SLES at different pH values is compared. Overall, the data are in very good agreement with results obtained from a range of other *in vitro* and *in vivo* studies.

As a straightforward and relatively rapid approach to screen formulations for their impact on skin-barrier integrity, the skin impedance method has also been used to evaluate the harshness of cleansing formulations such as soap bars and syndets, shower gels with or without harshness-reducing skin-conditioning ingredients, shaving preparation formulations, hand dishwash formulations, baby wash products, etc. Again, the results correlate and are consistent with other *in vitro* biophysical and *in vivo* clinical studies[78]. In summary, these results demonstrate that skin impedance measurements can be used as a direct, quantitative method for characterizing skin-barrier integrity for a wide range of skin-cleansing formulations.

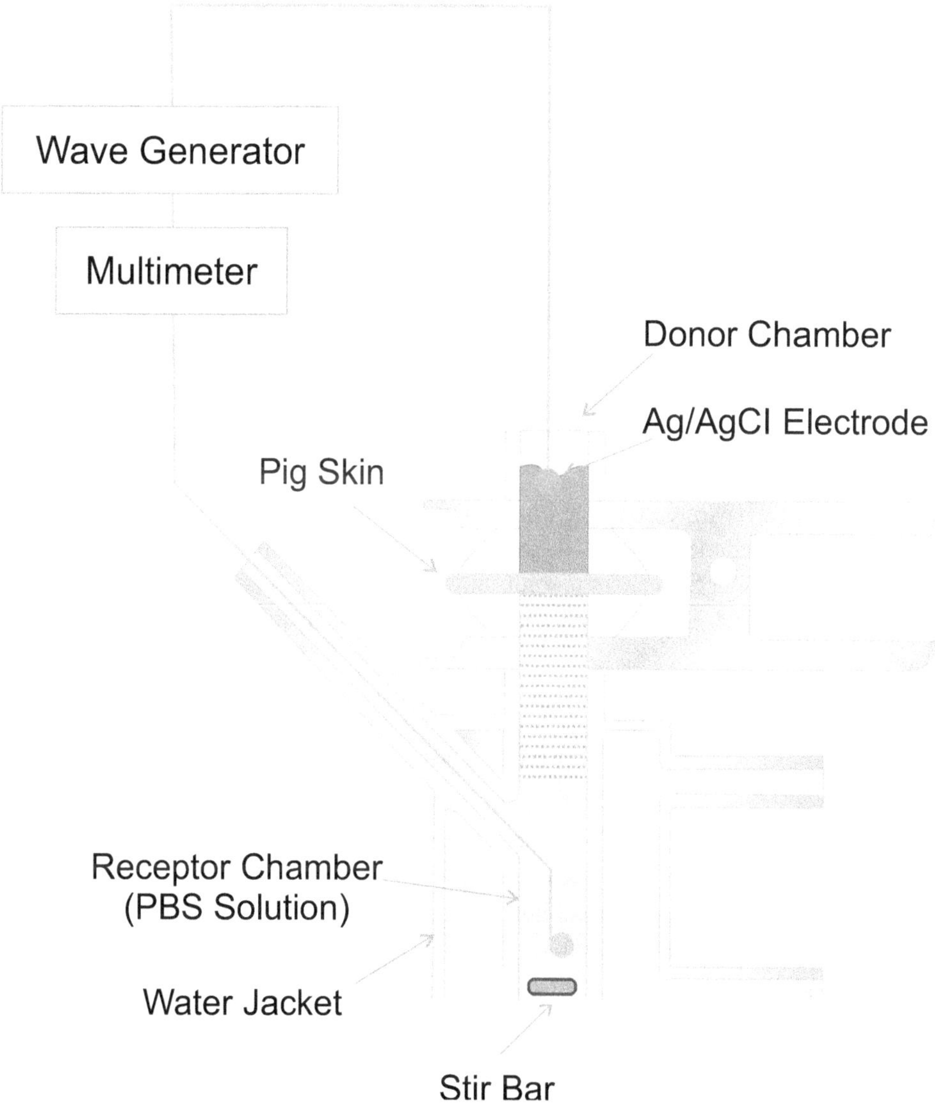

Figure 1. Experimental setup of the Franz diffusion cell to measure pig skin electrical impedance *in vitro*[54]. Pig skin is secured between the donor and the receptor compartments with the SC side facing upwards. An AC sinusoidal signal is applied across the skin. The electric current is measured and the skin impedance can be calculated by Ohm's law.

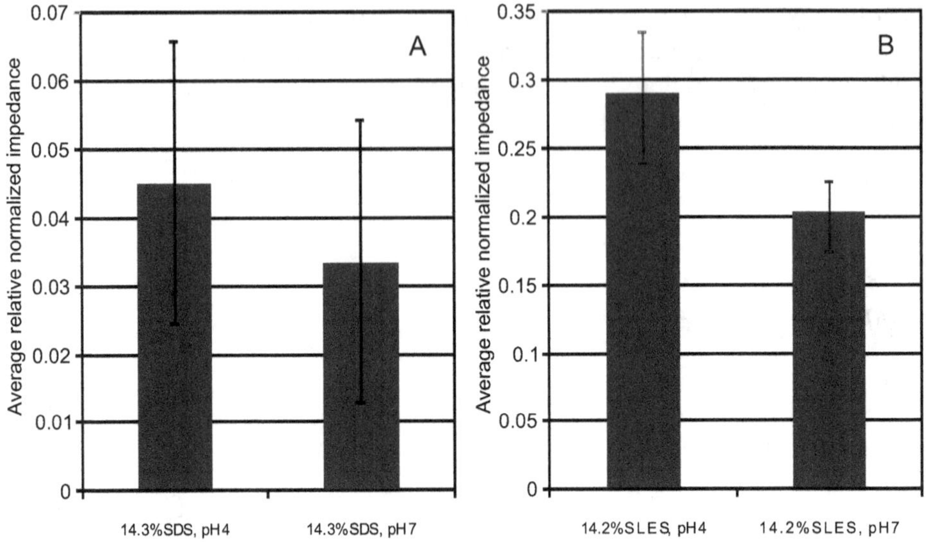

Figure 2. (A) Average relative normalized impedance (the higher, the less damage to the skin barrier and the milder the surfactant system is) versus the SDS solution pH when the porcine skin samples are exposed to 14.3% SDS surfactant solution with different pH values for five hours at room temperature; (B) Average relative normalized impedance versus SLES solution pH when the skin samples are exposed to 14.2% SLES surfactant solution with different pH values for five hours at room temperature[54]. Note the scale in the two plots is different.

4. Mechanical behavior of skin

The skin is a material that demonstrates both elastic and plastic characteristic behavior (viscoelasticity). The mechanical and material properties of skin (e.g., SC stress, after-wash tightness, elasticity, and friction) are affected by exposure to surfactants or other stimuli. Surfactant damage causes dry skin and loss of elasticity, which often leads to cracking of the skin[1]. However, very little is currently understood about this subject since multiple skin layers, including *stratum corneum*, viable epidermis, and dermis are involved.

Most instruments designed to assess the mechanical behavior of skin (*in vivo*) apply a known stress to the skin and measurement of the resulting strain, which can be monitored in different ways. By applying a sinusoidal stress to the skin surface, the viscoelastic characteristics and complex modulus of skin can be studied both *in vivo* and *in vitro* with a gas-bearing electrodynamometer[79–81]. Torsion devices (such as Dermal Torque Meter from Dia-Stron) were developed to study the elasticity parallel to the skin surface by measuring volumetric deformation after applying a twisting force[82–83]. Suction systems, on the other hand, were designed to measure the elasticity perpendicular to the skin surface[84]. These systems measure vertical deformation or stretching and the recovering of skin based on the electrical capacitance of skin (examples include DermaFlex from Cortex Technologies and BTC 2000 from DermaLab) or by using optical systems (e.g., Cutometer from Courage & Khazaka) to measure skin's elevation into a probe due to suction pressure[85]. A device based on shockwave propagation (Reviscometer from Courage & Khazaka) was developed to study skin viscoelesticity (specifically in the SC) by measuring the resonance running time of an acoustical shockwave[86]. This approach is very sensitive and able to differentiate between cosmetic treatments, and has been correlated to consumer perception[87].

As a thin film material, the SC can be investigated by using *in vitro* methods based on biomechanics, dynamic mechanical analysis (DMA), and wafer curvature techniques[88–89]. The drying stress under various conditions such as temperature, relative humidity, and topical cosmetic treatments can be compared and differentiated.

Changes in skin smoothness and friction by surfactants and other cosmetic products can be characterized by a friction meter[90–91]. Currently the Newcastle Friction meter is the only commercially available instrument for this evaluation.

5. Bioengineering methods to measure water flux and water content of skin

Water plays a very important role in physically and biologically maintaining healthy skin. At the same time, a key function of the SC is to act as a semi-impermeable membrane barrier to retain and keep water from leaving the body. Water flux and water content of the outer skin, therefore, are excellent indicators of skin-barrier integrity.

Over the last several decades many noninvasive biophysical and bioengineering instruments have been developed to objectively and quantitatively characterize various skin conditions (skin moisturization, skin diseases, skin aging, sun-mediated stress, etc.) as well as to evaluate skin protection and repair by cosmetic products.

There exists a concentration gradient in the SC, which decreases from the boundary with the viable epidermis to the outermost layers of the surface. This water diffusion flux depends on skin permeability, as well as on the water activity gradient between the human body and the external environment. More hydration at the SC surface will lead to a smaller concentration gradient and a lower transepidermal water loss (TEWL) value[92]. TEWL measurements can be taken to determine water flux by passive diffusion through the SC layer and can be considered as a measure of skin's intrinsic barrier properties. Higher TEWL values normally indicate a damaged or ineffective SC barrier due to chemical (such as surfactant) exposure or diseased skin conditions.

There are two TEWL measurement techniques: open-chamber and closed-chamber. The most known commercially available open-chamber TEWL meters are the Tewameter, ServoMed Evaporimeter, and DermaLab TEWL systems. Due to the vulnerability to disturbance from environmental air movements for the open-chamber systems, the measurements have to be conducted in a well-controlled laboratory environment and subjected to strict testing guidelines. It should be noted, however, that these instruments are quite reliable when used properly[93–95]. Currently closed-chamber TEWL meters that are free from environmental impact are becoming more popular since they are feasible for common workplace and dermatological laboratories. There are two different closed-chamber TEWL instruments available on the market. The VapoMeter from Delfin is a portable and battery-powered unit based on the unventilated concept while AquaFlux from Biox is a bench-top, AC-powered unit based on the condenser-chamber concept[96–97]. TEWL measurements have been used to study and predict skin irritancy following exaggerated surfactant exposure procedures, and the results show a positive correlation between TEWL measurements and visual assessment of skin condition[66, 72, 98–100].

Several instrumental methods have been developed to measure skin hydration and the SC water content (skin surface moisture change) by measuring skin permeability to an alternating electric field. Depending on instrument designs, different signals and parameters can be obtained. NOVA Dermal Phase Meter (based on impedance measurements, which are related to resistance to the flow of alternating current), Skicon200 skin surface hygrometer from IBS and Skin Sensor from DermaLab (based on high-frequency conductance measurements), and Corneometer (based on capacitance measurements) from Courage & Khazaka are among the most popular instruments that are portable and easy to use[37, 41, 66, 69, 98]. Measurements of skin hydration using these devices to study surfactant-skin interactions have been reported and, again, a good correlation between these results and visual dryness/irritation grading has been shown[29, 101–103].

It has to be noted that although TEWL is related to the water content on the skin surface, measurements of TEWL and skin hydration do not always directly correlate. It has been reported that visible skin dryness correlates well with low levels of skin hydration but is not always accompanied by an increase in TEWL readings[24]. In fact, TEWL indicates whether the skin-barrier integrity is physiologically or biologically broken down, which is not a prerequisite for skin dryness, while skin hydration provides information about the physical condition of the skin surface layers. Nevertheless, if the skin is too dry, the surface may physically break down and crack, causing barrier damage and ultimately leading to higher TEWL.

Washing procedures also affect skin/SC pH, which is correlated with skin/SC hydration. The pH of normal skin is between 4 and 6. This acidic environment of the skin surface is very important for maintaining epidermal barrier function and the restoration of the damaged skin barrier. Higher pH has been observed for skin under pathological conditions or after exposure to detergents[33, 104]. The skin/SC pH can be measured by a commercially available instrument (glass electrode) skin pH meter PH 900. However, the concept of SC pH is somewhat problematic, as normal SC does not have free water.

To obtain useful and reliable information regarding the interaction between surfactant-based products and skin, and to better understand the effect of surfactants on skin-barrier function to support strong claim substantiation, it is highly recommended to combine measurements that include several electrical probe methods and TEWL measurements[105].

b. Surfactant-lipid interactions

Skin-barrier function resides primarily in the heterogeneous organization of ordered lipid lamellae of the *stratum corneum*. Surfactant-lipid interactions play a critical role in damaging skin-barrier function and in repairing the barrier after cleansing stress.

Although it is possible to study lipid behavior in intact skin or isolated SC, the complicated structure of the SC and the inherent variability of biological samples make the detailed analysis of lipid phase behavior in real SC lipid organization very challenging[106]. A widely employed approach for investigating skin-barrier biophysics is to use model lipid systems that consist of a mixture of free fatty acid (FFA), ceramides (CER), and cholesterol (CHO) to mimic the SC lipid structure/phase and anticipate its barrier function. Such lipid models of the SC barrier have been widely used and validated by many studies using diverse biophysical experimental methods[107–111]. While the model lipid system is certainly not the same as the lipid composition and organization in the SC, this approach is a simple and useful starting point in which the major SC lipid classes are represented.

1. Differential scanning calorimetry (DSC)

DSC investigates the changes in the liquid-crystal organization of the lipids (from SC or lipid model) by monitoring the shift of molecular structural transition temperature (the melting temperature T_m or the glass transition temperature T_g). Fluidity and disordered arrangement of lipid structure and selective lipid extraction induced by surfactant application can be studied by DSC[112–114].

2. Vibrational spectroscopy (FT-IR)

Fourier Transformed Infrared (FT-IR) spectroscopy measures the vibrational energies (wavelength and intensity) of molecules by light absorption in the infrared range. The IR spectra are affected by neighboring molecular environments and can be used to provide powerful and simultaneous information on both intra- and intermolecular interactions in lipid model systems as well as isolated SC or even skin *in vivo*[115–117]. This technique is very sensitive to molecular composition, structure, and interactions between neighboring molecular components. Lipid chain dynamics, chain packing/organization, conformational order and structure (gel, crystalline, liquid crystalline), fluidity (molecular interactions in lipid bi-layers), domain formation, and phase behavior (orthorhombic, hexagonal, disordered or liquid) in model lipid systems with various compositions can be quantitatively examined since certain IR spectra regions of the SC or SC lipids are very sensitive to these parameters. Figure 3 contains typical FT-IR spectra of a lipid model system at different temperature ranges. Typically one would examine the symmetric CH_2 stretching/rocking (νsCH) around wavenumber 2850 cm^{-1}, and/or CD_2 symmetric stretching/rocking (νsCD) parameters for fatty acid around wavenumber 2090 cm^{-1}. For illustration, Figure 4 contains a plot of the position of the CH_2 stretching band as a function of temperature, allowing us to elucidate the phase behavior of a selected lipid system. The νsCH mode is very suitable for probing the behavior of ceramide chains since it is an intense and relatively narrow band with very limited cholesterol interference[43]. The νsCD mode on the other hand comes only from the fatty acid component and can be used to probe the conformational order of fatty acid through the behavior of the deuterated acyl chains[118].

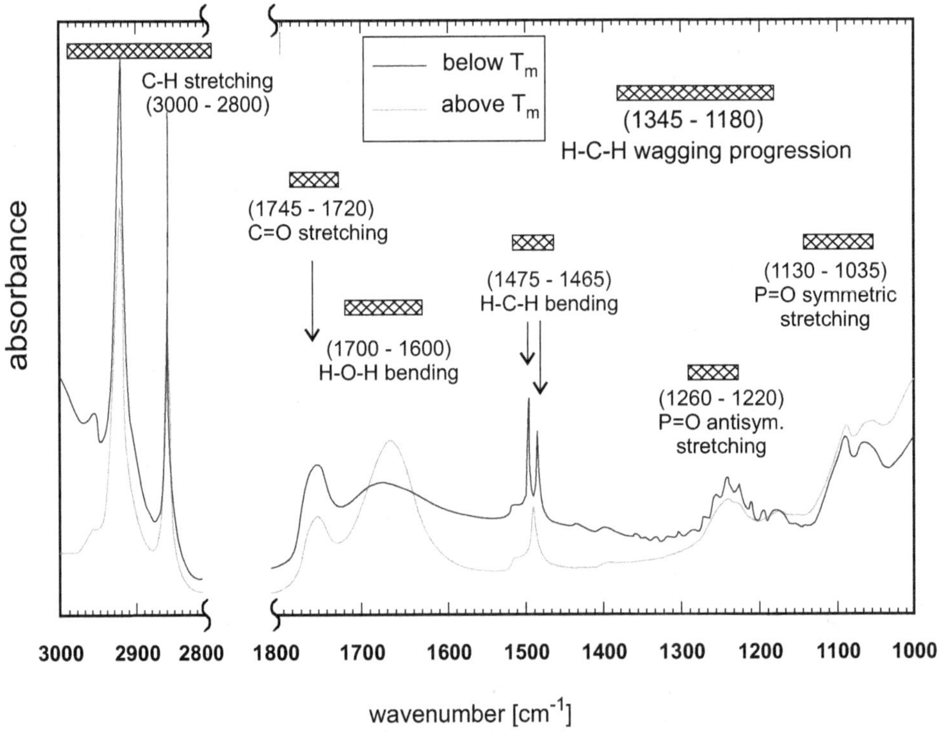

Figure 3. Typical FT-IR spectra of a lipid structure at different temperature ranges 119.

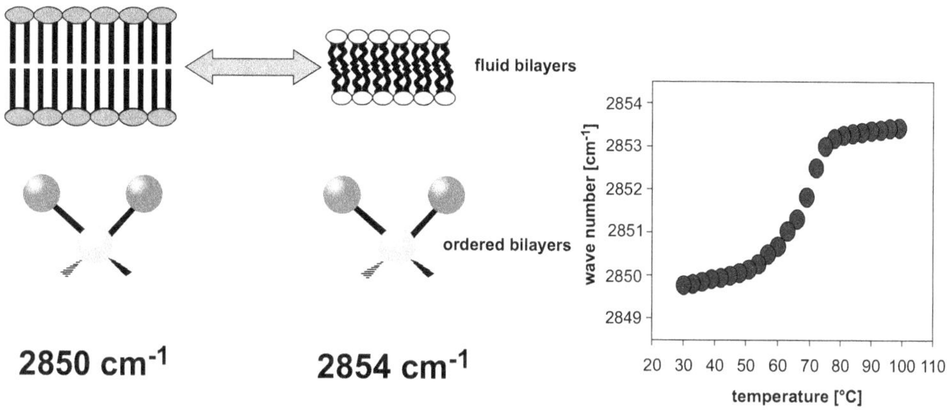

Figure 4. SC lipid conformation order (i.e., bi-layer fluidity) can be determined from the peak position of the symmetric CH_2 stretching mode of the lipid chains from the IR spectra of the SC[9, 119].

FTIR spectroscopy has been applied extensively to study the interactions between surfactants and *stratum corneum* lipids[9, 24, 69, 120]. *In vivo* and *in vitro* attenuated total reflectance Fourier-transform infrared (ATR-FTIR) and transmission-mode IR spectroscopy of skin, isolated SC, or lipid model systems can be used to examine the characteristics of the SC and/or SC lipids (fluidity and integrity of lipid domains) following surfactant exposure and sequential tape striping[9, 24, 120–122]. Integrity of the intercellular lipid domains and damage to SC lipid barrier bi-layer by surfactant exposure as well as recovery can thus be investigated. The effect of pH of the surfactant systems on the SC barrier integrity can also be determined. ATR-FTIR can be used to investigate delivery and monitor deposition (mapping or imaging) of skin-beneficial ingredients (*in vivo*) in skin-cleansing formulations, which correlates well with electrical measurements[41, 69]. With the help of tape stripping, one may determine the distribution profile of molecular components deposited or topically applied across the SC. For isolated *stratum corneum*, transmission-mode FT-IR can be used to study damage and restoration of the skin barrier *in vitro*[109,123].

3. *Quartz crystal microbalance (QCM)*

The quartz crystal microbalance (QCM) detects very small changes in mass via a piezoelectric mechanism and has been broadly utilized as a physical, chemical, electrochemical, and biochemical sensing tool in various applications[124]. As a simple mass measuring technique with nanogram resolution, it can accurately monitor *in situ* subtle surface coverage changes including penetration and diffusion of molecules, and monolayer sorption onto thin films. This oscillator technology is straightforward and convenient to use, especially for complicated solid-liquid interfacial phenomena.

For skin penetration studies, particularly with a focus on SC lipids, the SC mass change is normally very subtle while the skin system is very heterogeneous and complicated. Hence, accurately detecting mass changes due to penetration of exogenous molecules through the SC layer, or studying the effect of chemical penetration on SC lipid phase behavior and structure is very challenging. When experimentally feasible, QCM provides a more sensitive and quantitative approach to such problems than traditional gravimetric measurements[19–20, 32].

Recently, water vapor uptake and surfactant sorption onto SC lipid model layers cast on a quartz crystal were studied using the QCM technique[32, 125–126]. In a very recent article, *in vitro* water vapor uptake and surfactant absorption onto skin lipid model films were quantitatively studied using the QCM[111]. Figure 5 outlines this technique for measuring surfactant adsorption to a model lipid system. The results show that barrier properties of the lipid model system may be damaged by surfactant absorption, as well as by long-term water exposure, due to alterations to the lipid film structure. Surfactant absorption is found to be concentration dependent even beyond its critical micelle concentration (CMC). QCM results for different surfactant systems are consistent with reported clinical data in showing that a clinically milder surfactant, such as sodium lauryl ether sulfate (SLES), does not perturb the film as much as a clinically harsh surfactant, such as sodium dodecyl sulfate (SDS), as shown in Figure 6. These results indicate that this experimental approach is valid and valuable in understanding the effect of surfactants on skin-barrier lipid organization, and hence skin-barrier function.

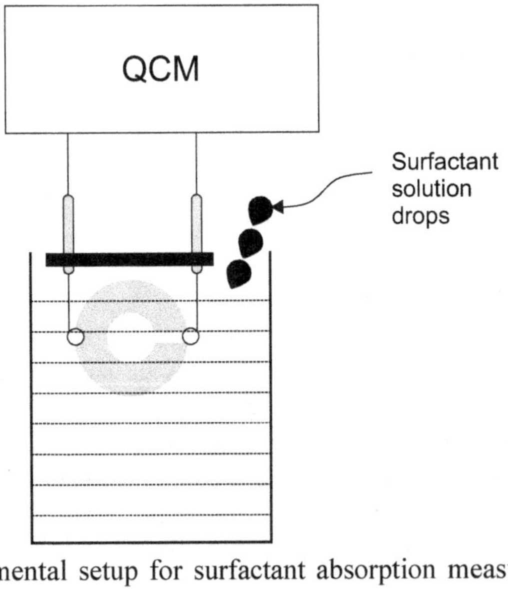

Figure 5. Experimental setup for surfactant absorption measurement of a lipid model coated QCM 111.

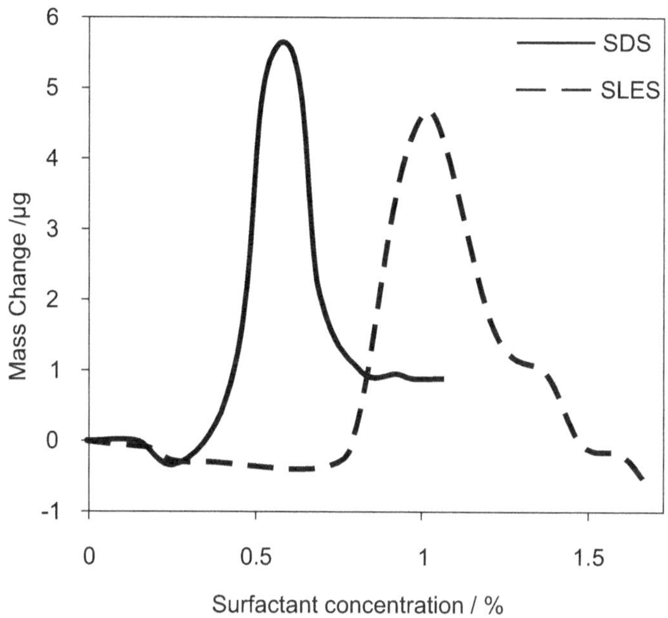

Figure 6. Comparison of QCM absorption profiles of model lipid systems in sodium lauryl ether sulfate (SLES) and sodium lauryl sulfate (SDS) solutions as a function of surfactant concentration[111]. The results show that surfactant absorption into the lipid matrix, and the associated water uptake, are significantly diminished in the case of SLES. Also almost double the concentration of SLES is needed to achieve the maximum mass increase.

c. Skin-protein interactions

Since proteins and surfactants are both amphiphilic materials, surfactant molecules would bind to proteins through interactions between both hydrophilic and hydrophobic groups in a stereochemically constant structure. This binding is dependent on the surfactant chemistry, concentration, temperature, pH, etc. The protein structure will become altered by surfactant binding and protein denaturation can be used as an indication of skin-barrier damage or irritation caused by surfactants. In fact, a correlation between surfactant-induced skin damage or irritation and the interactions of the surfactant molecules with *stratum corneum* proteins[127]. Various protein models (albumin such as BSA, NMF model, zein, etc.) have been used to study surfactant-protein interactions.

1. BSA denaturation test

As a globular protein, bovine serum albumin (BSA) contains 76% sequence identity with human albumin. The denaturation of BSA has been used as a model protein to human skin protein for harshness evaluation. Correlation between surfactant-induced BSA denaturation and skin roughness, after exposing to detergent solutions, was demonstrated[128–129].

Different parameters can be measured to study protein (BSA) denaturation by surfactants. Conductivity and zeta potential of the surfactant-BSA solution can be measured to measure the charge change of the mixing system[78, 130–131]. FTIR spectroscopy, and Raman spectroscopy, and DSC can be used to determine changes in protein secondary structure and investigate the thermal unfolding of BSA caused by surfactants in solution[78, 132–133]. Fluorescence spectroscopy studies have been applied to obtain information on the nature of protein-surfactant aggregates and to monitor changes in the tertiary structure induced by interactions with ionic surfactants, which can result in the exposure of tryptophan residues[134–135]. Since protein denaturation is normally accompanied by a rise in pH and changes in viscosity and surface tension, monitoring these parameters of the BSA solution with the addition of surfactant solution would provide some information about the configuration of BSA and the surfactant-protein interactions[130, 132, 136]. *In vitro* assays based on these parameters (e.g., pH rise) have been developed to predict potential of surfactant-induced skin irritation[137].

2. Zein solubility assay

Dissolution of zein, a protein from corn, can be measured in surfactant solutions to correlate surfactant-induced protein damage with soap harshness or skin irritation. Zein is a water-insoluble protein that becomes water soluble to some extent if it is denatured by surfactants. Theoretically, there is a positive correlation between zein solubility and skin harshness; the more zein that is solubilized, the higher is the tendency to irritate human skin. The study of surfactant interactions with insoluble proteins such as zein can yield valuable information about the effects of surfactants on skin and hair. Model experiments made with zein reveal that the ability of the surfactant to denature and solubilize this protein correlates very well with the dermal irritancy potential of the surfactant[138]. This material has been extensively used in the skin care industry as a model system to understand the effect of surfactants on skin, and as a measure of surfactant-protein interaction, and to predict and screen skin irritation tendency and harshness of soap or surfactant ingredients in skin-cleansing formulations[137, 139–140]

Various surfactant systems including mixing surfactant systems, as well as cleansing formulations (such as soap bars, clear shower gels, shaving preparation formulations, and hand dishwash formulations) with different ingredients have been studied with this zein solubility assay. The results correlate well with other *in vitro* methods and *in vivo* clinical test results.[78, 141] One example is shown in Figure 7, where dissolved zein concentration is plotted as a function of soap concentration[78]. As expected, dissolved zein concentration for milder synthetic Dove soap bar is significantly lower than that for other regular soap bars.

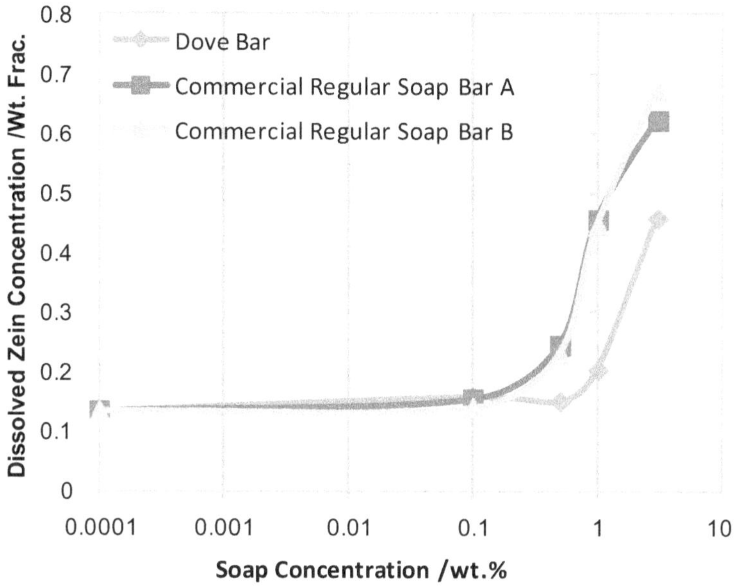

Figure 7. Zein solubility of various soap bars as a function of soap concentration.

3. NMF level measurements

Cleansing changes in NMF levels in SC can be measured *in vivo* by ATR-FTIR spectroscopy[142] and IR imaging with tape stripping[143].

By IR spectroscopic imaging and confocal Raman microspectroscopy[25, 144], information on the molecular composition and distribution of NMF components can also be obtained.

CONCLUSIONS

The objective of this chapter has been to provide an understanding of the various phenomena impacting the nature and degree of surfactant effects on skin during cleansing practices. Once these fundamentals have been understood, we then provide practical guidance to measurement methods that can be used to study surfactant-skin interactions and to thereby assess the effects of surfactants on skin-barrier integrity. By doing so, some aspects of surfactant damage to skin caused by cleansing products have also been discussed.

Skin structure is complicated, and all the mechanism of surfactant-skin interactions is not yet fully understood. Because of this, developing methods to assess the multiple facets of surfactant-skin interactions, and to comprehensively examine damage induced by surfactant-based cleansing products, remains challenging. Besides *in vivo* and clinical methods for human skin evaluation, the development of many noninvasive *in vitro* and instrumental methods in recent years has considerably increased the level of objective and quantitative performance discrimination for cleansing product screening. Yet each method only deals with one or a few of the many aspects of surfactant-skin interactions. Each specific method cannot be used as the sole method to accurately and comprehensively evaluate the harshness of cleansing formulations. Since no single methodology or approach has gained universal acceptance, a combination of many methods is recommended to provide a reliable assessment of the harshness of cleansing formulations and their impact on the integrity of the skin barrier[82]. Ideally, at this stage of our knowledge, choice of the measurement approaches, their combinations, and relative weighing, are of critical importance to providing guidance to formulators and experts in generating useful surfactant structure-efficacy information as well as useful claim substantiation.

ACKNOWLEDGMENTS

The authors would like to thank Timothy W. Gillece, Raymond Rigoletto, and Hani Fares, of Ashland Specialty Ingredients for their technical assistance in producing this manuscript. We also acknowledge the support of Ashland, Inc. and TRI-Princeton for allowing us to publish this work.

REFERENCES

1. Wickett R.R., Visscher M.O. Effect of topical treatments on irritant hand dermatitis in health care workers. Am. J. Infection Control 2006; 34 S2: S98–110.
2. Madison K.C. Barrier function of the skin: “La Raison d’Être” of the epidermis. J. Invest. Dermatol. 2003; 121: 231–240.
3. Elias P. Stratum corneum defensive functions: an integrated view. J. Invest. Dermatol. 2005; 125: 183–200.
4. Johnson A.W. Overview: fundamental skin care--protecting the barrier. Dermatol. Therapy 2004; 17: 1–5.
5. Elias, P.M. Epidermal lipids, barrier function and desquamation. J. Invest. Dermatol. 1983; 80: 44s–49s.
6. Silva C.L., Topgaard D., Kocherbitov V., Sousa J.J.S., Pais A.A.C.C., Sparr E. Stratum corneum hydration: phase transformations and mobility in stratum corneum, extracted lipids and isolated corneocytes. Biochim. Biophys. Acta 2007; 1768: 2647–59.
7. Flach C.R., Mendelsohn R., Rerek M.E., Moore D.J. Biophysical studies of model stratum corneum lipid monolayers by infrared reflection-absorption spectroscopy and Brewster angle microscopy. J. Phys. Chem. B 2000; 104: 2159–65.

8. Bouwstra J.A., Gooris G.S., Dubbelaar F.E.R., Ponec M. Phase behavior of lipid mixtures based on human ceramides: coexistence of crystalline and liquid phases. J. Lipid Res. 2001; 42: 1759–70.

9. Ananthapadmanabhan K.P., Lips A., Vincent C., Meyers F., Caso S., Johnson A., Subramanyan K., Vethamuthu M., Rattinger G., Moore D.J. pH induced alterations in stratum corneum properties. Int. J. Cosmet. Sci. 2003; 25: 103–12.

10. Prottey C., Ferguson T. Factors which determine the skin irritation potential of soaps and detergents. J. Soc. Cosmet. Chem. 1975; 26: 29–46.

11. Moore P.N., Puvvada S., Blankschtein D. Challenging the surfactant monomer skin penetration model: penetration of sodium dodecyl sulfate micelles into the epidermis. J. Cosmet. Sci. 2003; 54: 29–46.

12. Karande P., Jain A., Mitragotri, S. Relationships between skin's electrical impedance and permeability in the presence of chemical enhancers. J. Controlled Release 2006; 110: 307–13.

13. Rawlings A.V., Matts P.J. Stratum corneum moisturization at the molecular level: an update in relation to the dry skin cycle. J. Invest. Dermatol. 2005; 124: 1099–110.

14. Rawlings A.V. Dry and xerotic skin conditions. in: Skin Moisturization, Leyden J.J., Rawlings A.V. (editors), Marcel Dekker, New York, NY, 2002: 119–143.

15. Blank I.H. Factors which influence the water content of the stratum corneum. J. Invest. Dermatol. 1952; 18: 433–40.

16. Blank I.H. Further observations on factors which influence the water content of the stratum corneum. J. Invest. Dermatol. 1953; 21: 259–71.

17. Rhein L.D., Robbins C.R. Fernee K., Cantore R. Surfactant structure effects on swelling of isolated human stratum corneum. J. Soc. Cosmet. Chem. 1986; 37: 125–39.

18. Rhein L.D. Review of properties of surfactants that deter- mine their interactions with stratum corneum. J. Soc. Cosmet. Chem. 1997; 48: 253-74.

19. Faucher J.A. Goddard E.D. Interaction of keratinous substrates with sodium lauryl sulfate: I. sorption. J. Soc. Cosmet. Chem. 1978; 29: 323–37.

20. Faucher J.A. Goddard E.D. Interaction of keratinous substrates with sodium lauryl sulfate. II. permeation through stratum corneum. J. Soc. Cosmet. Chem. 1978; 29: 339–52.

21. Ghosh S., Blankschtein D. The role of sodium dodecyl sulfate (SDS) micelies in inducino skin barrier perturbation in the presence. J. Cosmet. Sci. 2007; 58: 109–33.

22. Rhein L.D., Simion F.A., Hill R.L., Cagan R.H., Mattai J., Maibach H.I. Human cutaneous response to a mixed surfactant system: role of solution phenomena in controlling surfactant irritation. Dermatologica 1990; 180: 18–23.

23. Blake-Haskins J.C., Scala D., Rhein L.D., Robbins C.R. Predicting surfactant irritation from swelling response of a collagen film. J. Soc. Cosmet. Chem. 1986; 37: 199–210.

24. Ananthapadmanabhan K.P., Moore D.J., Subramanyan K., Misra M., Meyer F. Cleansing without compromise: the impact of cleansers on the skin barrier and the technology of mild cleansing. Dermotol. Therapy 2004; 17: 16–25.

25. Caspers P.J., Lucassen G.W., Carter E.A., Bruining H.A., Puppels G.J. In vivo confocal Raman microspectroscopy of the skin: noninvasive determination of molecular concentration profiles. J. Invest. Dermatol. 2001; 116: 434–42.

26. Ananthapadmanabhan K.P., Subramanyan K., Rattinger G.B. Moisturizing cleansers. in: Skin Moisturization, Leyden J.J., Rawlings A.V. (eds), Marcel Dekker, New York, NY, 2002: 405–32.

27. Imokawa G., Akasaki S., Minematsu Y., Kawai M. Importance of intercellular lipids in water-retention properties of the stratum corneum: induction and recovery study of surfactant dry skin. Arch. Dermatol. Res. 1989; 281: 45–51.

28. Froebe C.L., Simion F.A., Rhein L.D., Cagan R.H., Kligman A. Stratum corneum lipid removal by surfactants: relation to in vivo irritation. Dermatological 1990; 181: 277–83.

29. Fulmer A.W., Kramer G.J. Stratum corneum lipid abnormalities in surfactant-induced dry scaly skin. J. Invest. Dermatol. 1986; 86: 598–602.

30. Loden M. The simultaneous penetration of water and sodiumlauryl sulfate through isolated human skin. J. Soc. Cosmet. Chem. 1990; 41: 227–33.

31. Ananthapadmanabhan K.P., Meyers C.L., Aronson M.P. Binding of surfactants to stratum corneum. J. Soc. Cosmet. Chem. 1996; 47: 185–200.

32. Okahata Y., Ebato H. Absorption behaviors of surfactant molecules on a lipid-coated quartz-crystal microbalance. An alternative to eye-irritant tests. Anal. Chem. 1991; 63: 203–07.

33. Gfatter R., Hackl P. Braun F. Effects of soap and detergents on skin surface pH, stratum corneum hydration and fat content in infants. Dermatology 1997; 195: 258–62.

34. Barry B.W. Mode of action of penetration enhancers in human skin. J. Controlled Release 1987; 6: 85–97.

35. Rhein L.D. In vitro interactions: biochemical and biophysical effects of surfactants on skin. In: Surfactants in Cosmetics, 2nd edition, Rieger M.M., Rhein L.D. (eds), Marcel Dekker, Inc., New York, NY, 1997: 397–426.

36. Warner R.R., Boissy Y.L., Lilly N.A., Spears M.J., McKillop K., Marshall J.L., Stone K.J. Water disrupts stratum corneum lipid lamellae: damage is similar to surfactants. J. Invest. Dermatol. 1999; 113: 960–6.

37. Thune P. The effects of detergents on hydration and skin surface lipids. Clinics in Dermatology 1996; 14: 29–33.

38. Bouwstra J.A., Dubbelaar F.E.R., Gooris G.S., Weerheim A.M., Ponec M. The role of ceramide composition in the lipid organisation of the skin barrier. Biochim. Biophys. Acta 1999; 1419: 127–36.

39. Rawlings A.V., Harding C.R., Watkinson A., Chandar P., Scott I.R. Humectants. In: Leyden J.J., Rawling A.V. (eds), Skin Moisturization, Marcel Dekker, Inc., New York, NY, 2002: 245–66.

40. Bouwstra J.A., Ponec M. The skin barrier in healthy and diseased state. Biochim. Biophys. Acta 2006; 1758: 2080–95.

41. Brancaleon L., Bamberg M.P., Sakamaki T., Kollias N. Attenuated total reflection–Fourier transform infrared spectroscopy as a possible method to investigate biophysical parameters of stratum corneum in vivo. J. Invest. Dermatol. 2001; 116: 380–6.

42. Rawlings A.V., Watkinson A., Rogers J., Mayo A.-M., Hope J., Scott I.R. Abnormalities in stratum corneum structure, lipid composition and desmosome degradation in soap-induced winter xerosis. J. Soc. Cosmet. Chem. 1994; 45: 203–20.

43. Velkova V., Lafleur M. Influence of the lipid composition on the organization of skin lipid model mixtures: an infrared spectroscopy investigation. Chem. Phys. Lipids 2002; 117: 63–74.

44. Laugel C., Yagoubi N., Baillet A. ATR-FTIR spectroscopy: a chemometric approach for studying the lipid organization of the stratum corneum. Chem. Phys. Lipids 2005; 135: 55–68.

45. Saad P., Moore D.R., Moore D.J., Menon G., Flach E., Flach C.R., Mendelsohn R. Quantitative IR spectroscopy studies of changes in lipid dynamics and organization in isolated stratum corneum exposed to basic pH. Biophysical Journal 2010; 98: 275a.

46. Plasencia I., Norlen L., Bagatolli L.A. Direct visualization of lipid domains in human skin stratum corneum's lipid membranes: effect of pH and temperature. Biophysical Journal 2007; 93: 3142–55.

47. Kitagawa S., Yokochi N., Murooka N. pH-dependence of phase transition of the lipid bilayer of liposomes of stratum corneum lipids. Int. J. Pharmaceutics 1995; 126: 49–56.

48. Moore D.J., Caso S., Vincent C., Ananthapadmanabhan K.P. pH induced alterations in stratum corneum properties. J. Am. Academy of Dermatology 2004; 50 (Suppl. 1): 33.

49. Misra M., Shi S., Vincent C., Ananthapadmanabhan K.P. Surfactant- and pH-induced ultrastructural changes in stratum corneum. J. Am. Academy of Dermatology 2005; 52 (Suppl. 1): 40.

50. Sznitowska M., Janicki S., Baczek A. Studies on the effect of pH on the lipoidal route of penetration across stratum corneum. J. Controlled Release 2001; 76: 327–35.

51. Lee G., Swarbrick J., Kiyohara G., Payling D.W. Drug permeation through human skin. III. Effect of pH on the partitioning behavior of a chromone-2-carboxylic acid. Int. J. Pharmaceutics 1985; 23: 43–54.

52. Murahata R.I., Aronson M.P. The relationship between solution pH and clinical irritancy for carboxylic acid-based personal washing product. J. Soc. Cosmet. Chem. 1994; 45: 239–46.

53. Fluhr J.W., Kao J., Jain M., Ahn S.K., Feingold K.R., Elias P.M. Generation of free fatty acids from phospholipids regulates stratum corneum acidification and integrity. J. Invest. Dermatol. 2001; 117: 52–8.

54. Lu G., Moore D.J. Study of surfactant–skin interactions by skin impedance measurements. Int. J. Cosmet. Sci. 2012; 34: 74–80.

55. Serup J. EEMCO guidance for the assessment of dry skin (xerosis) and ichthyosis: clinical scoring systems. Skin Res. Tech. 1995; 1: 109–14.

56. Pierard G.E. EEMCO guidance for the assessment of dry skin (xerosis) and ichthyosis: Evaluation by stratum corneum strippings. Skin Res. Tech. 1996; 2: 3–11.

57. Beradesca E. and the EEMCO Group. EEMCO guidance for the assessment of stratum corneum hydration: Electrical methods. Skin Res. Tech. 1997; 3: 126–32.

58. Rogiers V. EEMCO guidance for the assessment of transepidermal water loss in cosmetic sciences. Skin Pharmacol. Appl. Skin Physiol. 2001; 14: 117–28.

59. Parra J.L., Paye M. EEMCO guidance for the in vivo Assessment of Skin Surface pH. Skin Pharmacol. Appl. Skin Physiol. 2003; 16: 188–202.

60. Pierard G.E. EEMCO guidance to the in vivo Assessment of Tensile Functional Properties of the Skin. Skin Pharmacol. Appl. Skin Physiol. 1999; 12: 352–62.

61. Pierard G.E. EEMCO guidance for the assessment of skin colour. J. Euro. Acad. Dermato-Venereol. 1998; 10: 1–11.

62. Berardesca E., Leveque J.L., Masson P. EEMCO guidance for the Measurement of Skin Microcirculation. Skin Pharmacol. Appl. Skin Physiol. 2002; 15: 442–56.

63. Leveque J.L. EEMCO guidance for the assessment of skin topography. Euro. Acad. Dermato-Venereol. 1999; 12: 103–14.

64. Imokawa G. Surfactant mildness. In: Surfactants in Cosmetics, Rieger M.M., Rhein L.D. (eds), Marcel Dekker, New York, 1997: 427–71.

65. Babulak S.W., Rhein L.D., Scala D.D., Simion F.A., Grove G.L. Quantitation of erythema in a soap chamber test using the minolta chroma (reflectance) meter: comparison of instrumental results with visual assessments. J. Soc. Cosmet. Chem. 1986; 37: 475–9.

66. Wilhelm K.-P., Freitag G., Wolff H.H. Evaluation of the acute human irritation model by noninvasive techniques. J. Am. Acad. Dermatol. 1994; 30: 944–9.

67. Obata M., Tagami H. A rapid in vitro test to assess skin moisturizers. J. Soc. Cosmet. Chem. 1990; 41: 235–41.

68. Barel A.O., Lambrecht R., Clarys P., Morrison B.M., Paye M. A comparative study of the effects on the skin of a classical bar soap and a syndet cleansing bar in normal use conditions and in the soap chamber test. Skin Res. & Tech. 2001; 7: 98–104.

69. Moore D.J., Orofino S., Antonopoulos P. Maintaining moisturization from rinse-off products. HAPPI 2006; 11: 77–81.

70. Batt M.D., Fairhurst E. Hydration of the stratum corneum. Int. J. Cosmet. Sci. 1986; 8: 253–64.

71. Garber C.A., Nightingale C.T. Characterizing cosmetic effects and skin morphology by scanning electron microscope. J. Soc. Cosmet. Chem. 1976; 27: 509–31.

72. Misra M., Ananthapadmanabhan K.P., Hoyberg K., Gursky R.P., Prowell S., Aronson M. Correlation between surfactant-induced ultrastructural changes in epidermis and transepidermal water loss. J. Soc. Cos. Chem. 1997; 48: 219–34.

73. Warner R.R., Stone K.J., Boissy Y.L. Hydration disrupts human stratum corneum ultrastructure. J. Invest. Dermatol. 2003; 120: 275–84.

74. Zhang G., McMullen R., Moore D.J. Unpublished data, 2011.

75. Waters K.A. The effects of surfactants on penetration across the skin. Int. J. Cosmet. Soc. 1993; 15: 260–70.

76. Ghosh S., Blankschtein D. Why is sodium cocoyl isethionate (SCI) mild to the skin barrier? - An in vitro investigation based on the relative sizes of the SCI micelles and the skin aqueous pores. J. Cosmet. Sci. 2007; 58: 229–44.
77. Ghosh S., Hornby S., Grove G., Zerwick C., Appa Y., Blankschtein D. Ranking of aqueous surfactant-humectant systems based on an analysis of in vitro and in vivo skin barrier perturbation measurements. J. Cosmet. Sci. 2007; 58: 599–620.
78. Lu G., Moore D.J. Unpublished data, 2011.
79. Finlay B. Dynamic mechanical testing of human skin in vivo. J. Biomechanics 1970; 3: 557–68.
80. Christensen M.S., Hargens C.W., Nacht S., Gans E.H. Viscoelastic properties of intact human skin: instrumentation, hydration effects, and the contribution of the stratum corneum. J. Invest. Dermatol. 1977; 69: 282–6.
81. Matts P., Goodyear E. A new instrument to measure the mechanical properties of human stratum corneum in vivo. J. Cosmet. Sci. 1998; 49: 321–33.
82. Kajs T.M., Gartstein V. Review of the instrumental assessment of skin: effects of cleansing products. J. Soc. Cosmet. Chem. 1991; 42: 249–71.
83. Agache P.G., Monneur C., leveque J.L., Rigal J. Mechanical properties and Young modulus of human skin in vivo. Arch. Dermatol. Res. 1980; 269: 221–32.
84. Diridollou S. In vivo model of mechanical properties of human skin under suction. Skin Res. Tech. 2000; 6: 214–21.
85. Murray B.C., Wickett R.R. Sensitivity of Cutometer data to stratum corneum hydration level. A preliminary study. Skin Res Technol. 1996; 2: 101–6.
86. Ruvolo E.C., Stamatas G.N., Kollias N. Skin viscoelasticity displays site- and age-dependent angular anisotropy. Skin Pharmacol. Physiol. 2007; 20: 313–21.
87. Dahlgren R.M., Elsnau W.H. Measurement of skin condition by sonic velocity. J. Soc. Cosmet. Chem. 1984; 35: 1–20.
88. Levi K., Weber R.J., Do J.Q., Dauskardt R.H. Drying stress and damage processes in human stratum corneum. Int. J. Cosmet. Sci. 2010; 32: 276–93.
89. Levi K., Dauskardt R.H. Application of substrate curvature method to differentiate drying stresses in topical coatings and human stratum corneum. Int. J. Cosmet. Sci. 2010; 32: 294–8.
90. Prall J.K. Instrumental evaluation of the effects of cosmetic products on skin surfaces with particular reference to smoothness. J. Soc. Cosmet. Chem. 1973; 24: 693–707.

91. Nacht S., Close J.-A., Yeung D., Gans E.H. Skin friction coefficient: changes induced by skin hydration and emollient application and correlation with perceived skin feel. J. Soc. Cosmet. Chem. 1981; 32: 55–65.

92. Blank I.H., Moloney J., Emslie A.G., Simon I., Apt C. The diffusion of water across the stratum corneum as a function of its water content. J. Invest. Dermatol. 1984; 82: 188–94.

93. Rogiers V., Houben E., De Paepe K. Transepidermal water loss measurements in dermato-cosmetic sciences. in: Bioengineering of the Skin: Water and the Stratum Corneum, 2nd ed., Fluhr J., Elsner P., Berardesca E., Maibach H.I. (eds), CRC Press, Boca Raton, FL 2005: 63–76.

94. Kalia Y.N., Pirot F., Guy R.H. Homogeneous transport in a heterogeneous membrane: water diffusion across human stratum corneum in vivo. Biophys. J. 1996; 71: 2692–700.

95. Rodrigues L., Pinto P., Galego N., Silva d, Pereira L. Transepidermal water loss kinetic modeling approach for the parameterization of skin water dynamics. Skin Res. Technol. 1999; 5: 72–80.

96. Imhof R.E. Methods and equipment for measuring vapor flux from surfaces. US Patent 6439028 (2000).

97. Imhof R.E., Xiao P., De Jesus M.E.P., Ciortea L.I., Berg E.P. New developments in skin barrier measurements. in: Skin Moisturization, 2nd edition, Rawling A.V., Leyden J.J. (eds), Informa Healthcare, New York, NY, 2009: 463–79.

98. Wilhelm K.P., Cua A.B., Wolff H.H., Maibach H.I. Surfactant-induced stratum corneum hydration in vivo: prediction of the irritation potential of anionic surfactants. J. Invest. Dermatol. 1993; 101: 310–5.

99. Smith H.R., Rowson M., Basketter D.A., McFadden J.P. Intra-individual variation of irritant threshold and relationship to transepidermal water loss measurement of skin irritation. Contact Dermatitis 2004; 51: 26–9.

100. Lukacovic M.F., Dunlap F.E., Michaels S.E., Visscher M.O., Watson D.D. Forearm wash test to evaluate the clinical mildness of cleansing products. J. Soc. Cosmet. Chem. 1988; 39: 355–66.

101. Agner T., Serup J. Skin reactions to irritants assessed by non-invasive bioengineering methods. Contact Dermatitis 1989; 20: 352–9.

102. Tagami H., Kanamaru Y., Inoue K., Suehisa S., Inoue F., Iwatsuki K., Yoshikuni K., Yamada M. Water sorption-desorption test of the skin in vivo for functional assessment of the stratum corneum. J. Invest. Dermatol. 1982; 78: 425–8.

103. Imokawa G., Akasaki S., Kawamata A., Yano S., Takashi N. Water retaining function in the stratum corneum and its recovery properties by synthetic pseudo-ceramides. J. Soc. Cosmet. Chem. 1989; 40: 273–85.

104. Fluhr J.W., Bankova L., Elias P. Stratum corneum pH and ions↓distribution and importance. in: Bioengineering of the Skin: Water and the Stratum Corneum (2nd ed.), Fluhr J.W., Elsner P., Berardesca E., Maibach H.I. (eds), CRC Press, Boca Raton, FL, 2005: 27–47.

105. Wilson D., Berardesca E., Maibach H. In vivo transepidermal water loss and skin surface hydration in assessment of moisturization and soap effects. Int. J. Cosmet. Sci. 1988; 10: 201–11.

106. Kessner D., Ruettinger A., Kiselev M.A., Wartewig S., Neubert R.H.H. Properties of ceramides and their impact on the stratum corneum structure. Skin Pharmacology and Physiology 2008; 21: 58–74.

107. Kitson N., Thewalt J., Lafleur M., Bloom M. A model membrane approach to the epidermal permeability barrier. Biochemistry 1994; 33: 6707–15.

108. Bouwstra J.A., Thewalt J., Gooris G.S., Kitson N. A model membrane approach to the epidermal permeability barrier: an X-ray diffraction study. Biochemistry 1997; 36: 7717–25.

109. Mendelsohn R., Rerek M.E., Moore D.J. Infrared spectroscopy and microscopic imaging of stratum corneum models and skin. Phys. Chem. Chem. Phys. 2000; 2: 4651–7.

110. Rowat A.C., Kitson N., Thewalt J.L. Interactions of oleic acid and model stratum corneum membranes as seen by 2H-NMR. Int. J. Pharm. 2006; 307: 225–31.

111. Lu G., Gillece T.W., Moore D.J. Study of water vapor and surfactant absorption by lipid model systems using the quartz crystal microbalance. Chem. Phys. Lipids 2011; 164: 259–65.

112. Golden G.M., McKie J.E., Potts R.O. Role of stratum corneum lipid fluidity in transdermal drug flux. J. Pharm. Sci. 1987; 76: 25–8.

113. Baby A.R., Lacerda A.C., Velasco M.V., Lopes P.S., Kawano Y., Kaneko T.M. Evaluation of the interaction of surfactants with stratum corneum model membrane from Bothrops jararaca by DSC. Int. J. Pharm. 2006; 317: 7–9.

114. Lanke S.S.S., Kolli C.S., Strom J.G., Banga A.K. Enhanced transdermal delivery of low molecular weight heparin by barrier perturbation. Int. J. Pharm. 2009; 365: 26–33.

115. Moore D.J., Rerek M.E. Insights into the molecular organization of lipids in the skin barrier from infrared spectroscopy studies of stratum corneum lipid models. Acta Derm. Venereol. Supp. 2000; 208: 16–22.

116. Rerek M.E., Moore D.J. Skin lipid structure: insights into hydrophobic and hydrophilic driving forces for self assembly using IR spectroscopy. in: Surfactants in Personal Care Products and Decorative Cosmetics, 3rd ed., Rhein L.D., O'Lenick A., Schlossman M., Somasundaran P. (eds), CRC Press, Boca Raton, FL, 2007: 189–209.

117. Mendelsohn R., Flach C.R., Moore D.J. Determination of molecular conformation and permeation in skin via IR spectroscopy, microscopy, and imaging. Biochem. et Biophys. Acta 2006; 1758: 923–33.

118. Moore D.J., Rerek M.E., Mendelsohn R. Lipid domains and orthorhombic phases in model stratum corneum: evidence from Fourier transform infrared spectroscopy studies. Biochem Biophys Res Commun. 1997; 231: 797–801.

119. Moore D.J. Unpublished work, 2008.

120. Saad P., Flach C.R., Walters R.M., Mendelsohn R. Infrared spectroscopic studies of sodium dodecyl sulphate permeation and interaction with stratum corneum lipids in skin. Int. J. Cosmet. Sci. 2012; 34: 36–43.

121. Bommannan D., Potts R.P., Guy R.H. Examination of stratum corneum barrier function in vivo by infrared spectroscopy. J. Invest. Dermatol. 1990; 95: 403–8.

122. James-Smith M.A., Hellner B., Annunziato N., Mitragotri S. Effect of surfactant mixtures on skin structure and barrier properties. Annals of Biomedical Engineering 2011; 39: 1215–23.

123. Pensack R.D., Michniak B.B., Moore D.J., Mendelsohn R. Kinetic/structural studies of barrier reformation in intact stratum corneum following thermal perturbation. Applied Spectroscopy 2007; 60: 1399–404.

124. Marx K.A. Quartz crystal microbalance: a useful tool for studying thin polymer films and complex biomolecular systems at the solution-surface interface. Biomacromolecules 2003; 4: 1099–120.

125. Lee D., Ashcraft J.N., Verploegen E., Pashkovski E., Weitz D.A. Permeability of model stratum corneum lipid membrane measured using quartz crystal microbalance. Langmuir 2009; 25: 5762–6.

126. Lee M.H., Lim B., Kim J.W., An E.J., Lee D. Effect of composition on water permeability of model stratum corneum lipid membranes. Soft Matter 2012; 8: 1539–46.

127. Ananthapadmanabhan K.P. Protein-surfactant interactions. in: Interactions of Surfactants with Polymers and Proteins. Goddard E.D, Ananthapadmanabhan K.P. (eds.), CRC Press, Boca Raton, FL, 1993: 319–365.

128. Gelamo E.L., Silva C.H.T.P., Imosato H., Tabak M. Interaction of bovine (BSA) and human (HSA) serum albumins with ionic surfactants: spectroscopy and modeling. Biochim. Biophys. Acta 2002; 1594: 84–99.

129. Imokawa G., Sumura K., Katsumi M. Study on skin roughness caused by surfactants. II. Correlation between protein denaturation and skin roughness. J. Am. Oil Chem. Soc. 1975; 52: 484–9.

130. Ghosh S., Banerjee A. A multitechnique approach in protein/surfactant interaction study: physicochemical aspects of sodium dodecyl sulfate in the presence of trypsin in aqueous medium. Biomacromolecules 2002; 3: 9–16.

131. Ruiz-Pena M., Comas-Rojas H., Rodriguez-Calvo S. Perez-Gramatges A. Self-association behaviour of protein: surfactant systems in alcohol/water mixtures. IEEE Proc.-Nanotechnol. 2005; 152: 177–81.

132. Wei X., Chang Z., Liu H. Influence of sodium dodecyl sulfate on the characteristics of bovine serum albumin solutions and foams. J. Surfactants and Detergents 2003; 6: 107–12.

133. van de Weert M., Haris P.I., Hennink W.E., Crommelin D.J. Fourier transform infrared spectrometric analysis of protein conformation: effect of sampling method and stress factors. Anal. Biochem. 2001; 297: 160–9.

134. Lu R.-C., Cao A.-N., Lai L.-H., Xiao J.-X. Effect of anionic surfactant molecular structure on bovine serum albumin (BSA) fluorescence. Colloids and Surface A: Physicochem. Eng. Aspects 2006; 278: 67–73.

135. Hazra P., Chakrabarty D., Chakraborty A., Sarkar N. Probing protein-surfactant interaction by steady state and time-resolved fluorescence spectroscopy. Biochem. Biophys. Res. Comm. 2004; 314: 543–9.

136. Tavss E.A., Eigen E., Kligman A.M. Anionic detergent-induced skin irritation and anionic detergent-induced pH rise of bovine serum albumin. J. Soc. Cosmet. Chem. 1988; 39: 267–72.

137. Morrison B.M., Paye M. A comparison of three in vitro screening tests with an in vivo clinical test to evaluate the irritation potential of antibacterial liquid soaps. J. Soc. Cosmet. Chem. 1995; 46: 291–9.

138. Pezron I., Galet L., Clausse D. Surface interaction between a protein monolayer and surfactants and its correlation with skin irritation by surfactants. J. Colloid Interface Sci. 1986; 180: 285–89.

139. Lips A., Ananthapadmanabhan K.P., Vathamuthu M., Hua X.Y., Yang L., Vincent C., Deo N., Somasundaran P. Role of surfactant micelle charge in protein denaturation and surfactant-induced skin irritation. in: Surfactants in Personal Care Products and Decorative Cosmetics, 3rd ed., Rhein L.D., O'Lenick A., Schlossman M., Somasundaran P. (Eds), CRC Press, Boca Raton, FL, 2007: 177–88.

140. Ruso J.M., Deo N., Somasundaran P. Complexation between dodecyl sulfate surfactant and zein protein in solution. Langmuir 2004; 20: 8988–91.

141. Putterman G.J., Wolejsza N.F., Wolfram M.A., Laden K. The effect of detergents on swelling of stratum corneum. J. Soc. Cosmet. Chem. 1977; 28: 521–32.

142. Lu G., Zhang G., Moore D.J. Unpublished data, 2011.

143. Moore D.J., Bi X. The application of infrared spectroscopic imaging to skin delivery: visualizing molecular localization in formulations and in skin. in: Science and Applications of Skin Delivery Systems, Wiechers J.W. (ed.), Allured Publishing Corporation, Carol Stream, IL, 2008: 49–59.

144. Zhang G., Moore D.J., Mendelsohn R., Flach C.R. Vibrational microspectroscopy and imaging of molecular composition and structure during human corneocyte maturation. J. Invest. Dermatol. 2006; 126: 1088–94.

PART 11.2

IMAGING TECHNIQUES AND ANALYSIS FOR QUANTIFICATION OF SKIN APPEARANCE

Author

Roger L. McMullen, Ph.D.
Principal Scientist
Materials Science Department
Ashland, Inc.
Bridgewater, NJ 08807

Adjunct Professor
School of Natural Sciences
Fairleigh Dickinson University
Teaneck, NJ 07666

ABSTRACT

Imaging technologies have become increasingly important in the evaluation of cosmetic ingredients and their effects on skin. This need has been greatly fueled by requirements for the technical evaluation of the effects of new ingredients and formulations intended for use in anti-aging, skin whitening, pore size reduction, and anti-acne products. This chapter provides an in-depth focus of imaging technologies that are utilized to evaluate the appearance of skin from the outside as well as to look inside the skin to assess its overall health state. In addition to obtaining a vast description of instrumentation and techniques used for such applications, the reader will also gain insight into the fundamental physical principles underlying these technologies.

In the last two decades, a number of imaging modalities have been developed to provide quantitative assessment of the skin's topographical structure. Commercial instrumentation based on fringe projection techniques is now available and provides us with a close-up three-dimensional view of the skin's surface, which is especially useful for quantifying furrows and pores. Other skin imaging technologies have also advanced by leaps and bounds, especially in the area of polarized light and fluorescence photography, which are commonly used in conjunction with image analysis techniques. In fact, it is now quite common for laboratories to carry out multi-spectral multi-modal imaging, which combines polarized light, fluorescence, and other modes of photography under one umbrella.

Novel thermal imaging technologies allow us to gather temperature distribution maps of skin, providing us with anatomical differentiation as well as the ability to focus on specific areas of interest that have undergone treatment with active cosmetic ingredients. Below the surface of skin, great strides have also been made in the evaluation of the skin's internal structure. Examples of techniques useful in this regard include, but are not limited to, reflectance confocal microscopy and ultrasonography. There have been many advances in these imaging techniques over the past 10–15 years that have been coupled with a flurry of *in vivo* studies. In fact, many of these technologies are used to carry out important evaluation of skin lesions, both benign and malignant, as well as other important phenomena that occur in skin.

In this chapter we also discuss high-resolution microscopy methods, which in many respects have started to reach their maturity and offer many insights into phenomena that occur in skin. Equally important, image-processing and analysis techniques that are associated with all of these imaging technologies provide us with quantitative descriptions of skin-related measurements. This is especially true for histological and immunofluorescent staining techniques, which are exceptionally useful to monitor the effects of skin care active ingredients. In most cases, treatment of skin with active ingredients leads to the upregulation or downregulation of specific proteins and other biomolecules as measured in cell culture systems *in vitro* and in the various morphological components of skin as monitored *in vivo* or *ex vivo*. Traditionally, histological and immunofluorescent images were qualitatively assessed by a researcher or pathologist. Thanks to advances in image analysis software, such evaluations can be achieved quantitatively. The overall goal of this chapter is to touch upon many important facets of this technology and provide the reader with a general overview and the current state-of-the-art.

TABLE OF CONTENTS

11.2.1 SKIN SURFACE IMAGING AND ANALYSIS

Skin topography is an extremely important component of the consumer's sensorial experience, mostly perceived by visual observation and touch. Since the stratum corneum is the outermost layer of skin, it is the first part of the integument seen by the observer. The stratum corneum is comprised of corneocytes, which exfoliate from the skin. The exfoliation pattern depends on the overall health state of the skin. For example, in dry, scaly skin, corneocytes tend to exfoliate in large clusters. This is known as scaling and is frequent in dry skin as well as many common dermatological diseases, such as psoriasis. On the other hand, in smooth, moisturized skin corneocytes will shed off in much smaller clusters, ideally as individual cells. Skin ashing is a term frequently used to describe skin characterized as dry with decreased luster properties.[1] The skin's microrelief pattern also contributes significantly to its topography. Fine grooves (furrows) intersect with each other, forming many types of shapes including squares, rectangles, triangles, rhomboids, and trapezoids that contribute to the skin's glyphic patterns. Glyphic patterns provide the skin with the necessary flexibility to accommodate various ranges of motion, especially in the joint regions. Glyphic patterns should be distinguished from wrinkles, which are genetically determined and develop during adulthood as a result of dermal matrix deterioriation.[2] The formation of wrinkles can be accelerated by various environmental factors including exposure to solar radiation. In addition to the stratum corneum and its components, there are a number of appendages (e.g., hair and pores) in skin that also contribute to its three-dimensional landscape.

In this section of the chapter, we describe many of the methods used to measure skin topography. These include polarized light photography, skin replica methods, and fringe projection techniques. In addition, we examine various factors associated with quantification of pore appearance, which contribute greatly to skin topography, especially in the facial region. Lip health is another area of great importance to the consumer and therefore of great interest to cosmetic scientists attempting to improve its appearance. For this reason, we discuss several techniques to measure not only lip properties, but also the influence of both cosmetic and active ingredient treatments. A detailed discussion of lip structure can be found elsewhere in this book in the major section on substrates.

Other imaging techniques have also been used to a great extent to characterize various features of skin. For example, ultraviolet reflectance photography is used to better visualize areas of hyper- and hypopigmentation in skin. Fluorescence reflectance microscopy is also capable of generating pertinent information about internal structures of skin, such as collagen, horn, porphyrins (due to acne vulgaris), etc. The emergence of these techniques over the last two decades has led to the development of commercially available instruments to conduct multi-spectral multi-modal facial imaging.

a. Polarized light photography

Surface and subsurface features of the skin can be accentuated with polarized light photography.[3,4] Important surface features measured by polarization photography consist of wrinkles, furrows, and pores. Subsurface features, on the other hand, include erythema, vascular lesions (e.g., portwine stains, rosacea, etc.), and pigmented lesions.[5] Polarized light photography has been employed in clinical dermatology and for the evaluation of personal care products for more than two decades.

Before delving into the particularities of polarization photography, there are a few principles of optics that should be considered. There are two types of light reflection: specular and diffuse reflection. **Specular reflection** is associated with glare and has a shiny appearance, which in the case of skin results from direct reflection from the outermost surface of the stratum corneum. The angle of incidence equals the angle of reflection in specular reflection, similar to the phenomenon that occurs when light reflects from a smooth surface. A familiar example of this in nature is when one observes a lake with a mountain in the background with the mountain's reflection projected on the smooth lake's surface. In skin, only about 4–7% of the incident light on the surface of skin undergoes specular reflection.[6]

Diffuse reflection, on the other hand, is light scattered at various angles due to imperfections at the surface where the angle of reflection is not equivalent to the angle of incidence. Light also penetrates into the skin where it may be absorbed by melanin and other chromophores, or it interacts with other structures such as collagen fibers causing the light to scatter (changing its orientation of polarization) prior to reflecting back outside of the skin. This latter process is known as backscattering and accounts for approximately 93–96% of incident light that interacts with skin.[6]

During polarization photography, the diffuse and specular components can be separated using linear polarization filters. Normally, one filter is placed in front of the light source and the other is mounted on the lens. In our laboratory, we typically use polarization paper that can be cut to size in order to cover the light source. When the polarizers are aligned parallel to each other we observe specular reflection, similar to the image of volar forearm skin shown in Figure 1a. Notice the accentuation of the surface features and crosshatched nature of furrows by maintaining the same degree of polarization of light that illuminates the subject and is read by the camera sensor.

In contrast, orienting the polarizing filters perpendicular to one another allows us to view diffuse scattering (see Figure 1b). Images obtained of skin in this manner will contain information resulting from the backscattering phenomenon, especially that caused by vascularization. These images were obtained from a relatively young individual (35 years old) with Fiztpatrick Type II skin, little history of photo-damage, and from a region of the body (volar forearm) that is generally protected from UV rays.

(a)

(b)

Figure 1: Photographic images of the volar forearm of a subject with Fitzpatrick Type II skin; age 35. Polarizers were placed in front of the illumination light source and the lens. (a) Image obtained with polarizers oriented parallel to each other. (b) Image obtained with polarizers oriented perpendicular to each other (cross polarizers). The small dark spot in the middle of the field of view is a marking reference point.

In addition to qualitative visual observation of the images, typically one would quantify various features in the image. This is especially true in the case of the image obtained with parallel polarizers. Normally, one is interested in the density and directionality of the furrows in a given image. Usually, computer-generated algorithms or image-processing and analysis software are utilized to isolate the furrows from the original image. In Figure 2, several typical steps are shown using commercially available software (Image Pro Plus and Adobe Photoshop) in order to isolate the furrows so that further measurements can be made.

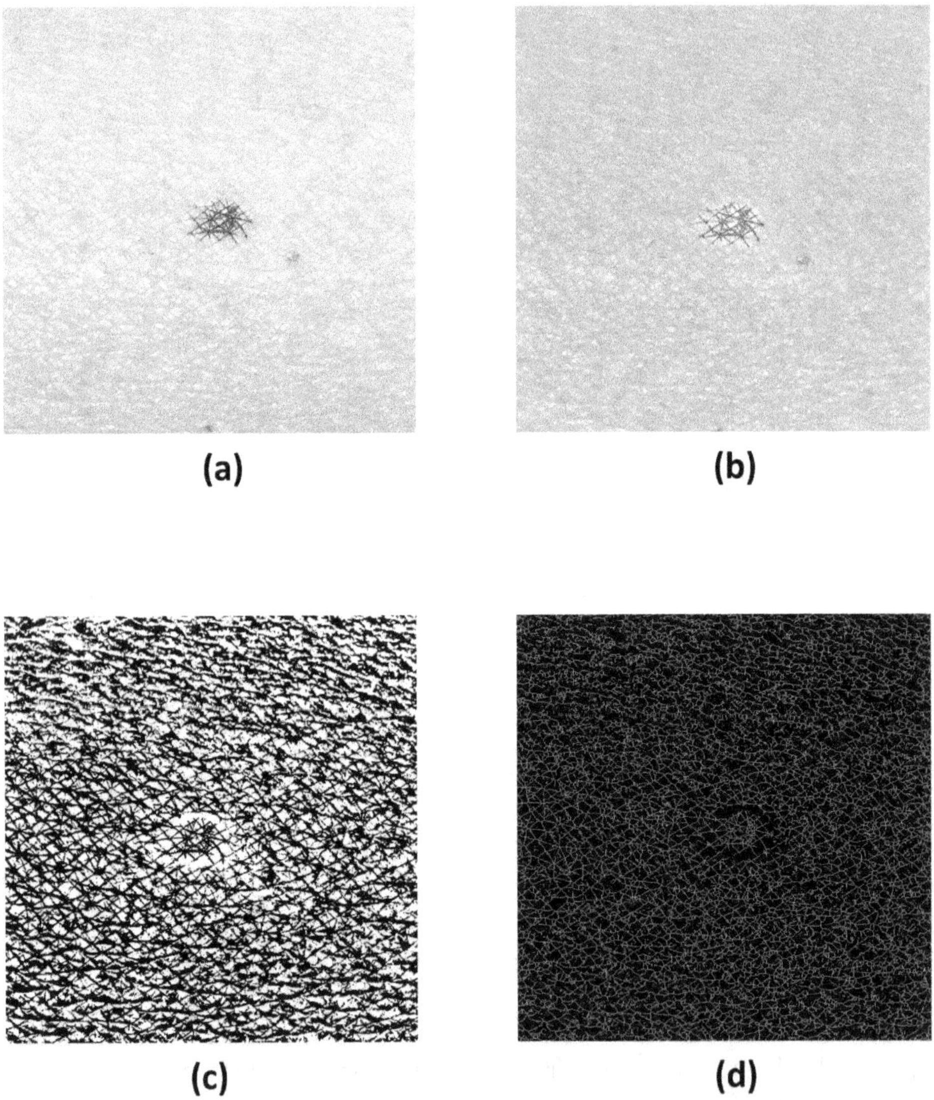

Figure 2: (a) Image from Figure 1a subjected to a series of image-processing steps to isolate furrows including: (b) flattening and conversion to grayscale, (c) sharpening and contrast adjustment, and (d) inversion and skeletonization.

The mounting of illuminating lights is a key factor in obtaining properly lit images. The very first systems used for this purpose consisted of a flash unit fixed in the hot shoe mount of the camera. Later, more sophisticated flash housing units were developed, placing two light sources on each side of a macro lens. The camera and lighting system shown in Figure 3 is a typical macrophotography flash system manufactured by Nikon. Similar systems are also available through other camera manufacturers, such as Canon. In these systems, polarization paper can be cut-to-size and inserted underneath the front cover of the speed light. A linear polarization filter can also be mounted directly on the lens. In more recent years, a multipurpose system known as the Visia Complexion Analysis (VISIA-CR, Canfield Scientific, Fairfield, NJ) was developed allowing researchers to conduct visible light, polarized light, UV reflectance, and fluorescence reflectance photography (www.canfieldsci.com). These other modes of photographic investigation and the multi-spectral multi-modal facial imaging system are described in the sections below.

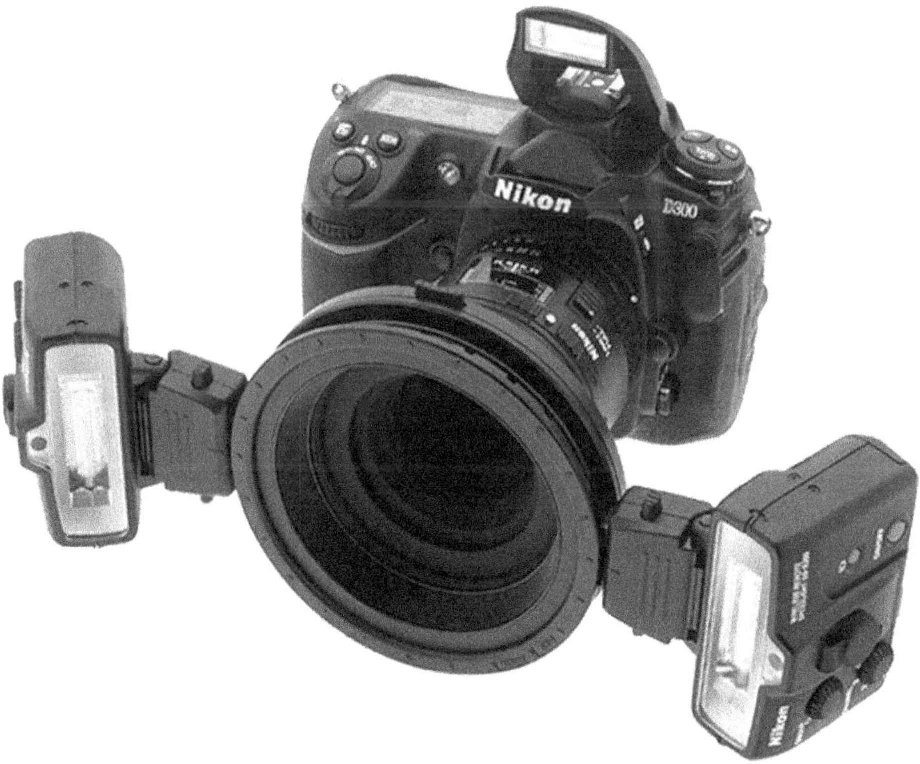

Figure 3: Photograph of a Nikon DLSR (Model D300), which contains the Nikon R1 Wireless Close-Up Macro Speedlight Flash System.

b. Imaging Techniques with Skin Replicas

Skin replica techniques are among the oldest of the trade.[7] They are relatively quick procedures that are easy to carry out, and they provide very useful information about the surface structure of the skin. To a large extent, innovative instruments capable of noninvasive (noncontact) three-dimensional imaging have captured the spotlight and in many cases have become the preferred method of topographical analysis of skin. However, these instruments are often very costly and not available to most laboratories. Thus, researchers still find utility for replicas in the analysis of skin topography.[8,9] Skin replicas can capture topographic features such as deep wrinkles, furrows, pores, and, even, droplets of sweat beads.[10,11] Utilizing digital imaging techniques, replicas may be imaged and, subsequently, analyzed with image analysis software.

The most common skin replica experiments are carried out using a dental impression material made of vinyl polysiloxane (Silflo, Flexico Developments Ltd., Potters Bar, UK) in combination with a solvent thinner and catalyst. These materials are available through CuDerm Corporation (Dallas, TX; www.cuderm.com) and are used in conjunction with a replica locator. Silflo is mixed with catalyst, usually 1 mL of the impression material with 1 drop of catalyst, and then poured into a replica locator, which is placed at the site of interest on the skin. The ensuing polymerization reaction results in a paste that hardens with time.

Historically, replicas were analyzed by taking a photograph with a film-based SLR camera or by conducting profilometry. It should be noted that the obtained replica is a negative impression of the skin surface. However, in many cases researchers take an additional step and create a positive impression of the mold. In the case of contact or laser profilometry, one can generate a three-dimensional image of the surface. Contact profilometry generates a topographic map of the surface by rastering a stylus on the positive impression.[12,13] Laser profilometry, on the other hand, operates on the principle of laser triangulation, does not require contact with the sample, and generates a three-dimensional image of the replica by performing vertical (z-axis) measurements of the height while scanning in the lateral directions (x- and y-axes).[14] Depending on the desired level of magnification, scanning electron microscopy could also be used to capture surface details of replicas.[15,16] Nowadays, most groups perform the analysis on the negative impression rather than going through the additional step of generating a positive impression. In part, this is due to advances in image-processing techniques, which allow for the inversion of the negative impression image.

With the most common analysis, a digital image of the replica may be obtained by mounting a digital SLR camera (containing a macro lens) above the sample. A typical setup would include a macro copy stand that includes a camera mount and, in some cases, illumination lights (see Figure 4). If illumination lights are not provided with the system a remote flash system can be used with the camera (Nikon and Canon provide macro flash units that serve this purpose fine). Fiber optic illuminators are also often employed. Regardless of the light source, the replica must be illuminated with oblique light at an optimal grazing angle of 25°. Another alternative for imaging the replica is to use a flatbed scanner. This technology allows high resolutions to be obtained and provides greater depth of field imaging than that available with a standard macro lens used in combination with a DSLR camera.

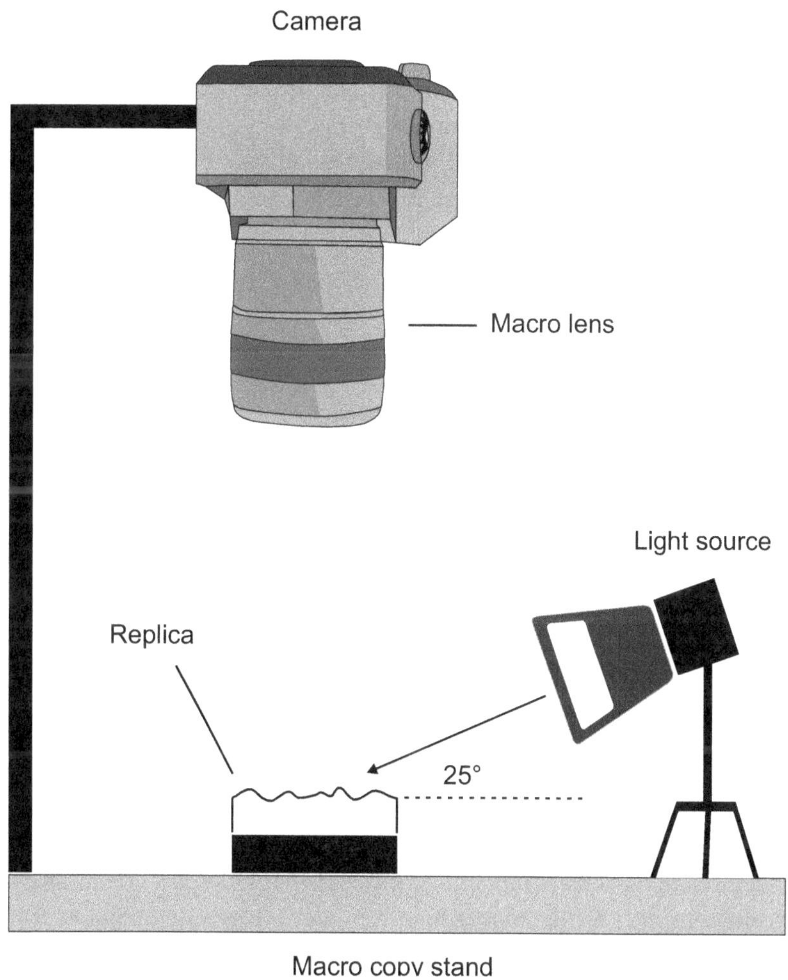

Figure 4: Illustration of a macro copy stand that includes a camera, macro lens, and illumination source to provide oblique lighting of a skin replica.

Skin replicas are usually analyzed to determine the degree of roughness and density of wrinkling of the skin. It has been most successfully used to measure photo-damaged skin and premature aging of skin subjected to tobacco smoke.[9,10] A typical replica analysis would be carried out on the perioribital region adjacent to the eye. From the generated image one may perform optical profilometry in which the light intensity of the furrows is measured. Important parameters include the average depth of the furrow, variance between the altitude of the highest peak and lowest peak of the furrows, and the density of furrows.[9]

Skin replica analysis can also be extended to other phenomena in skin, such as monitoring sudoriferous behavior. As an example, Figure 5 contains a skin replica image (obtained with a flatbed scanner) of the volar forearm of an individual exposed to a high-temperature environment (45°C) for 30 min to induce sweating. Small protruding beads of sweat on the surface of the skin result in dark areas in the image, which can be isolated and quantified using several image-processing and analysis techniques. In this way, the number of active sweat glands per given area can be quantified.

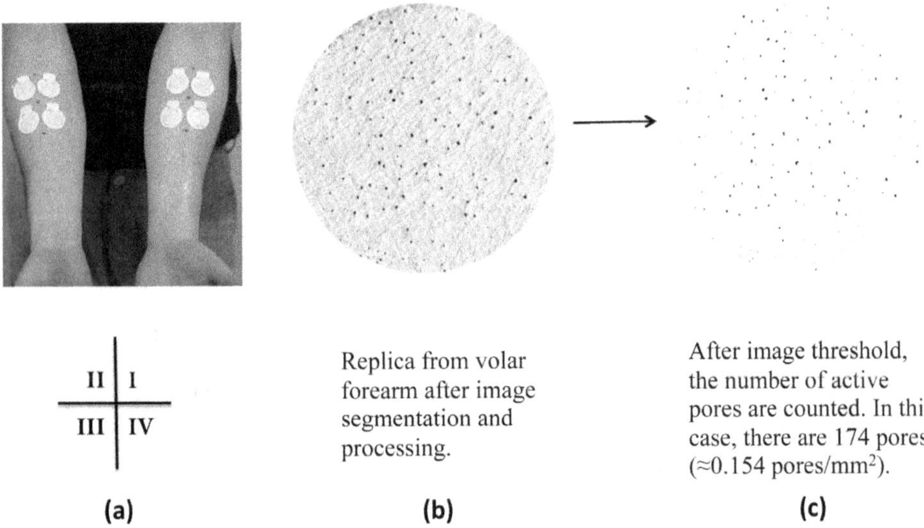

Figure 5: (a) Photograph of the volar forearms of a subject containing replica rings arranged in a four-quadrant layout. (b) Digital image of a cast from the volar forearm region along with (c) its image-processed counterpart containing isolated sweat profusions on a white background (counted). Reprinted from McMullen et al. with permission from the Society of Cosmetic Chemists, © 2013.[17]

c. Fringe Projection Methods to Measure Skin Topography

In addition to replica methods and photography, **skin topography** is also frequently measured using **fringe projection** methods. As shown in Figure 6, a digital projector is employed to project a phase-shifting fringe pattern on an object of interest.

Meanwhile, an image of the fringe pattern on the three-dimensional object is obtained with a camera. Due to surface topography, the fringe pattern is deformed and can be analyzed by a computer algorithm allowing for the generation of a three-dimensional image. For evaluating the surface features of skin the two most popular commercially available instruments are the PRIMOS® (GFMesstechnik GmbH, Teltow, Germany) and DermaTOP® (EOTECH SA, Marcoussis, France) systems.[19] The principal difference between the two instruments is the manner in which the fringe patterns are produced. In the PRIMOS® system, fringe patterns are generated with micro-mirrors while the DermaTOP® system utilizes a template to generate the shadows.[18,20] Optimally, the DermaTOP® FOV HE-25 system performs a measurement on a 20 × 15 mm^2 field of view with 2 μm vertical resolution, 15 μm lateral resolution, and 1 s acquisition time. On the other hand, the PRIMOS® premium system gathers data from a 24 × 14 mm^2 field of view with 2.4 μm vertical resolution, 24 μm lateral resolution, and 70 ms acquisition time.[21] The reader should note that these specifications are only for two specific models. It should be mentioned that each company has a series of instruments with various specifications.

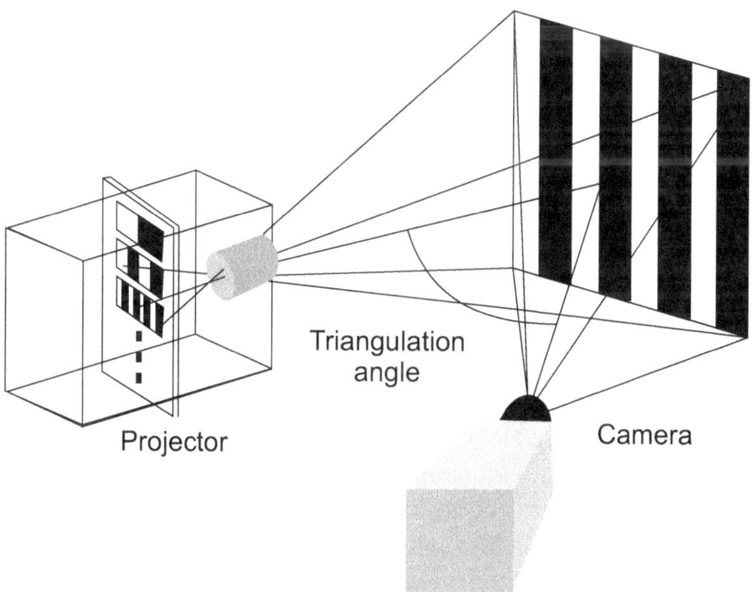

Figure 6: Schematic of a fringe projection (interferometry) profilometer. Reproduced from Lagarde et al. with permission by John Wiley & Sons, © 2002.[18]

Fringe projection techniques are used to measure skin topography directly *in vivo* and also *in vitro* using skin replicas. Skin topography, also referred to as skin relief or texture, is an important feature of the skin that reveals its state of health. Most studies focus on measuring skin roughness and other topographical features, such as wrinkles and furrows.[22] In addition, these techniques may be also utilized to monitor the skin's health state as associated with lesion malignancy, laser remodeling, radiation treatment, treatment with cosmetic products, and hydration state of the skin.[21] For illustration, Figure 7 demonstrates the use of the DermaTOP® system to monitor the difference between the temple skin (periorbital region obtained with a replica technique) of two subjects, one 73 years old and the other 23 years old. The deep furrow in the middle of the three-dimensional plot can clearly be discerned in the elderly subject (septuagenarian). On the other hand, in the vicenarian (23-year-old) pores are the dominant feature as there are no discernible deep wrinkles or furrows.

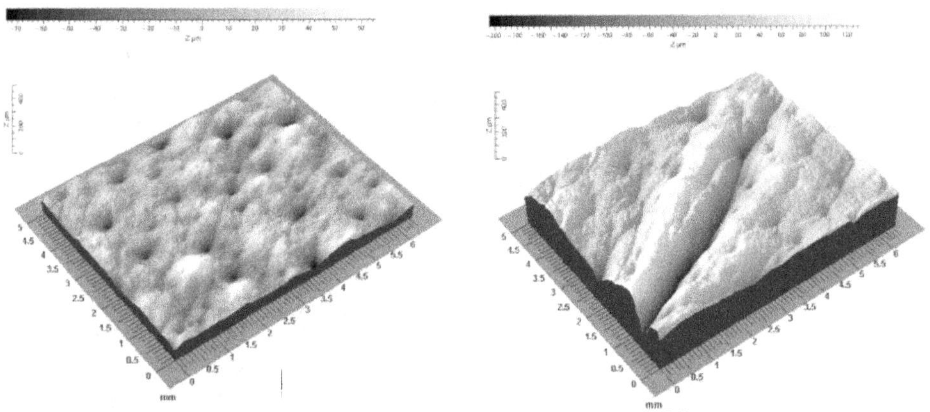

Figure 7: Three-dimensional image of the temple (periorbital region) of (a) a 23-year-old and (b) 73-year-old subject. Reprinted from Lagarde et al. with permission from John Wiley & Sons, © 2005.[22]

For further illustration, Figure 8 contains three-dimensional representations (in two-dimensions) of the furrow distribution in the volar forearm region of both subjects (also of a skin replica), along with image analysis markings to quantify the anisotropy of the furrows (i.e., the quantity of furrows oriented in different directions). In the vicenarian subject, it is clear that the furrows form a crosshatched structure where the level of isotropy is high while in the septuagenarian subject the orientation of the furrows is more anisotropic. Findings from these studies can be summarized as follows. Roughness, peak-trough amplitude, and anisotropy of the furrows decrease with age. The density of the furrows, on the other hand, decreases with age.[22] Other important skin surface parameters that can be measured with fringe projection devices include the maximum roughness (R_m), the mean roughness (R_a), mean depth of roughness (R_z), and waviness (W_t).[23] Overall, these techniques are being employed by many different laboratories around the world as newer, more portable devices are becoming available.

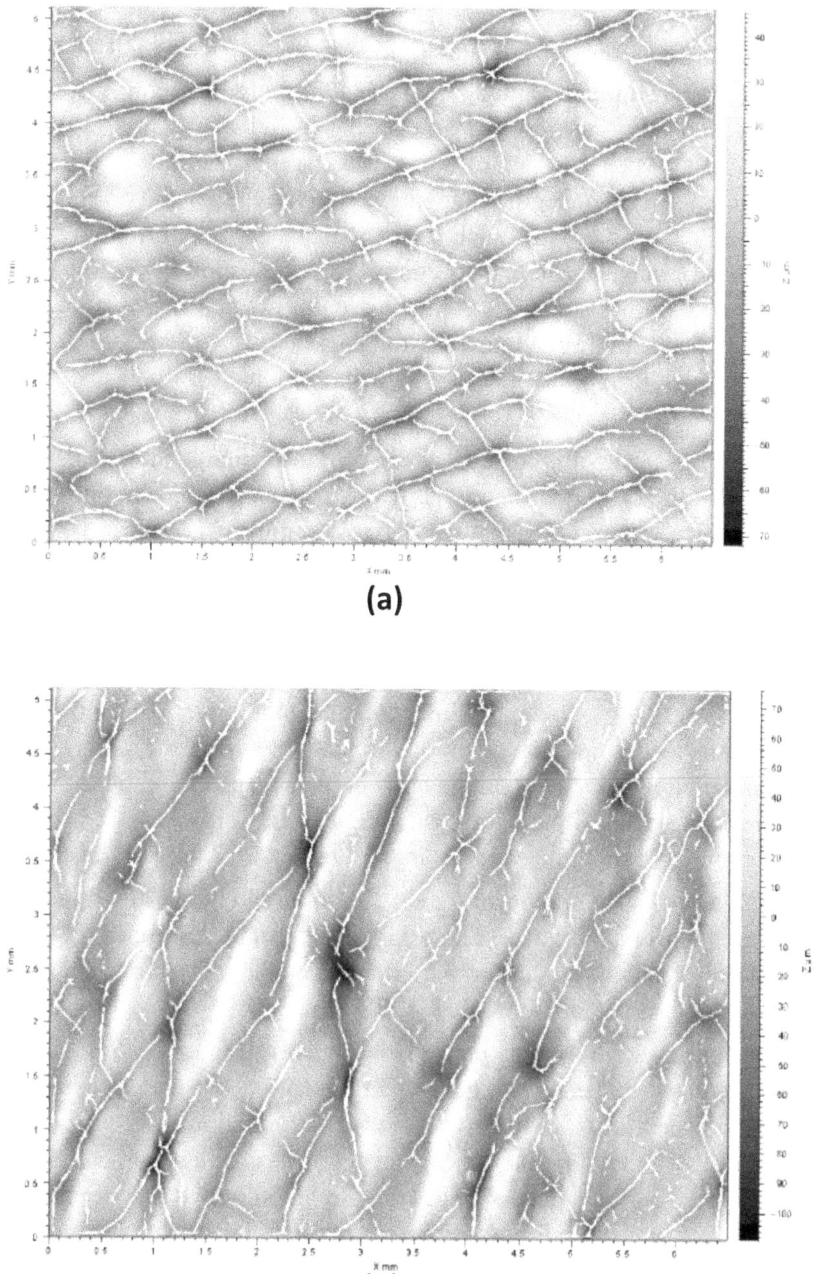

Figure 8: Two-dimension representation of a three-dimensional image of the volar forearm of (a) a 23-year-old and (b) 73-year-old subject. Furrow markings generated by an image analysis package are shown. Reprinted from Lagarde et al. with permission from John Wiley & Sons, © 2005.[22]

d. Pore Measurements

Over the last decade, increasing attention has been given to the topic of skin pores—also often referred to as facial pores. In this case, the term "pore" evolved from the lay population to describe an opening in the skin associated with a pilosebaceous unit, which consists of the sebaceous gland and hair follicle. These "pores" are clearly evident to the human eye and are especially visible in certain anatomical regions of the body, such as the face, where they often present themselves in areas adjacent to the nasal region. Such pores are generally associated with excessive sebum production.[24] In most cultures, the visible appearance of these pores is undesirable for many individuals, and for this reason, there have been considerable efforts in recent years by the personal care industry to develop products that reduce pore size.

Not to be confused with pilosebaceous pores, sudoriferous pores also open up at the surface of the skin. Eccrine glands secrete a clear isotonic solution of sweat on the skin's surface to provide an evaporative cooling apparatus for the body. The gland is connected to the surface of the skin by means of the eccrine duct—a long tubular structure. These pores are located on the top of furrow ridges in skin and are not visible by the naked eye. On the other hand, facial pores associated with pilosebaceous units are generally much larger. They can be classified into three different types: visible skin pores (0.1–0.6 mm^2), enlarged skin pores (0.3–0.6 mm^2), and blackhead embedded pores (tonality is lower than the rest of the skin surface).[25] It should be noted, however, that there is not a universal agreement on the classification of pores. There are also such classifications as invisible pores (< 0.04 mm^2), visible pores (0.04–0.07 mm^2), and enlarged pores (> 0.07 mm^2).[26]

Surprisingly, there has not been a great deal of research investigating the nature of facial pores until recent years. The origin and formation of pores is dependent upon a variety of factors including hereditary factors, seborrhea, acne, comedogenic xenobiotics, aging, and chronic UV light exposure.[27]

Recent studies suggest that pore size is greatly influenced by gender and sebaceous activity—males tend to have greater quantities of pores, possibly due to greater androgen activity.[25] In females there is no correlation linking age with pore size or quantity. On the other hand, while acne-prone skin tends to contain greater quantities of pores, there appears to be no correlation between severities of acne and pores.[25] From a different perspective, treatments intended to reduce the size of facial pores are primarily concentrated in the dermatological arena and include topical retinoid therapy, chemical peeling, and laser therapy.

Quantitative Assessment of Pore Size and Quantity

Assessment of pore size and quantity may be achieved utilizing several different imaging techniques. The most basic of these include visual grading, macrophotography, and evaluation of silicone replicas. Visual grading may be completed in the presence of a panelist or utilizing a photograph. In most cases, it is imperative to correlate visual grading to one of our quantitative techniques. Macrophotography is a rapid, noninvasive strategy for quantifying pores; however, it is very difficult to obtain reproducible results due to challenges with illumination conditions. Nevertheless, utilizing a carefully controlled facial positioning and lighting system, one may accurately count the number of pores and their size. These can be estimated from the area measurements of two-dimensional photographs. Figure 9 contains a photograph obtained with an optical image analyzer called Facial Stage (Facial Stage DM3, Moritex Saitama, Japan). The original photograph and its image-processed counterpart are shown in the figure. The yellow circles in Figure 9c, the enlarged processed image, are representative of facial pores.

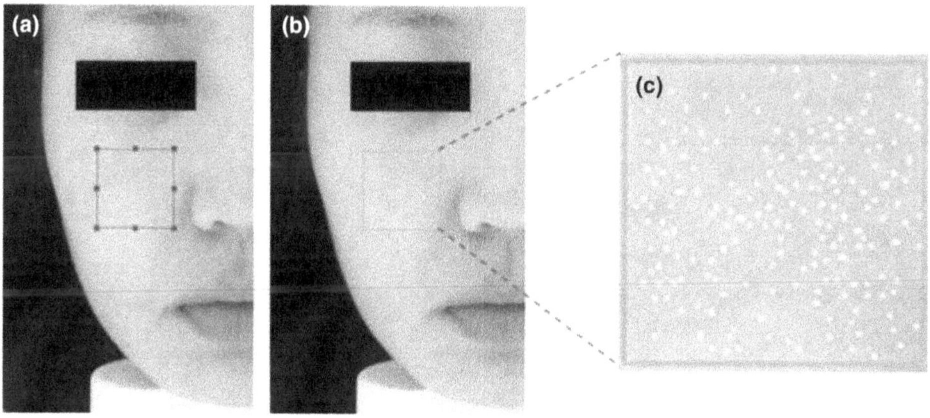

Figure 9: Image of visible skin pores obtained with the Facial Stage optical image analyzer illustrating (a) the origal image, (b) processed image, and (c) enlarged region of the selection in (b). Reprinted from Kim et al. with permission of John Wiley & Sons, © 2014.[26]

As already mentioned, silicone replicas are also a useful and inexpensive modality for quantifying pores, although special care must be taken to ensure extremely precise quantities of the silicone resin are combined with the hardening catalyst. Since this is a kinetic reaction, timing is of the utmost importance. Differences in the thickness or flow properties of the silicone-catalyst mixture during application to the skin will affect the polymer's ability to penetrate deep into the pore. To reiterate, silicone replicas can be evaluated by generating macrophotographic images in the presence of oblique light. Alternatively, one may utilize a flatbed scanner to generate the digital images. Our laboratory's experience is that both techniques work equally well.

Fringe projection techniques that generate three-dimensional images of the skin surface topography are also used for quantifying pores and provide an estimate of pore volume. An example of skin pore measurement with this technique is provided in Figure 10 utilizing the PRIMOS® premium system. Studies of pore volume with this instrument demonstrated very good correlation with visual grading by trained panelists, illustrating the contribution of pore volume to the overall appearance of facial pores.[26] Stereoimaging with an optical topometer is also a viable route for quantifying pores.[28]

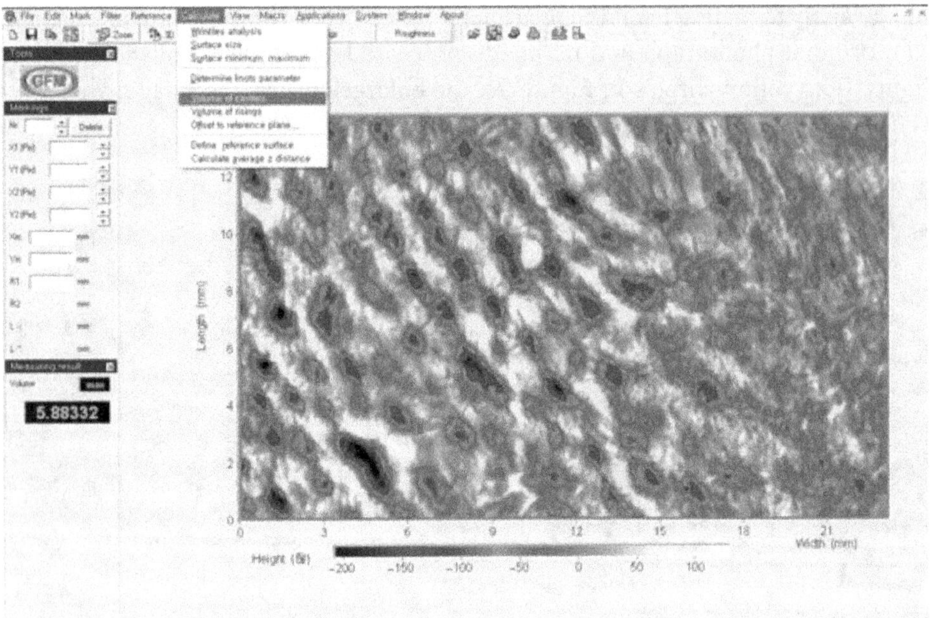

Figure 10: Analysis of pore volume with the PRIMOS premium system. Reprinted from Kim et al. with permission from John Wiley & Sons, © 2014.[26]

Confocal laser scanning microscopy may also be used to investigate the dimensions of pores.[29] While this technique is extremely valuable for investigating the anatomy of the pore, it is not the instrument of choice for quantifying attributes of large numbers of pores due to its limited imaging area. Nevertheless, pertinent information relating the fine morphological structure of skin with pores is invaluable and may provide avenues for future research focused on the reduction of pore size.

e. Skin Thermography

The ability to measure the temperature distribution and changes in skin is extremely useful not only from a practical point of view, but also for a more profound understanding of processes occurring within the skin. Skin thermography, or digital infrared imaging, affords the researcher such an avenue to explore various phenomena involving the state of health of the skin. Infrared cameras are designed to measure infrared radiation in the short- to mid-wave (3–5 μm) and long-wave (7–14 μm) regions of the electromagnetic spectrum. These devices essentially measure the emitted energy of the sample. Kirchoff's law provides us with a general relationship between emitted (E), transmitted (T), and reflected (R) energy:

$$E+T+R=1 \quad (1)$$

In many circumstances, the transmitted energy is close to zero and E+R=1. In general, objects that are good emitters are poor reflectors and good reflectors are poor emitters. Not surprisingly, E=1 in the case of a black body—something that absorbs all incident electromagnetic radiation—while most objects in nature result in E<1. In the case of skin, it is both a good absorber of energy and also a good emitter, where E=0.98. In contrast, aluminum foil is a good reflector (R=0.98), but a poor emitter (E=0.02). Nevertheless, skin is a very good object for conducting thermography measurements.

The use of infrared thermography in the medical field has expanded significantly in recent years due to the increasing availability of infrared cameras. Such studies provide data related to inflammatory conditions (injuries, infections, etc.) as well as vascular activity (angiogenesis, varices, etc.). Typically, infrared images, or thermograms, of skin represent thermal energy emission stemming from the outermost portion of the epidermis down to the dermis, roughly 5 mm deep.

In the personal care arena, there are also various applications of infrared thermography. For example, it can be utilized to monitor skin surface temperature when conducting antiperspirant efficacy studies. In a study described in the literature, subjects were first acclimatized in an environmentally controlled room at 28°C and 40% RH for 30 min, and then placed in a sauna at 45°C and 30% RH for an additional 60 min.[17] During the test, axillae sweating and eccrine sweat pore activity was monitored by gravimetric analysis and a skin replica technique; however, infrared thermography was utilized to monitor the overall anatomical temperature distribution of each subject. Figure 11 contains a series of images obtained for one of the subjects upon entry into the environmental room, then after 30 min in the room, followed by a period of time spent in the sauna chamber. In Figure 11a, the overall surface temperature of the skin is lower than in Figures 11B–11D. This phenomenon occurred because the subject was acclimatized in an office for several hours beforehand at a much lower temperature than in the environmental room. After 30 min in the environmental room (Figure 11B), the surface temperature of the subject begins to increase, especially in the rostral (facial) region and the superior torso. After 10 min in the sauna (Figure 11C), the peak temperature is reached at the rostral region, superior torso, and lower limbs. The subject begins to sweat profusely after 10 min in the sauna, resulting in an overall cooling effect over all surfaces of the integument as shown in Figure 11D. Subsequent images were obtained at 30, 40, and 50 min, which demonstrated similar behavior as that observed at 20 min. In summary, these data demonstrate that the 30-min acclimatization in the environmental room followed by the first 10 min in the sauna chamber is sufficient to bring the subject to a state of profuse sweating, which can be monitored from that point onward by other tests, such as gravimetric analysis and skin replica techniques.

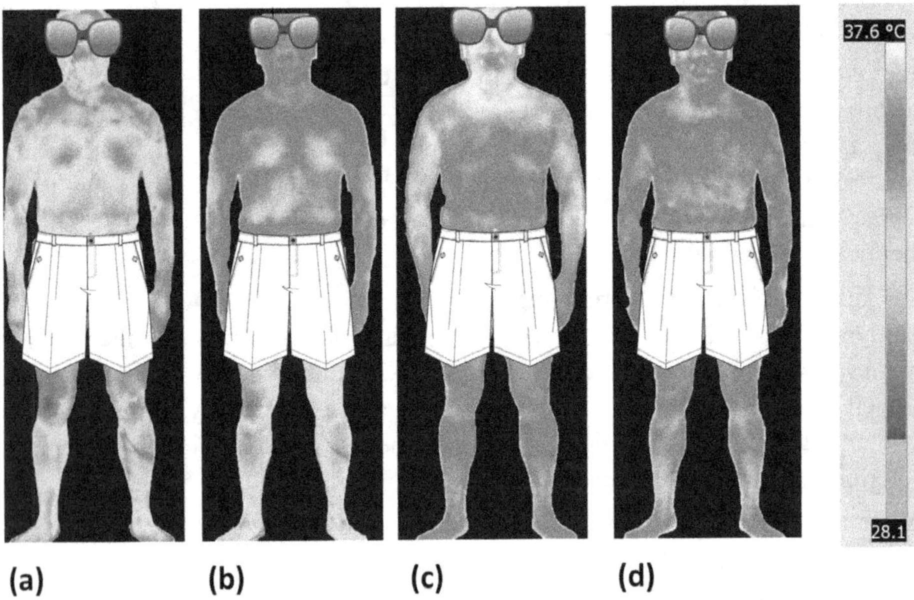

Figure 11: Infrared thermograms of a subject undergoing antiperspirant studies. Images were obtained to monitor the global temperature distribution of the subject during the test. Images were collected upon (a) entry into the environmental room, (b) after 30 min acclimatization in the environmental room, and after (c) 10 min and (d) 20 min in the sauna. The scale for all of the images is provided on the right and ranges from 28.1°C to 37.6°C. Precise measurements of temperature can be made at every pixel in the image. Reprinted from McMullen et al. with permission from the Society of Cosmetic Chemists, © 2013.[17]

Infrared thermography may also be used to monitor the skin's response to environmental stress, such as exposure to hot and cold temperatures. For example, one may wish to investigate the use of an active ingredient to mitigate the skin's response to stress. To carry out such an experiment, one would treat skin with an active ingredient-containing vehicle in the form of a cream at a dose of 2 mg/cm^2 to the inner forearm of subjects twice per day. After 3 weeks, baseline readings should be obtained and subjects could be subjected to stress first with a heating pad for 10 min followed by cold pad stress for 10 min (see Figure 12). After application of stressors, thermograms may be obtained every 2–3 minutes for 1 hour. Figure 13 contains an example of a baseline reading and one obtained after exposure to both hot and cold stresses. Since there may be some temperature gradient due to vascularity, care must be taken to obtain temperature readings from selected regions of the images.

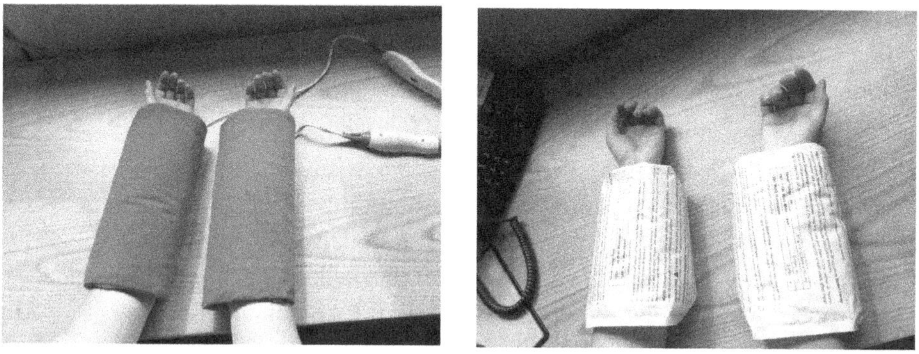

(a) (b)

Figure 12: Application of (a) hot and (b) cold pads used to induced stress in skin.

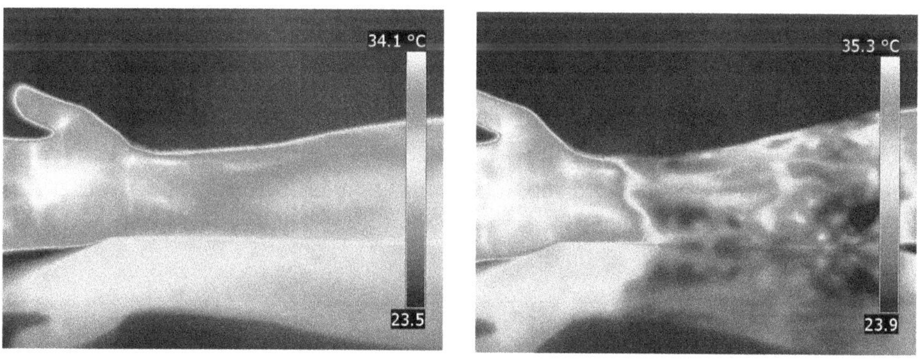

(a) (b)

Figure 13: Infrared thermograms of the volar forearm comparing (a) a baseline reading versus (b) the arm after it had undergone a hot and cold stress cycle. Images kindly provided by Mihaela Gorcea, Ashland, Inc.

f. Ultraviolet (UV) Reflectance Photography

Skin pigmentary disorders, such as melasma, vitiligo, and hypopigmentation, as well as disorders resulting from photo-damage, are commonly detected with **UV light photography**.[30] This mode of photography is based on the photo-physical properties of melanin, which absorbs much greater in the UV region of the electromagnetic spectrum than the visible region. Therefore, pigmented and depigmented lesions are more discernible than they would be using visible light photography.[31] In fact, the use of UV light photography in dermatology has been in practice for many years. Using Wood's lamp, which provides broad UVA spectral output with a maximum at 365 nm, dermatologists have been diagnosing pigmentary disorders since the early part of the twentieth century.[32,33] This technique is especially useful for monitoring photo-damage or melasma in subjects with Fitzpatrick Skin Types I–III in the case of hyperpigmentation. On the other hand, it readily views hypopigmentation disorders, such as vitiligo, in subjects with Fitzpatrick Skin Types V and VI.

In general, UV photography is conducted with the same type of cameras employed for light photography with some modifications. In order to carry out such experiments, one should employ a camera that is sensitive to UV light. In film photography, high-speed (e.g., ISO 1600) black-and-white film is used due its enhanced sensitivity to the otherwise weak UV signal, and because color film contains a UV-absorbing protective coating. At present, most digital SLRs can be modified so that the CCD or CMOS sensor is sensitive to UV light. Digital SLRs contain a UV and IR filter pack that only allows visible light to reach the sensor. This can be removed by a specialty camera shop and replaced by a UV transmitting filter in front of the sensor (providing a dedicated UV camera) or over the lens.[34] Lenses that are able to transmit UV light are readily available, and most macro lenses (made of fluorite and quartz glass) that are used for dermatological photography are suitable for this purpose. Finally, xenon flashes are a good source of UV light as long as the flash diffusers are removed from the flashes (these attenuate UV light) and replaced with UV pass filters.[31] The strategic positioning of several flashes around the subject's face is key to obtaining proper illumination conditions.

By definition, UV photography infers that one is working in the spectral range of 300–400 nm. However, in dermatology the combination of UV and fluorescence photography are often carried out in conjunction with each other. In this case, UV (300–400 nm) and visible (due to fluorescence) light is captured in the final image. In any event, UV images of skin provide a sensitive technique for the localization of melanin.

g. Fluorescence Reflectance Photography

Based on similar principles as UV reflectance photography, fluorescence reflectance photography refers to photographic images that are generated by illuminating the skin with UV light (either broad band 300–400 nm or a narrower band in this range) and then capturing an image in the visible region of the electromagnetic spectrum. In this modality, incoming UV light is absorbed by chromophores, which then fluoresce at longer wavelengths. This type of photography was pioneered at Massachusetts General Hospital by Nik Kollias and colleagues in the mid-1990s to evaluate acne as well as hyperpigmentation in photo-damaged skin.[31,35] In their experiments, chromophores were excited in skin by placing a UV band pass and an IR block filter over the illuminating flashes, allowing only a broad band of UVA light (340–380 nm) to reach the skin's surface. As shown in the diagram in Figure 14, the reflected light from skin passes through a UV block filter before arriving to the sensor (or film) in the camera. In this way, we only view visible light resulting from skin fluorescence.

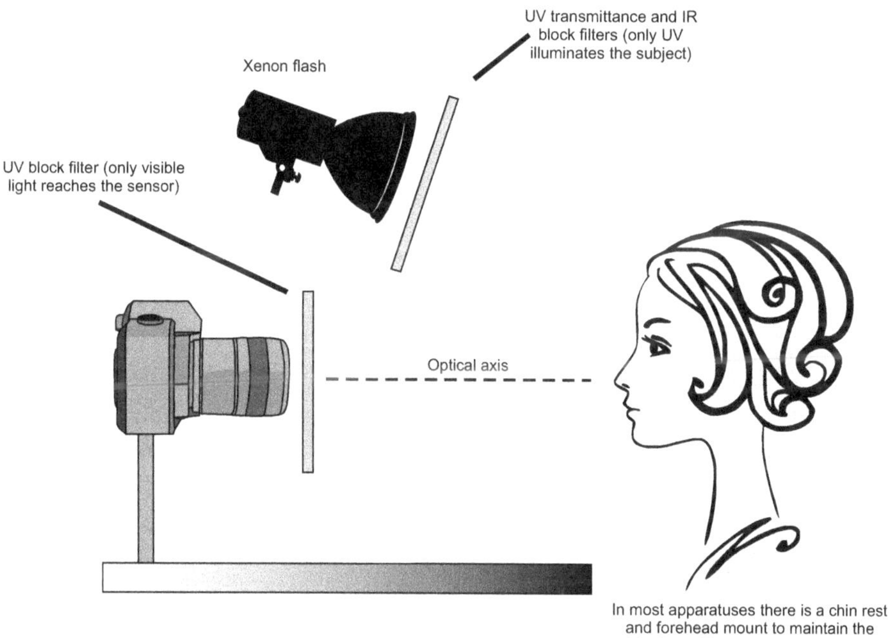

Figure 14: Diagram of a typical apparatus used for conducting fluorescence reflectance photography.

The illuminating UVA light, centered at about 365 nm, results in absorption of light by melanin (dark in the image) as well as by collagen, which results in fluorescence at 420 nm due to collagen cross-links in skin. In the acquired image, fluorescence due to collagen appears bright, while dark is representative of the presence of melanin. In the evaluation of acne vulgaris, fluorescence occurs due to protoporphyrin IX produced by *Propionibacterium acnes* in open comedones, follicles, and inflammatory lesions.[35]

h. Multi-Spectral Multi-Modal Facial Imaging

Within the last two decades, sophisticated imaging systems have been developed to collect **clinical** (standard white light), **cross-polarized** (diffuse reflectance), **porphyrin fluorescence**, **horn fluorescence**, **collagen fluorescence**, and **excitation light images**.[36] One of the most commonly used imaging systems in dermatological and cosmetic research to capture such images is the VISIA-CR system manufactured by Canfield Scientific (Fairfield, NJ). Utilizing a professional DSLR camera in combination with xenon strobe lights and various filters, images are obtained and then processed with image-processing and analysis software.

Figure 15 contains various images collected with the VISIA-CR system. The standard white light image can be used to analyze furrows, wrinkles, and other topographical and surface textural features of the skin. The diffuse reflectance image, obtained with crossed-polarizers, provides information about backscattered light. This is light that enters the skin, becomes scattered and depolarized, and then exits the skin. Before exiting the skin, the light interacts with skin's internal structures, such as melanin, collagen, hemoglobin, and carotenoids. Diffuse reflectance images provide us with information related to skin pigmentation, erythema, infiltrates, and blood vessels.[4] In fact, the use of cross-polarization photography has been applied to study erythematic inflammatory lesions in acne vulgaris.[3] It should be noted, however, that erythema is observed with much more facility in fair-skinned individuals (Fitzpatrick Types I and II) than those with a darker complexion.

A key feature of the VISIA-CR and related technologies is the capability to resolve fluorescent images resulting from fluorescence of important biochemical components in skin in an automated fashion. Fluorescent photography has been used extensively in the evaluation of acne vulgaris. Table 1 identifies the various filters that are used in the VISIA-CR system to obtain fluorescence images corresponding to specific biochemical features in the image.

Table 1. Excitation and band pass filters in the VISIA-CR system allowing for the visualization of various features in skin.

	Excitation filter	Captured emission image
Porphyrin	405 nm ± 10 nm	Long pass filter (≥ 620 nm)
Horn	405 nm ± 10 nm	Band pass filter (540 nm ± 40 nm)
Collagen	405 nm ± 10 nm	Band pass filter (450 nm ± 40 nm)

As stated in the previous section, porphyrin fluorescence corresponds to protoporphyrin IX produced by the bacteria *Propionibacterium acnes*, which is present in acne vulgaris–afflicted skin. The porphyrin image is red (see Figure 15d) and the brighter orange-red fluorescence, especially noticeable around the nasal region, is attributed to protoporphyrin IX. Cutaneous horn is an outward growth on the skin surface that is characterized by its keratin content and its similarity to hard keratin structures, such as nails. It is typically observed in patients with acne vulgaris and also in other individuals in areas of the skin typically exposed to the sun, such as the back of the hands and the face. Due to the presence of keratin in horn, excitation at 405 nm results in green fluorescence emission that is captured at a band centered at 540 nm. The green fluorescence image is shown in Figure 15e, with the darkest shades of green in the image corresponding to horn. In the current case, these are observed in the cheek region of an acne vulgaris–afflicted patient in the form of small acne lesions. Collagen fluorescence images obtained with the VISIA-CR have a blue tone due to emission centered at 450 nm. Collagen cross-links are believed to be the source of the fluorescence, although there is some debate in the literature that additional photo-physical studies of collagen are required to better understand its fluorescence.[37] Nevertheless, in dermatological fluorescence photography this phenomenon can be used as an indicator of the skin health state. For example, in acne vulgaris patients, the development of acne lesions can lead to areas where collagen growth is disrupted. In the image in Figure 15f, darker shades of blue in the image correspond to damaged collagen. Likewise, it is well known that photo-damage results in lower fluorescence intensity of collagen cross-links in skin.[38]

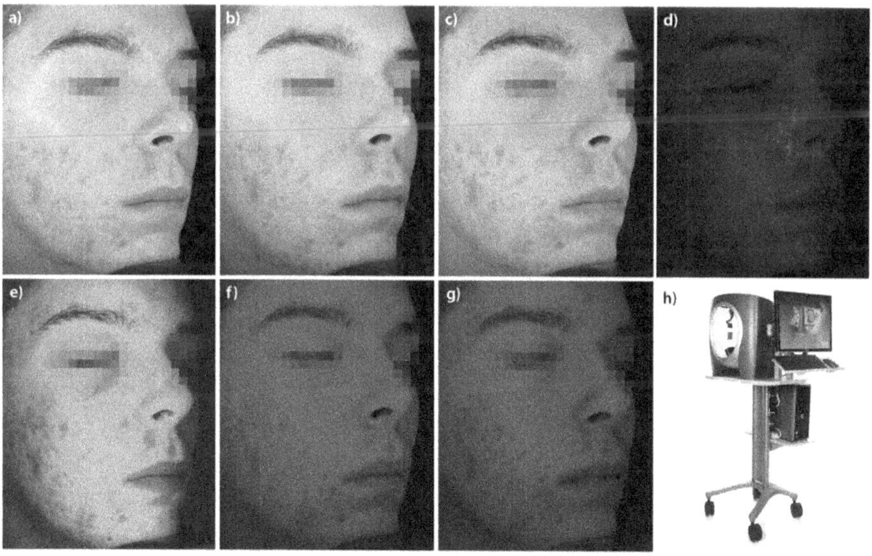

Figure 15: Facial images of an acne vulgaris patient generated with the VISIA-CR multi-spectral multi-modal facial imaging system: (a) standard white light image (clinical photograph), (b) standard white flat-lit image (analysis image), (c) cross-polarized image (diffuse reflectance image), (d) porphyrin fluorescence image, (e) horn fluorescence image, (f) collagen fluorescence image, (g) excitation image, and (h) VISIA-CR imaging system. Images kindly provided by Canfield Scientific (Fairfield, NJ).

i. Photographic Analysis of Lips

Imaging techniques are frequently used to evaluate lips; often examining the efficacy of active ingredients or the cosmetic properties of lip products. Often, the evaluation of lipsticks is the first product assessment to come to mind. Typically, product developers are interested in obtaining a quantitative measure of the **color**, **gloss**, **covering power**, **long-lasting effects**, and **streakiness**.[39,40] Traditional color measurements of lips are carried out by reflectance spectrophotometry in the visible region of the electromagnetic spectrum or by reflectance stimulus colorimetry. While these methods are accurate assessments of the lips' color, they are hindered by the small sampling area—generally on the order of mm^2 to cm^2—and because they require contact with the substrate.

Photographic image analysis, on the other hand, allows noninvasive evaluation of the products on the lips and the ability to analyze larger areas. A major challenge with utilizing imaging techniques for the lips is the ability to carefully control lighting conditions and the positioning of the subject. For lipstick and makeup applications, one should utilize a lighting control system that corresponds to daylight (e.g., CIE Illuminant D65) and a suitable table mount for the subject to position the face, such as an opthalmic table (similar to the assembly in Figure 14).[39,41] In any event, reproducibly positioning the subject's facial region is especially challenging as contours, anatomical features, and even changes in facial expressions can affect the way light interacts with the skin surface. Researchers must also decide other factors associated with light sources, such as the use of polarized light to enhance specular reflection or soft light to visualize diffuse reflection. During the course of a day, the consumer can experience of variety of lighting conditions. On a sunny day, direct sunlight causes strong highlights and shadows, corresponding to adjacent specular and diffuse regions on the lips. In contrast, an overcast sky produces more even illumination and a more even tone. Indoors, lighting may also present a variety of situations depending on the light source and if diffusers (commonly found in office environments) are placed in front of or below the light source.

The actual determination of color by image analysis is another unique challenge in which careful calibration procedures must be employed. One study conducted with lipsticks demonstrated the utility of photographically generated images to yield color values in line with that obtained with well-established spectrophotometric and colorimetric techniques.[39] However, this requires a color extraction procedure by applying algorithms to the R, G, and B values obtained from the digital photographs.

j. Hyperpigmentation Measurements of Skin

The development of age spots, hyperpigmentation, and melasma are all forms of melanogenesis. A great deal of research has been completed in this area as many institutions strive to design ingredients that lighten skin. This is especially true for the Asian market where much of the population suffers from the development of age spots. Age spots develop in the facial region and can be quantified by digital photography in combination with image analysis. Such measurements require reproducible lighting and positioning systems so that serial measurements can be conducted in order to follow the effects of a given treatment regimen. The ultraviolet reflectance photography and multi-spectral multi-modal facial imaging techniques described in the sections above can be employed to quantify hyperpigmentation. Quantifying age spots can be quite challenging and for this reason there is considerable interest in developing reproducible methods to measure spots on the face.[42]

k. Imaging of Cellulite

Cellulite has a high rate of occurrence and is usually found in the buttocks and thigh regions of females. It has a number of medical descriptors—including adiposis edematosa and orange peel syndrome—and is caused by protrusions of fat into the dermis. The formation of cellulite results in a very uneven disposition of the skin surface, which can be captured by generating topographic maps of the surface utilizing fringe projection techniques.[43] Photographic imaging is also a reasonable alternative, although special care must be taken to illuminate the buttocks or thigh region reproducibly in all areas. This may be achieved by utilizing a circular illumination system that surrounds the leg and is coupled to a photographic recording device.[44] Insights into the internal structure of cellulite-afflicted skin have been achieved with ultrasonography, magnetic resonance imaging, optical coherence tomography, and reflectance confocal microscopy.[43] Applications of these methods to study various phenomena in skin are discussed in other sections of this chapter.

11.2.2 *IN VIVO* IMAGING OF INTERNAL FEATURES OF THE SKIN

So far, most of our discussion has centered on imaging surface features of skin. There are also many important phenomena that occur below the surface of skin that we may wish to visualize. In recent years, there has been a plethora of published research demonstrating the use of sophisticated instrumentation to gather information about processes occurring in the skin. The most commonly used techniques to carry out such analyses are laser Doppler perfusion, optical coherence tomography, magnetic resonance imaging (MRI), reflectance confocal microscopy, and ultrasonography. All of these techniques are employed to carry out *in vivo* skin measurements to: monitor blood flow in the case of erythema (laser Doppler diffusion); evaluate skin lesions, inflammatory diseases, and parasitic infestations (optical coherence tomography); measure skin thickness and identify skin lesions (ultrasonography); and for the evaluation of the constituents of the stratum corneum, epidermis, dermis (MRI and reflectance confocal microscopy).[45]

Unfortunately, this entire subject is too vast to review in the current text; however, we shall provide some insights into the use of reflectance confocal microscopy and ultrasonography—the most popular techniques—in the evaluation of the health state of the skin.

a. Reflectance Confocal Microscopy

Confocal laser scanning microscopy, also known as reflectance confocal microscopy, allows for the collection of high-resolution optical images. These images are collected at selected depths within the sample by a process known as optical sectioning. The images are gathered *en face* (horizontal rather vertical) as if one were looking down onto the skin from an aerial view. In the case of opaque samples (not allowing the penetration of light), one can generate a three-dimensional surface image of the specimen. For samples that are not opaque in which light is able to pass through them, such as the skin, interior structures may be imaged. The advantage of reflectance confocal microscopy, in contrast to normal light microscopy, is that the depth of focus is controlled and very limited for each lateral optical section. It is a noninvasive technique allowing for *in vivo* measurements, thereby providing information that would normally require histology. The use of reflectance confocal microscopy to study the skin has rapidly expanded in the last two decades, which can be primarily attributed to technological advances in instrument design. It is mostly used for the diagnosis of benign and malignant lesions associated with nonmelanoma and melanoma carcinomas as well as pigmentary disorders.[15,46-51] The methodology offers the researcher an inside view of the skin at the histological level, allowing one to perform examinations at the cellular level. Nevertheless, reflectance confocal microscopy offers much promise for applications in cosmetology. It has found use in measuring phenomena associated with photo-damage, chronological aging, pigmentary disorders, cellulite, hair biology, wounds, allergic dermatitis, and contact dermatitis.

The principle of reflectance confocal microscopy is illustrated in the diagram in Figure 16. The specimen is illuminated with infrared laser light, which by way of a beam splitter and condenser lens is focused on the sample. Light from the focal plane and out-of-focus planes is reflected towards the detector. However, the use of a pinhole aperture in front of the detector only allows light from the focal plane to reach the detector. In this way all extraneous light—not from the focal plane—will not take part in the formation of the optical section image. The laser light is focused on a small area of the sample. To generate an optical section the laser scans in the entire *x*- and *y*-plane. Multiple optical sections are obtained by adjusting the *z*- location of the focal plane. In this manner, one may generate thin optical section images of the skin, scanning from the stratum corneum interface down to the reticular dermis. For more details on this technique, specifically with reference to the skin, the reader is referred to Reference[51].

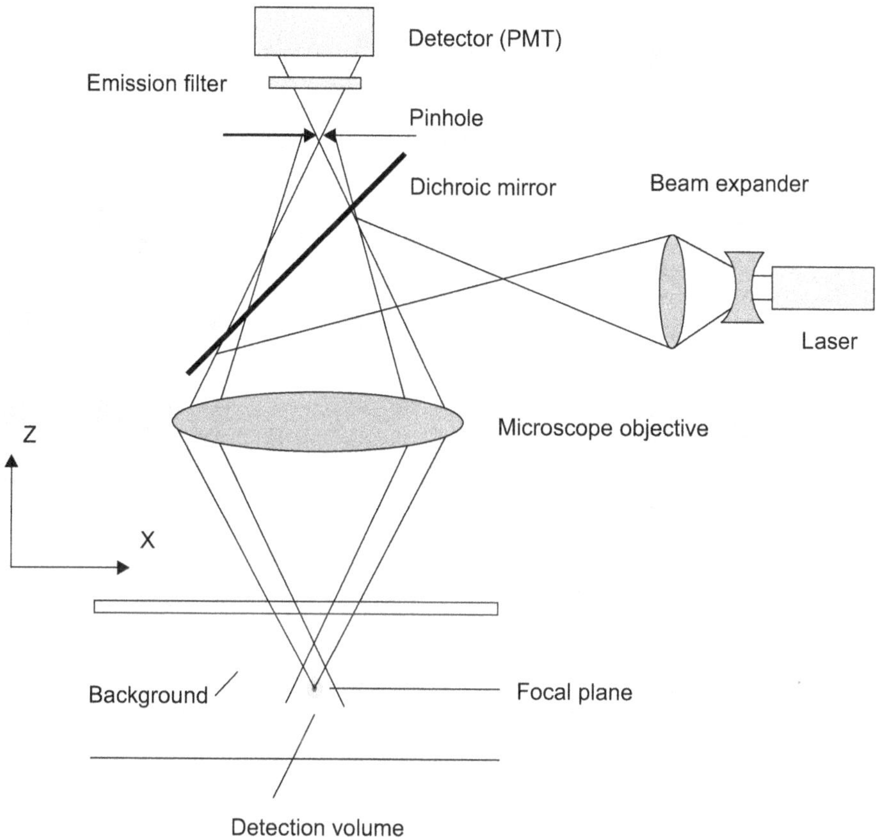

Figure 16: Diagram of a typical confocal scanning laser microscope. Reprinted with permission from Carl Zeiss.[52]

For illustration, a photograph of a confocal scanning laser microscope used quite frequently for the noninvasive *in vivo* evaluation of skin is provided in Figure 17. This particular system is a Vivascope 1500 manufactured by Lucid, Inc. (Rochester, NY). The optical resolution in the horizontal direction (*x*- and *y*-axis) is < 1.25 μm while the vertical resolution (*z*-axis) is < 5.0 μm. The field of view is 500 μm × 500 μm. The laser utilized in this system is 830 nm. As indicated in the figure, the probe on the optical head of the instrument is placed in contact with the skin. However, one must first prepare the site of examination by cleaning it with isopropyl alcohol, then applying an oil droplet to the instrument probe and ultrasound gel to the skin site. This approach increases image quality by avoiding large mismatches in refractive index that would otherwise be experienced by imaging directly in air.

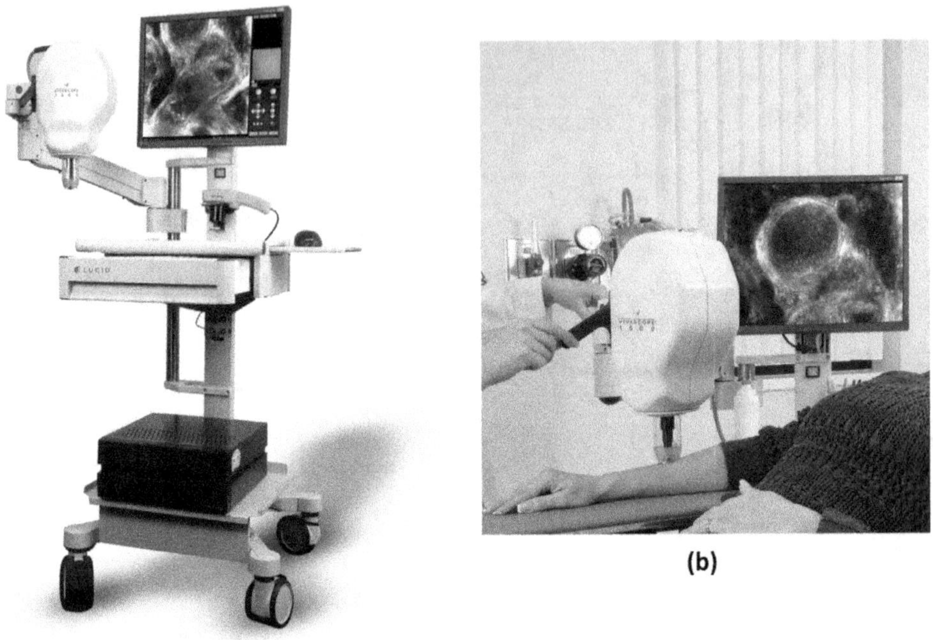

(a) (b)

Figure 17: Photograph of a common reflectance confocal microscope employed for *in vivo* skin measurements: (a) Vivascope 1500 manufactured by Lucid, Inc.; (b) close-up view of the instrument probe placed in contact with a subject. Photographs kindly provided by Lucid, Inc. (Rochester, NY).

When imaging the skin, the most striking features appear in images obtained from varying depths within the epidermis. Figure 18 contains images obtained at various depths in the skin starting with (a) the stratum corneum, which contains very bright features in the image. The very black areas in the image correspond to wrinkles and fissures in the skin that form part of its normal topography. The extraordinary brightness in this first image is due to the difference in the refractive index between the stratum corneum and the immersion medium (gel), which results in a great deal of backscattered light.[51] It should be noted that in confocal reflectance microscopy, contrast in the images occurs due to variations in refractive indices of organelles and ultrastructural components of the tissue, which in turn leads to variations in the degree of backscattered light. The polygonal-shaped corneocytes shown in the figure are 10–30 μm.

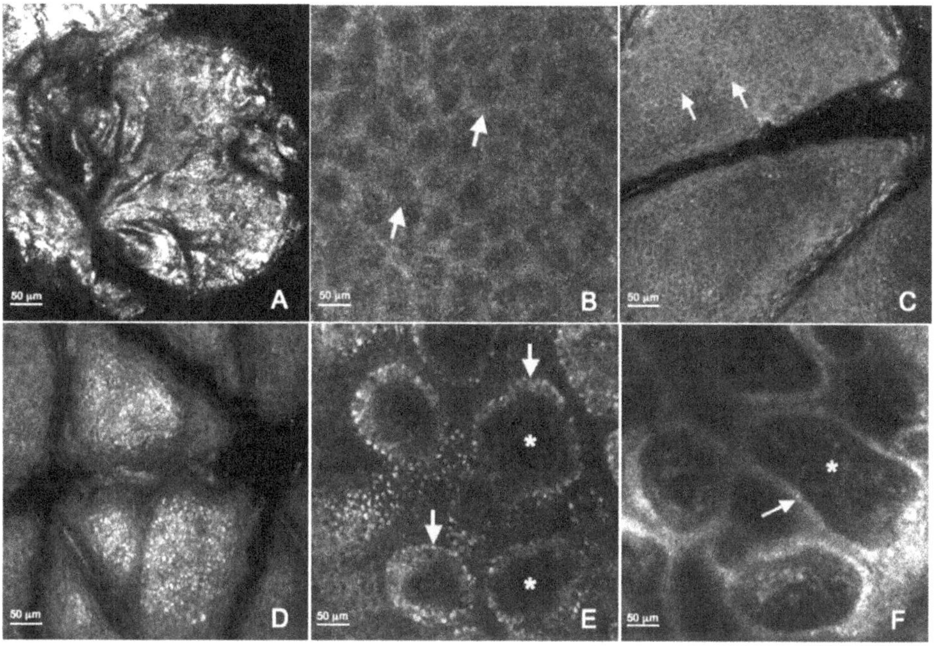

Figure 18: Reflectance confocal images of healthy skin. (a) Images of the stratum corneum are highly refractive (due to location at the air-skin interface). Dark in the image corresponds to folds. (b) A honeycomb structure of the keratinocytes is clearly apparent in the stratum granulosum. Cell nuclei (dark) are surrounded by cytoplasm (grainy). (c) Likewise, the individual cell structure of the stratum spinosum can be clearly discerned. (d) In the case of the stratum basal layer, cells are also clustered. The brightness in the image is due to the presence of both melanin and keratin. (e) Papillary rings (bright – arrow) due to keratinocytes surrounding dermal papillae (dark – asterisk) are found at the dermal-epidermal junction. (f) In the papillary dermis, one may discern reticular fibers associated with capillary vessels (asterisk) surrounded by bright rings (due to basal layer keratinocytes). Reprinted from Tavoloni Bragaa et al. with permission from OMICS Publishing Group, © 2012.[53]

Immediately below the stratum corneum, one may view (b) the stratum granulosum, which features a honeycomb pattern that consists of polygonal-shaped keratinocytes (25–35 μm) that are outlined by their faint cytoplasms that contain dark nuclei in the center of each cell. (c) The stratum spinosum also contains a honeycomb pattern and appears very similar in structure to the stratum granulosum, although the keratinocytes are smaller in this case. In (d) the basal layer, the basal cells (7–12 μm) are closely assembled together and appear much brighter due to the presence of both keratin and melanin in these cells. An image obtained from (e) the dermal-epidermal junction clearly identifies the presence of dermal papillae that can be identified as the dark regions (asterisks) surrounded by bright rings (arrows) due to basal keratinocytes. In the last image, one may view some features present in (f) the papillary dermis. Bright circles (arrow), representative of reticular fibers, surround capillary vessels (asterisk).[53]

To reemphasize, the power of confocal reflectance microscopy lies in its ability to noninvasively obtain *in vivo* images of the various strata of the epidermis extending down until the upper layers of the dermis. It provides us with pertinent information concerning a variety of disease states in skin. There has been an extensive amount of research over the last two decades investigating the skin with confocal reflectance microscopy, and continuing research in this area should help address many problems facing clinicians and researchers, both in the medical field as well as the personal care arena.

b. Ultrasonography

Ultrasound is an important diagnostic tool in general clinical medicine that allows clinicians to examine the health state of internal organs by the use of a noninvasive procedure. Over the last several decades, advances in ultrasound instrumentation have been developed allowing for the diagnosis of various skin conditions including benign and malignant skin tumors resulting from melanoma and nonmelanoma skin cancer as well as inflammatory diseases (e.g., psoriasis, morphea).[54] More recently, it is has also found use in lipoablation techniques (e.g., to eliminate cellulite) as well as collagen rejuvenation therapy in patients that have undergone surgical procedures.[55,56] Within the realm of the cosmetic industry, it is commonly used to measure skin thickness as well as to differentiate between chronologically aged and photo-damaged skin.[57] Overall, there has been a flurry of research utilizing ultrasound in the dermatologic community.[58] In addition to diagnosing skin ailments, the methodology has found extensive use as a research tool to investigate various phenomena confronting researchers of the skin.[59-63]

Ultrasonography techniques operate on the principle that high frequency sound waves generated by an ultrasound instrument propagate into the tissue and upon interaction with different physiological components return back to the instrument as echoes. The propagated wave is generated by a piezoelectric device, which converts electricity into sound waves, and the echo (reflecting from the tissue) is also detected by piezoelectric devices, which can also convert sound waves into electric signals. In practice, a ring is placed on the surface of the skin onto which a gel solution is placed. This limits the dissipation of sound waves into the air, which has much lower acoustic impedance than skin or water. In general medicine, frequency ranges of 2–15 MHz are used in ultrasound imaging. This frequency range is useful for imaging structures deep below the skin; however, for skin imaging higher frequencies must be employed. Typically, frequencies of 13.5–100 MHz are employed for imaging the skin, with most high-resolution imaging conducted at 20 MHz.[54] The higher the frequency, the higher is the resolution of tissue closer to the instrument transducers. However, this comes at a cost of imaging range, which decreases with increasing frequency. Extremely high frequencies (e.g., 500 MHz) have been employed to image *ex vivo* skin sections, although the high energy associated with these waves damages tissue and, therefore, is unsuitable for *in vivo* investigations.[64]

The basis of ultrasound measurement relies on the differences of how tissue reflects sound waves, which is greatly influenced by tissue composition and structure (e.g., vascularity and density). In skin, reflective differences can be ascertained for morphological structures based on their keratin, collagen, and water content. It is especially sensitive at the interface of such structures. In a typical B-mode scanning procedure—the preferred mode for skin studies—reflected sounds waves are transformed into two-dimensional luminosity images where low echo regions (hypoechogenic) are dark and high echo regions (echogenic) are light.[54]

For illustration, Figure 19 contains an ultrasound image of melanoma on the ventral forearm. The tumor (black oval structure—middle left) is clearly distinct as hypoechogenic from the surrounding tissue. The epidermis and dermis are clearly distinct in the echogram. In the dermis, the papillary (echo rich) can be differentiated from the reticular dermis. The subcutaneous region is echo poor. This is further illustrated in Figure 20 where we compare (a) undamaged skin with (b) skin that has experienced major photo-aging. The most apparent difference between these two echograms lies in the reticular dermis region, where many echo-poor regions can be found in photo-damaged skin corresponding to zones where connective tissue (e.g., collagen, elastin) has been degraded.

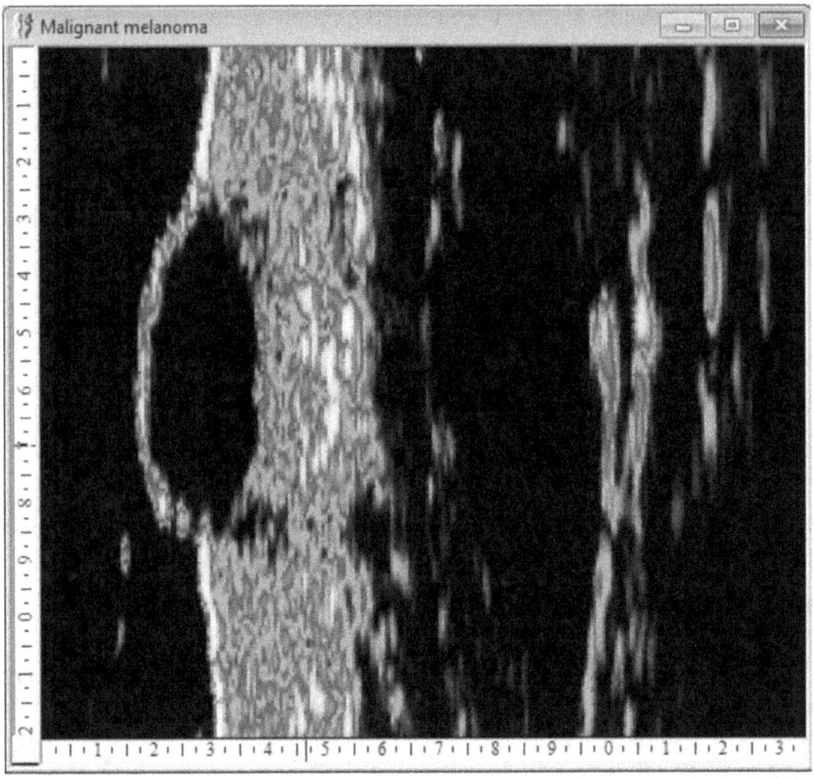

Figure 19: Echogram of a full-thickness section of skin containing a melanoma lesion. Image provided courtesy of Cortex Technology (Denmark).

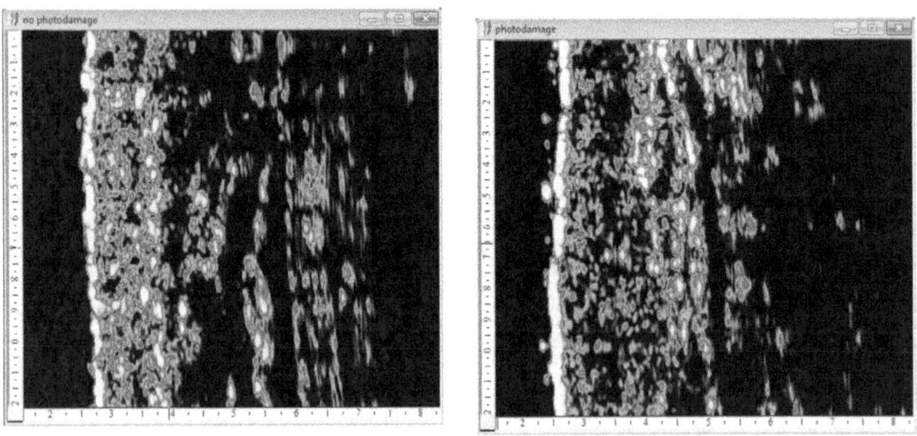

(a) (b)

Figure 20: Echograms of (a) undamaged and (b) photodamaged skin. Images provided courtesy of Cortex Technology (Denmark).

11.2.3 HIGH-RESOLUTION MICROSCOPIC TECHNIQUES FOR IMAGING SKIN

Often, in order to understand real-world phenomena one must delve into the realm of things not readily seen by the naked eye. Like most other tissues and organs, this is also true for skin. In addition to its morphological complexity, there are a number of anatomical structures that occur at the micron and submicron levels. Starting in order of resolving power for the imaging techniques presented in this section, our first discussion involves **reflected light microscopy**. Corneocytes are easily imaged from tape-stripping and cyanoacrylate surface biopsies with this technique. In addition to epi-luminiscence with visible light, we also discuss the application of **fluorescence microscopy** utilizing immunofluorescent staining techniques to the study of protein expression in skin. This is introduced in this section, but much of the associated detail is described in the final section of this chapter.

While light microscopy is less costly and requires less sample preparation, there are times when other modalities, such as scanning or transmission electron microscopy, are preferred. There are certainly advantages and drawbacks to each technique. For example, light microscopy is limited by depth of field, which can sometimes make it challenging when imaging topographical features of skin. In the case of most **scanning electron microscopy** studies, we are hampered by the requirement to coat the sample with a thin metal coating and to operate the instrument under high-vacuum conditions. However, recent advances in scanning electron microscopy technology allow for analysis at low-vacuum and normal climatic conditions (e.g., relative humidity). As discussed below, this offers us a lot of opportunities in the evaluation of the skin. **Transmission electron microscopy** is also an important means to investigate phenomena that occur in the skin. Below, we discuss several examples of its use to investigate the structure and function of skin. Finally, we touch upon some applications of **atomic force microscopy** to image and conduct surface roughness measurements of both individual corneocytes and thin sheets of stratum corneum.

a. Reflected Light Microscopy (Epi-illumination)

Reflected light microscopy, also known as **epi-illumination**, is the technique of choice when performing fluorescence microscopy or investigating samples in which we wish to study topography. In fluorescence microscopy, the sample is first treated with fluorescent dyes. Once in the microscope, the sample is illuminated with a well-defined band of light that corresponds to the wavelength where the dye absorbs light. Its fluorescence can then be monitored utilizing a filter that only allows light corresponding to the emission wavelength of the probe to pass through to the camera (Figure 21). Examples of studies completed with fluorescence microscopy (both *in vitro* with skin cell cultures as well as with thin sections of skin) can be found in the last section of this chapter on histology, immunofluorescence, and image analysis. In fluorescence microscopy the thin skin section or cell culture system is treated with a fluorescent dye; or a primary antibody along with a secondary antibody that contains a fluorescent probe covalently bound to its structure (the antibody technique is known as immunofluorescence). Whichever probe is utilized, the dye or the dye-antibody combination, these molecules will interact with some molecules in the skin section or cell culture system. Usually, immunofluorescence studies are carried out in order to monitor the upregulation or downregulation of a particular protein. Direct fluorescent dye staining (without the use of antibodies) is used to directly monitor the presence of certain molecules in skin cell cultures and skin sections. A typical example would be the use of Nile red, which is commonly employed to detect lipids (see the example in the last section of this chapter).

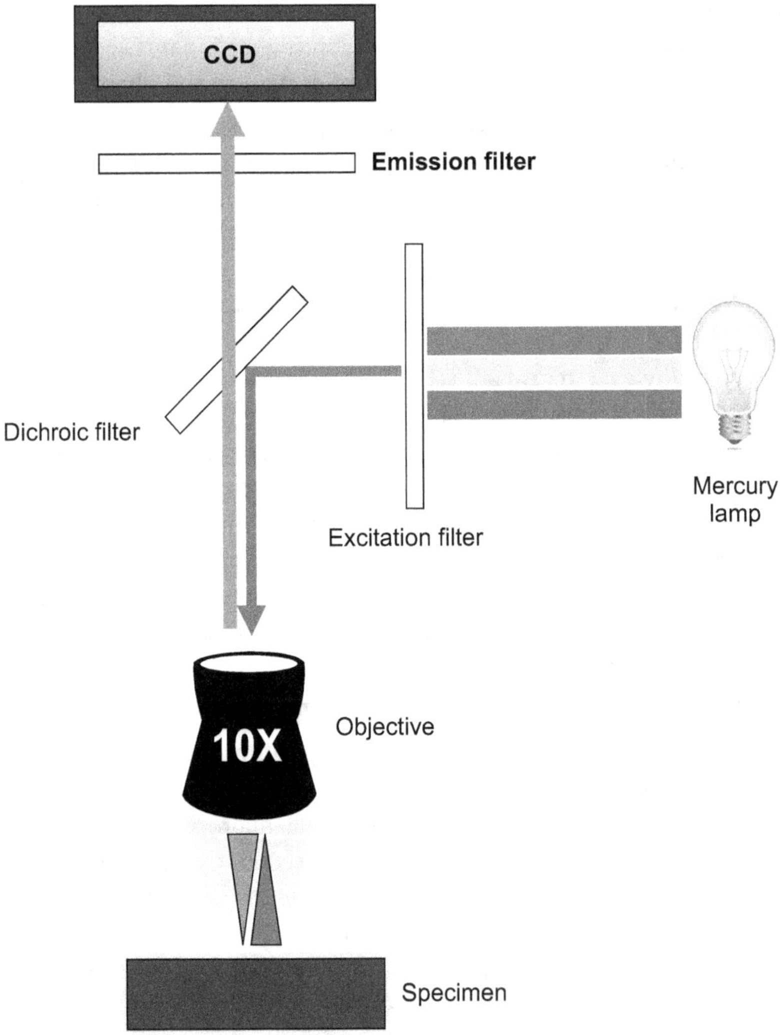

Figure 21: Schematic of a fluorescence reflectance microscope.

Typically, reflected light microscopy and fluorescence microscopy are distinguished from each other. In reflected light microscopy (nonfluorescence mode), the sample is illuminated from above with a wide band of visible light and an image is produced from the reflected light, both specular and diffuse. A key advantage to utilizing reflected light microscopy is the ability to resolve surface structural features. Unlike scanning electron microscopy, limited depth of field is a large hurdle with reflectance light microscopy. To circumvent this issue, many microscope manufacturers have designed mechanically controlled optical stages that allow the user to gather "stacks" of images. Multiple images are gathered along the *z*-axis, thus forming a "stack" of images. Essentially, each image (optical section) contains some element of the sample in focus. When all of the images are combined with a computer algorithm, only those elements in focus from each image are salvaged in the final composite image. Thus, by this means we greatly reduce limitations that are normally imposed by limited depth of field in reflected light microscopy. In "close-up" studies of the skin, this is particularly important due to its rich topographic structure.

A traditional reflected light microscope, such as that described in the preceding paragraph, is most useful for studying full-thickness *ex vivo* skin, thin histological sections of skin, or corneocytes. Full-thickness skin can sometimes be challenging, as it is not very flat and depth of field can be an issue. Histological sections of skin are normally treated with a dye that binds to specific entities, such as melanin, in skin. One such example is provided in the final section of this chapter where the Fontana Masson stain is used to detect melanin. *In vivo*, corneocytes can be removed from skin by tape stripping. The size of the corneocytes as well as various other dimensional parameters can be determined by image analysis. Examples of corneocyte images are provided in Figures 22–23. In this case, corneocytes were obtained by tape-stripping the volar forearm. In fact, the images actually show the bottom side of the corneocytes. As illustrated in Figure 22, corneocytes can be removed from the skin in clusters or as individual cells. This, of course, depends on the health state of the skin, its degree of hydration, and other factors. In this particular sample, most of the cells were removed in clusters. Image-processing and analysis procedures may be employed to determine the size and shape of the clusters. Figure 23 contains higher-magnification images of corneocytes obtained by the same method in the (a) dry and (b) wet state. Outlines of the corneocyte cells can be seen in Figure 23a due to the topographical nature of the specimen, which is presumably rougher in the dry state. In Figure 23b, the folds of corneocytes are more evident due to swelling in the wet state.

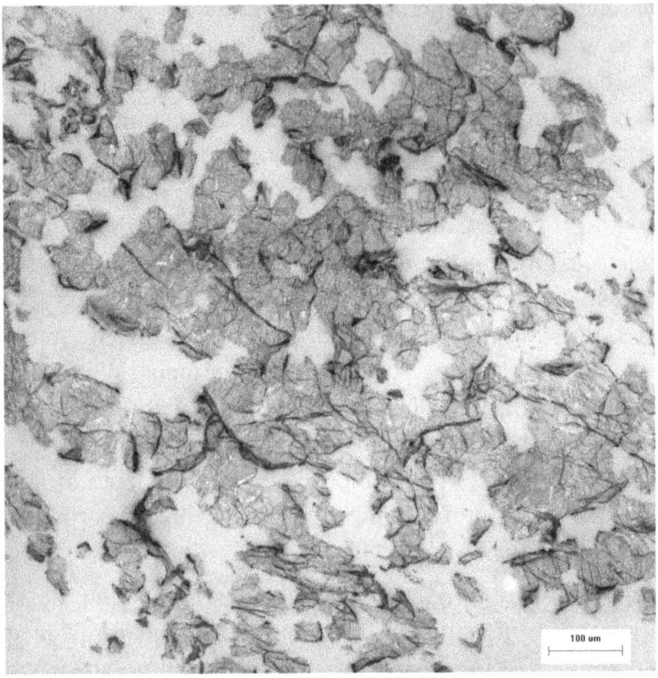

Figure 22: Optical image of corneocytes obtained by tape-stripping the volar forearm. Images were obtained with an Olympus BX-50 microscope with a 20x objective resulting in an overall magnification of 200x.

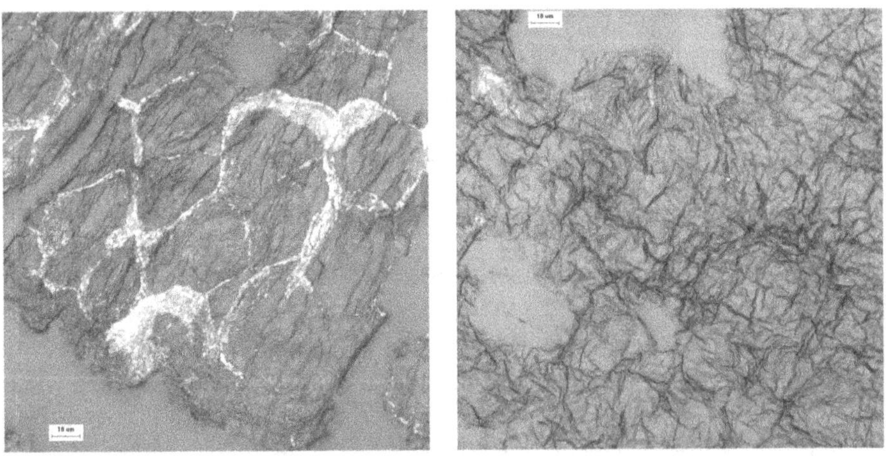

(a) (b)

Figure 23: Optical images of corneocytes obtained by tape-stripping the volar forearm in the (a) dry and (b) wet state. Images were obtained with an Olympus BX-50 microscope using a 100x objective resulting in an overall magnification of 1000x.

In a traditional reflected light microscope, it is not feasible to conduct *in vivo* measurements. There simply is not enough space between the translation stage and the objectives of the microscope. For this reason, many portable microscopes with the ability to capture *in vivo* readings have been developed in the last several decades (e.g., Scopeman). It is more challenging and costly to find such portable devices that can reach the resolution levels of traditional microscopes, which with a combination of objectives can attain up to 1500–2000x magnification. Nevertheless, such devices are important clinical and research tools that are used frequently due to their portability and ease of use.

b. Scanning Electron Microscopy (SEM)

Scanning electron microscopy (SEM) is a commonly used technique for examining the surface of samples. It is especially useful in cases where a large depth of field is required, such as that found in the skin. SEM has it downfalls as well. For example, most SEM instruments operate under high vacuum and require coating nonconductive samples with a thin layer (10 nm) of metal (e.g., gold, platinum, etc.) prior to analysis. The metal coating makes the surface conductive and prevents charging (white hot spots) on the surface. The principle of SEM is based on the use of an electron beam, either an electron gun or a tungsten filament source, which is focused through a series of electromagnetic lenses onto the sample. Electrons are either backscattered from the sample and collected with a backscattered electron detector or collected with a secondary electron detector. Images captured with the backscattered detector show differences in composition of the sample, while those captured with the secondary electron detector reveal morphology and topology. Most SEM images that we are accustomed to seeing are imaged using the secondary electron detector. In recent years, advances have been made in SEM instrument technology—ultimately leading to the development of the environmental SEM (ESEM)—allowing researchers to study biological samples at low pressure, in the wet state, and without metal plating.

Most of the work in the area of skin care related to SEM has focused on the evaluation of the outermost stratum corneum structure.[65,66] In most cases, SEM images are generated from positive casts constructed from skin replicas and examined for general topology and exfoliaton patterns of stratum corneum cells.[67] Corneocyte boundaries and points of tear or disengagement of stratum corneum cells from each other can easily be identified. In the more recent literature, the use of cryo-SEM shed light on the activity of moisturizing agents, specifically revealing that all stratum corneum cells are not hydrated to the same extent. In fact, centrally located corneocytes are more susceptible to hydration than those in the upper and lower regions of the stratum corneum.[68] Figure 24 contains representative cross-sectional images obtained for skin treated with various moisturizers. As illustrated in the figure, the stratum corneum can be broken down into three different zones of water uptake capacity. The upper and lower stratum corneum are nonswelling regions while the middle region has a greater capacity to swell. Overall, the cryo-SEM technique demonstrates the ability of SEM-based techniques to provide information not available with traditional SEM. Looking forward, both cryo-SEM and ESEM offer much promise in the evaluation of skin in terms of its health and to study the impact of novel ingredients and delivery technologies.

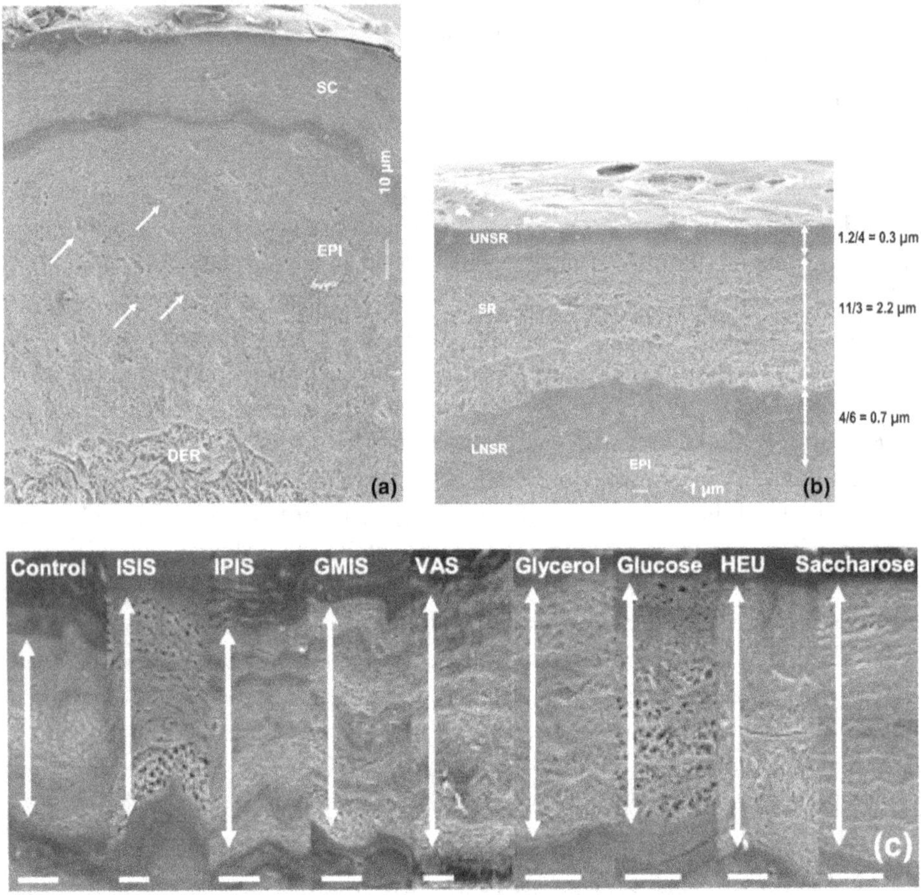

Figure 24: (a) Cryo-SEM image of a dermatomed skin cross-section equilibrated to 80% RH after cryo-fixation and cryo-planing. The stratum corneum (SC), viable epidermis (EPI), and dermis (DER) can clearly be distinguished. Arrows in the epidermis indicate the presence of keratinocyte nuclei. (b) The stratum corneum can be divided into three distinct regions based on its hydration properties: upper non-swelling region (UNSR), swelling region (SR), and lower non-swelling region (LNSR). (c) Cross sections of skin treated with various moisturizers: isostearyl isostearate (ISIS), isopropyl isostearate (IPIS), glyercol monoisostearate (GMIS), Vaseline (VAS – petrolatum), glyercol, glucose, hydroxyethyl urea (HEU), and saccharose. Reprinted from Caussin et al. with permission from John Wiley & Sons, © 2007.[68]

c. Transmission Electron Microscopy (TEM)

Many of the intricate details we know about skin structure have come about from **transmission electron microscopy** (TEM) studies. One need only to peruse some of the classic literature about skin structure and function to fully appreciate its contributions to the field.[69-71] Transmission electron microscopy is a remarkable high-resolution technique in which electrons are focused by electromagnetic lenses onto an extremely thin specimen and then arrive on the other side to create an image on the detector. The image projected on the detector depends on how the electrons interact with the thin specimen. The sample preparation in TEM is fairly involved and in most cases requires that the specimen be stained with vaporized heavy metals, such as osmium tetroxide or ruthenium tetroxide. For the most part, TEM has been used to elucidate the ultrafine structure of the epidermis, dermis, and skin appendages. Our current understanding of the process of cellular differentiation in the epidermis was made possible due to pioneering work with TEM. It is capable of imaging cellular organelles, macromolecules, and lipids with extremely high resolution. In fact, many of the details we know about stratum corneum lipid structure have come from TEM studies.[72] The current view of the organization of the structural proteins (elastin and collagen) of the dermis and dermal-epidermal junction are in part due to early studies conducted with TEM.[71] Regrettably, there are not as many research groups that specialize in TEM analysis of skin as there used to be; probably due to cumbersome sample preparation procedures and budgetary constraints. This is unfortunate, as many of the ingredients used in modern-day skin care formulations claim to modify the ultrafine structure of skin.

For illustration, Figure 25 contains a TEM image of (a) the viable epidermis and (b) stratum corneum stained with osmium tetroxide. Essentially, a portion of the stratum spinosum, stratum granulosum, and stratum corneum are shown in Figure 25a. The lowest stratum of skin (in this case stratum spinosum) is shown in the bottom left corner of the image, while the stratum corneum may be observed in the upper right corner. The stratum granulosum is sandwiched between them. It is difficult to discern the boundary between the stratum spinosum and stratum granulosum; however, one may notice the cell nuclei of one of the stratum spinosum layer keratinocytes in the bottom left of the image. The stratum granulosum is the area in the middle of the image that runs diagonally from the upper left corner of the image to the lower right corner. Keratohyalin granules, which contain profilaggrin, can be seen as electron-dense islands within this layer. In Figure 25b a higher magnification view of the stratum corneum is shown—in this case staining was carried out with ruthenium tetroxide. As evident in the image, ruthenium tetroxide is a better stain for picking up lipids. Figure 25c provides a closer look of the region indicated by the arrow in Figure 25b in which the arrangement of lipid bilayer lamellae in the stratum corneum can be clearly visualized. We should also note that the bright white regions in Figure 25b are an artifact of the staining procedure where the ruthenium tetroxide has digested portions of the corneocyte.

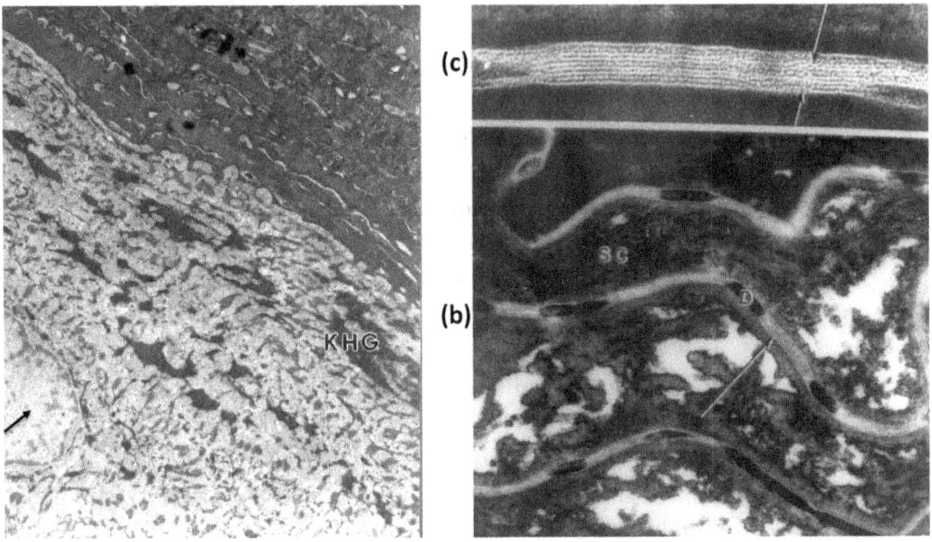

(a)

Figure 25: TEM images of various regions of the epidermis obtained from thin sections of human skin. In the first image (a) portions of the stratum spinosum, stratum granulosum, and stratum corneum are shown. In the bottom left corner of the image (arrow), one can discern the nucleus of a stratum spinosum keratinocyte. The region extending diagonally from the upper left corner to the lower right corner in the image corresponds to the stratum granulosum. Notable features in this layer are the keratohyalin granules (darkly stained regions). The stratum corneum is mostly confined to the upper right corner of the image. (b) A magnified view of the stratum corneum in which three corneocytes are separated by a thin light band corresponding to lipid lamellae. Dark regions along the lamellae correspond to desmosomes. (c) Higher magnification of the stratum corneum highlighting the lipid bilayer lamellae between corneocytes. Image (a) provided courtesy of Dr. Gopi Menon, Ashland, Inc. Images in (b) and (c) reprinted from Menon and Elias with permission from Springer, © 2001.[73]

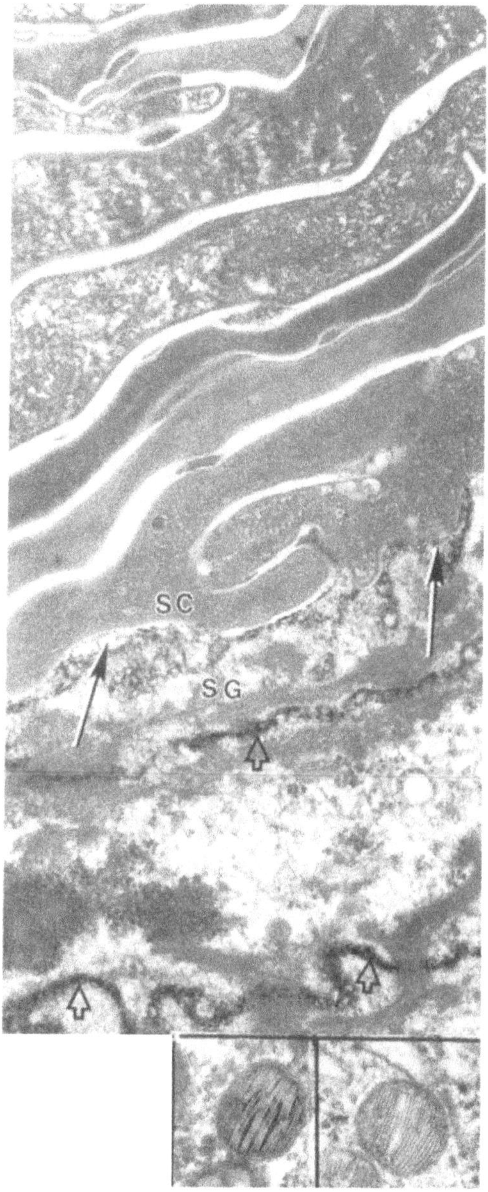

Figure 26: TEM image of a thin section of epidermis that underwent a tracer study. Colloidal lanthanum is an electron-dense tracer that leaves a dark trail in the image. It was injected in the dermis and can be seen migrating from the bottom to top of the epidermis through extracellular space in the viable epidermis. It does not reach the stratum corneum. The insets in the bottom right corner illustrate the ultrafine structure of lamellar bodies. Reprinted from Menon and Ghadially with permission from Wiley-Liss, © 1997.[74]

Another example of the use of TEM in the investigation of the epidermis is shown in Figure 26. In this case, a tracer study was carried out utilizing colloidal lanthanum. It is an electron-dense substance that upon injection into the dermis follows the nutritional supply line from the dermis up until the upper layers of the viable epidermis. The electron-dense tracer is present in the dark regions (indicated by the arrows) in extracellular space surrounding the keratinocyte. It stops its migration at the region of the stratum granulosum where the lamellar bodies are secreted. To provide further perspective, insets of the lamellar bodies (much higher magnification) are shown in the bottom right corner of Figure 26.

As an illustration of the use of TEM to investigate the properties of cosmetic ingredients, the image in Figure 27 contains a lipid barrier function enhancer sold under the trade name ProLipid 141 (Ashland, Inc.) which contains various ingredients: glyceryl stearate, behenyl alcohol palmitic acid, stearic acid, lecithin, lauryl alcohol, myristyl alcohol, and cetyl alcohol. The product was deposited onto a nylon membrane and allowed to dry. Close inspection of Figure 27 reveals lipid bilayer lamellae, which present themselves as light bands within the larger dark bands of the image. In this case, the sample was stained with ruthenium tetroxide, allowing for clear visualization of the lipid layers.

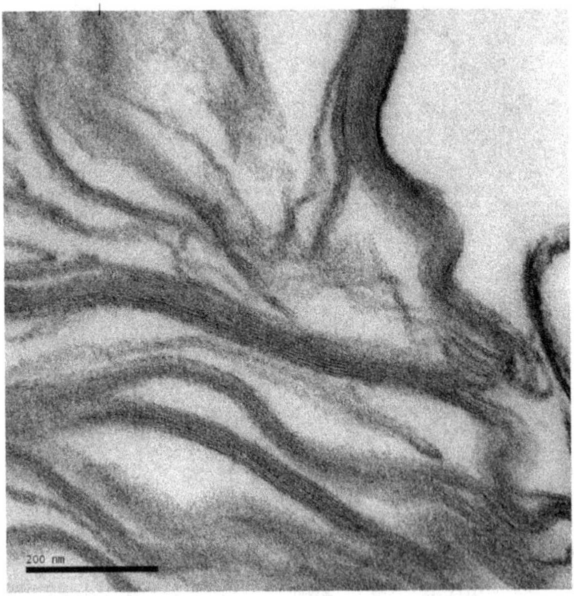

Figure 27: TEM image of a specialty ingredient product used in the cosmetic industry to fortify the stratum corneum lipid barrier. It is comprised of the following ingredients: glyceryl stearate, behenyl alcohol palmitic acid, stearic acid, lecithin, lauryl alcohol, myristyl alcohol, and cetyl alcohol. The product was dried on a nylon membrane. The lipid bilayer lamellae are evident as white bands within the black bands in the image. Image courtesy of Gopi Menon and David J. Moore, Ashland, Inc.

d. Atomic Force Microscopy (AFM)

Scanning probe microscopy (SPM) is a plethora of techniques used to study the surfaces of substrates. Most of the SPM modes are quantitative and operate by measuring the interaction of a stylus probe with the investigated specimen. **Atomic force microscopy** (AFM) is one of the techniques under this umbrella and consists of measuring the deflection of the cantilever portion of the stylus as the tip comes into contact with the sample.

As illustrated in Figure 28, a laser is reflected on the back of the cantilever, and as it moves in the *z*-direction due to topography of the sample, the position of the reflected laser on the photodetector is monitored. Therefore, by scanning in the *x*-*y* plane we can generate a three-dimensional image of the skin surface. One should be forewarned that imaging intact *ex vivo* skin is extremely challenging. Most AFM studies of skin have been carried out on individual corneocytes or isolated sections of skin.[75-77] After tape stripping, corneocytes can be isolated from the tape by dissolution in hexane and then mounted on an AFM stud. Various features of the corneocytes can be quantified including topology, rigidity, and friction.[76]

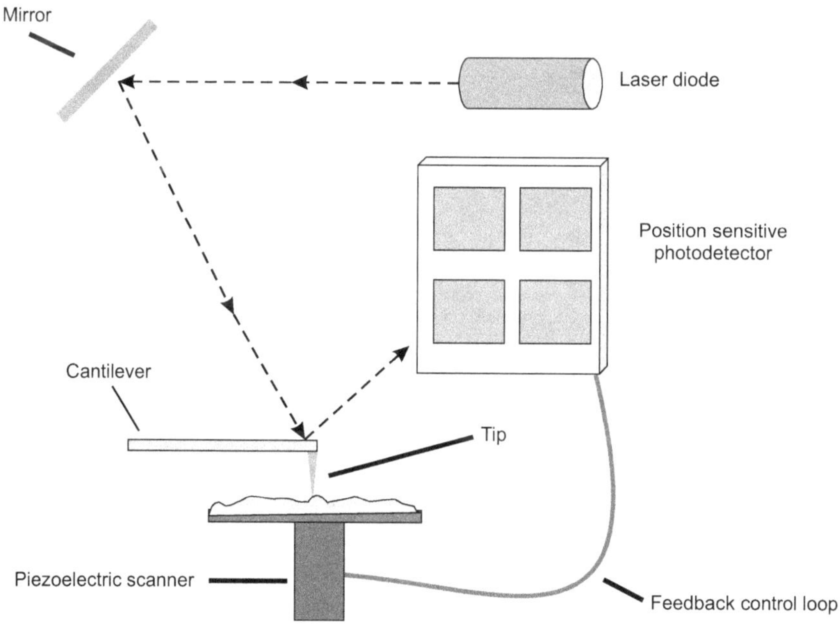

Figure 28: Schematic of a typical AFM instrument.

Figure 29 contains the images from (a) corneocytes obtained from the upper stratum corneum and (b) from the lower stratum corneum. Surface height measurements of the corneocytes (straight horizontal line in Figure 29) illustrate distinct topology for corneocytes obtained from the most superficial layers of stratum corneum, which have much rougher surfaces than corneocytes obtained from deeper layers. Differences in corneocyte topography have also been discerned for corneocytes isolated from distinct anatomical regions as well as samples obtained from subjects representing various age groups and individuals with pathologic skin conditions.[75] Other AFM studies have focused on characterizing structural proteins of skin, such as collagen, in terms of adhesion and elasticity.[78] A number of studies have also been conducted to better understand stratum corneum lipid organization, although these studies were carried out on lipid models of skin lipids.[79,80]

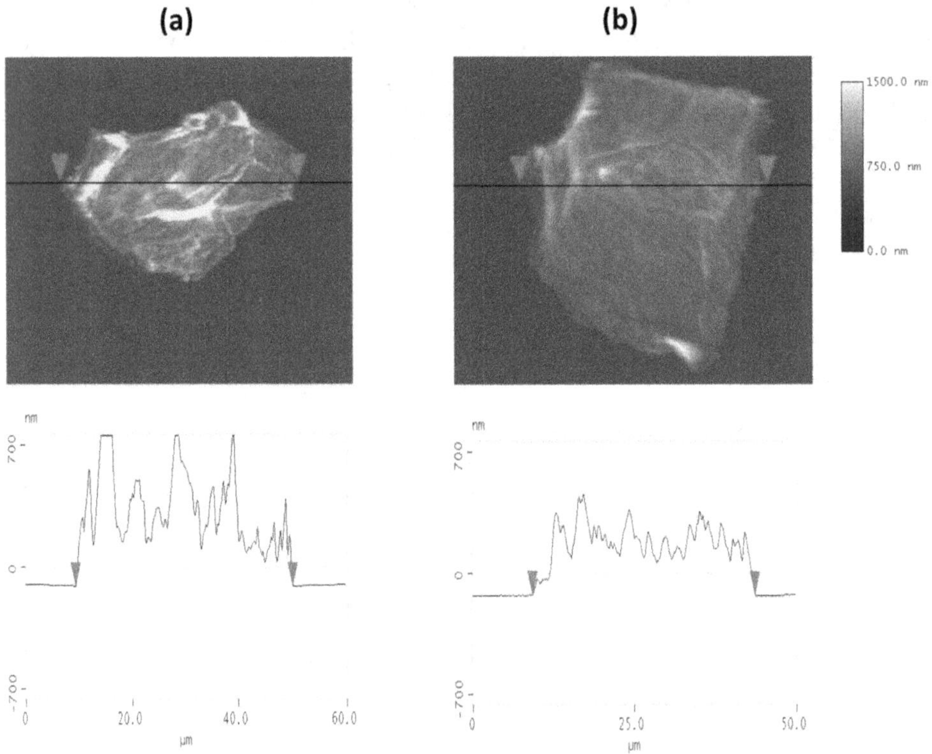

Figure 29: AFM images of corneocytes obtained from (a) superficial and (b) deeper layers of the stratum corneum. In each image a horizontal line is drawn to demonstrate the utility of height measurements, which are shown in the corresponding graphs below. Images kindly provided courtesy of Dr. Guojin Zhang, Ashland, Inc.

As already indicated, imaging intact skin is extremely difficult due to its extremely high roughness profile owed to furrows and fissures on the surface. In many circumstances, an AFM probe will twist on its side due to the height differences between peaks and valleys in the skin's topography. With care and precision, stratum corneum sheets can be isolated from *ex vivo* skin utilizing a trypsin digestion method.[81] Figure 30 contains an image of isolated porcine skin stratum corneum that was (a) treated with water or (b) treated with sodium dodecyl sulfate. A clear distinction can be made between the two samples. In the sodium dodecyl sulfate treated sample, the boundaries of individual corneocytes can clearly be discerned due to solubilization of skin surface structural lipids. In many instances, AFM is used as an imaging device. However, it should be emphasized that its true power is in quantitative measurements of micron- and nanoscale phenomena. For example, it would be extremely instructive to perform nano-indentation measurements with AFM, yielding modulus information and other pertinent information to better characterize skin—both to investigate contributions from various morphological features as well as to evaluate the influence of treatments. In any event, there are a number of scanning probe microscopy tools (or modes) that have not yet been explored in the investigation of skin. Hopefully, these technologies will help those researchers embarking on future imaging adventures with the skin.

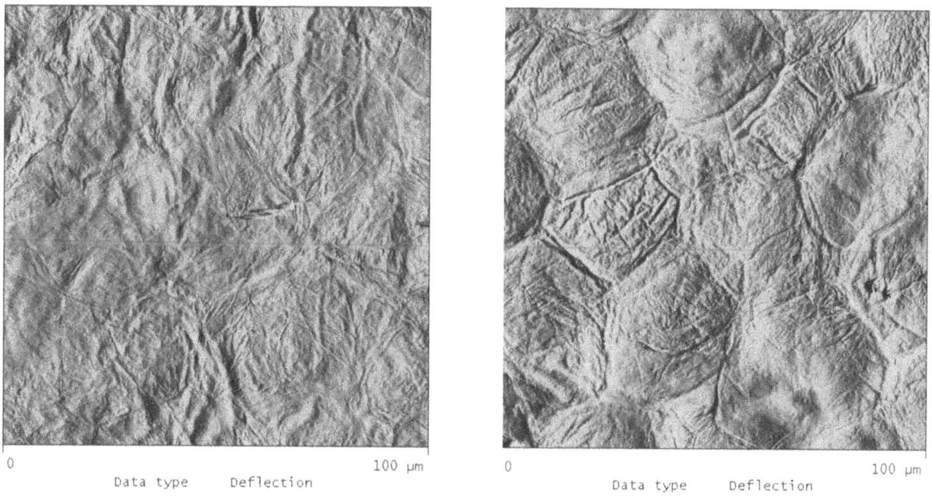

(a) (b)

Figure 30: AFM images of sheets of porcine stratum corneum treated with (a) H_2O and (b) 50 mM sodium dodecyl sulfate for 20 minutes. Images kindly provided courtesy of Dr. Guojin Zhang, Ashland, Inc.

11.2.4 IMAGE ANALYSIS TO QUANTIFY HISTOLOGICAL AND IMMUNOFLUORESCENT STAINING OF *EX VIVO* SKIN AND *IN VITRO* SKIN CELL CULTURES

Numerous *in vitro*, *ex vivo*, and *in vivo* tests exist for the determination of expression of biological molecules as related to skin immunological status, pigmentary changes, and skin aging. Often, these tests are carried out utilizing *in vitro* cell cultures, such as keratinocytes, fibroblasts and adipocytes, or with *ex vivo* skin. After a treatment protocol is administered, the substrate to be investigated may be treated with a histological stain, or an immunofluorescent dye, allowing certain features in the sample to be observed with an optical microscope. Typically, these features are the result of the interaction of the probe with biological molecules, which play a vital role in cellular function. Traditionally, qualitative comparison of images obtained from microscopes was the widely accepted analytical approach. However, the advent of image-processing and analysis methods offers great utility for conversion of microscope analysis from a qualitative to quantitative technique. In this section, we review how image analysis may be employed to quantitatively characterize data obtained from microscopic images of *in vitro* cultures of skin cells and thin sections of *ex vivo* skin. Through the use of various algorithms and image analysis techniques, specific features of interest in the image may be segmented and properly measured.[82-84]

In general, there are three typical steps involved in image analysis, which include image capture, segmentation, and measurement. Image capture involves the acquisition of an image, which, in the examples shown below, was obtained utilizing a light or fluorescence microscope equipped with a charge-coupled device (CCD). Segmentation consists of isolating objects of interest in an image that we wish to quantify. Some of the segmentation procedures discussed in this section consist of image threshold (conversion to binary image), color segmentation, or the use of image filters (e.g., Gaussian, Unsharpen mask, etc.). In terms of measurements, we are most interested in measuring the stained area in a given field of view, measuring the length of an object, and quantification of image histograms.

a. Measuring Pigmentation of Histological Skin Sections

The Fontana Masson staining technique is commonly employed to measure pigmentation effects such as skin whitening, tanning, and hyperpigmentation disorders. The staining procedure consists of treating a thin histological section of skin with silver nitrate ($AgNO_3$). As a result of treatment, $AgNO_3$ reacts with melanin to produce metallic silver (Ag) resulting in a black stain that can be visualized with a light microscope. Figure 31 contains photomicrographs of *ex vivo* skin sections that were treated with the Fontana Masson stain. The skin in Figure 31a was treated with a placebo, whereas that in Figure 31b was treated with a skin-whitening active ingredient. Upon visual inspection, one may deduce that less staining occurs in the active ingredient treated sample.

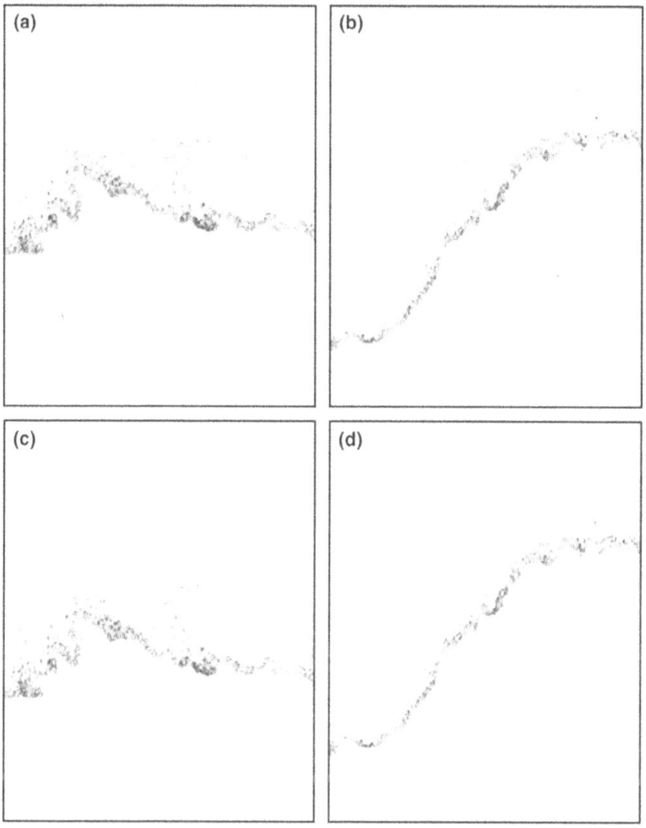

Figure 31: Photomicrographs of thin sections of skin stained with the Fontana Masson dye. Dark features in the images correspond to the amount of melanin present. Photomicrograph images for (a) placebo and (b) active ingredient treated samples are shown to demonstrate the skin whitening effect of an active ingredient. The placebo (c) and active ingredient (d) samples are then subjected to image-processing steps consisting of segmentation and grayscale conversion. Reprinted from McMullen et al. with permission from Society of Cosmetic Scientists and the Société Française de Cosmétologie, © 2010.[84]

A first step in the image analysis of the micrographs described above is to perform image segmentation. In this case, the image is segmented by isolating the epidermis on a white background by carefully selecting everything above the stratum basal layer up to and including the intact stratum corneum. The dermis and the layers of the stratum corneum that become dismembered (an artifact of the skin-sectioning technique) are removed so that their contributions are not considered in the analysis. The histogram of a grayscale image provides a distribution of the pixels in an image as a function of luminosity, in this case on a scale of 0–255. Histograms for both images (from Figures 31c and 31d) are shown in Figure 32. In each case, a large peak at high luminosity values is apparent in the histogram and corresponds to the white background in the images. In agreement with the histogram, the Area Under the Curve value obtained for the placebo (40 ± 7) is greater than that for the active ingredient (29 ± 7) treated sample. As we were interested in quantifying the dark features of the image that result from Fontana Masson staining, the Area Under the Curve was calculated within the limits of 0–175. The value of 175 was chosen after performing image thresholds to determine at which point in the histogram the dark features corresponding to the stain started to appear. Care must be taken when choosing this value as it can be influenced by experimental factors, such as light source intensity and quantity of stain employed. Therefore, it is advisable to calibrate the image analysis measurements, CCD, and microscope by taking an image of a photographic Macbeth card prior to each imaging session.

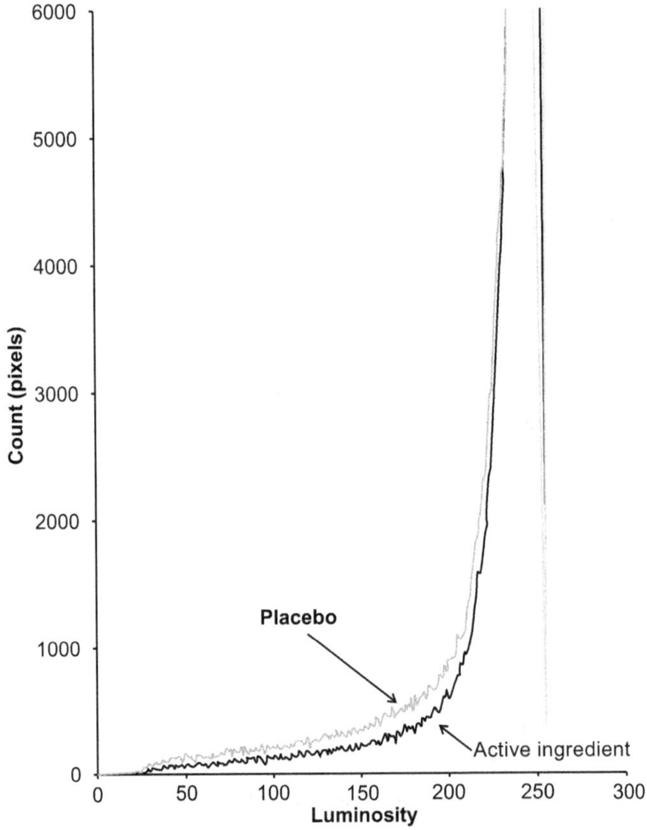

Figure 32: Image histograms corresponding to the processed images in Figures 31c and 31d. Reprinted from McMullen et al. with permission from Society of Cosmetic Scientists and the Société Française de Cosmétologie, © 2010.[84]

b. Immunofluorescence Staining Quantification in Fibroblast Cell Cultures

A common technique for the analysis of protein expression in cell culture systems is to utilize a primary antibody in conjunction with a fluorescent-labeled secondary antibody for fluorescence microscopy visualization. In the example provided, it is demonstrated how cytochrome c, in this case the antigen, can be detected by first using a primary antibody to bind to cytochrome c and a secondary antibody (containing a covalently attached fluorescent probe, Alexa Fluor 488) to bind to the primary antibody. Figure 33 contains fluorescent photomicrograph images of (a) control and (b) active ingredient treated samples of skin fibroblasts. The interest in monitoring cytochrome c expression is because of its function as an electron carrier in the electron transport chain present in the inner membrane of mitochondria. It has been shown that increasing the level of cytochrome c expression in the mitochondrial inner membrane results in a corresponding increase in the production of adenosine triphosphate (ATP), a critical source of energy for many cellular events. Comparison of the two images in Figure 33 reveals greater expression of cytochrome c in the active ingredient (Figure 33b) treated fibroblast cell culture system than the placebo (Figure 33a). As an alternative to the approach presented with the Fontana Masson staining experiment, the fibroblast images can be converted to grayscale images and then to binary images that contain only black and white, in which case white corresponds to the green fluorescent stain (see Figure 34). One may then determine the area occupied by white pixels and normalize this value to the number of cells present in the field of view.

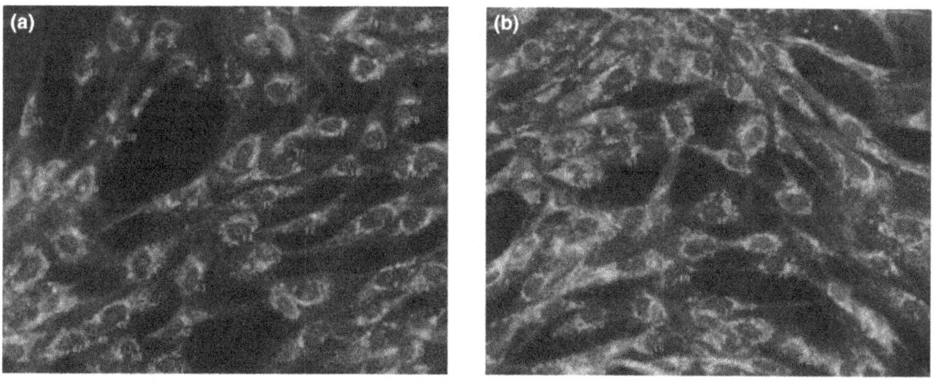

Figure 33: Fluorescent photomicrographs of fibroblasts treated with an antibody labelled with Alexa Fluor 488 to monitor mitochrondrial cytochrome c expression in (a) placebo and (b) active ingredient treated samples. The total number of cells present in the field of view was quantified. Reprinted from McMullen et al. with permission from Society of Cosmetic Scientists and the Société Française de Cosmétologie, © 2010.[84]

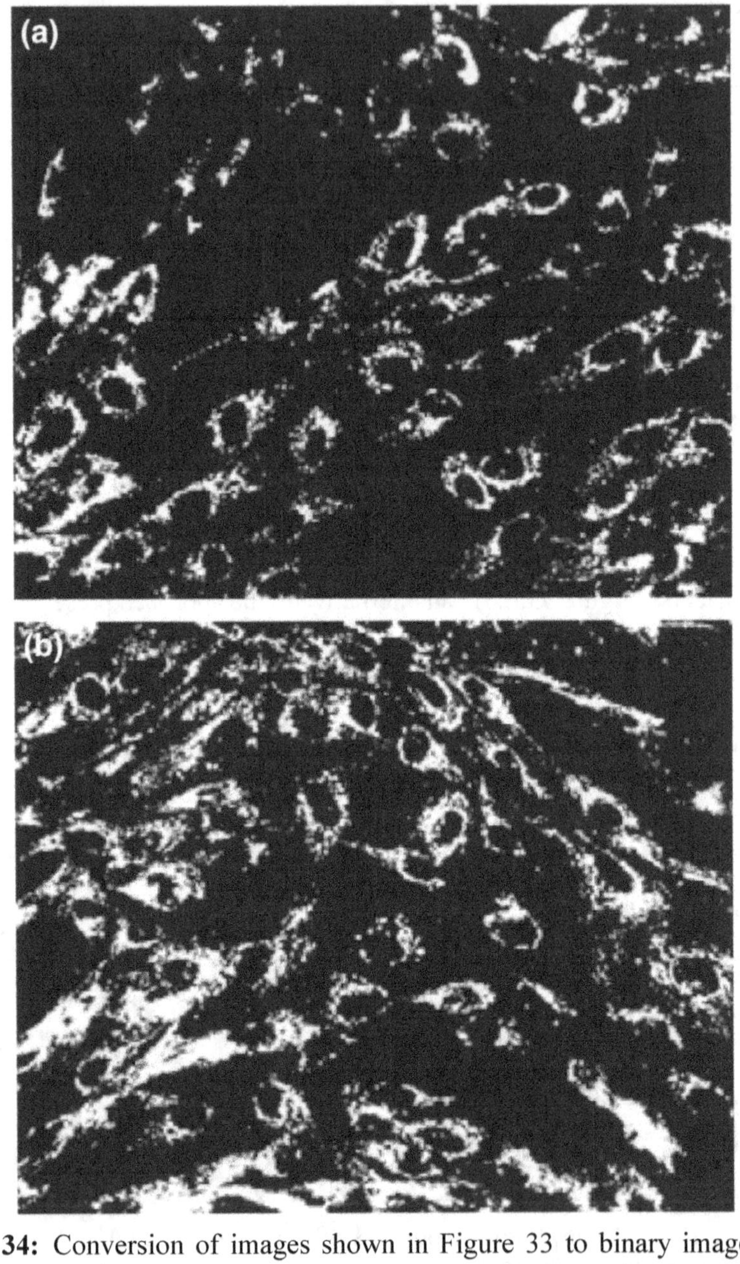

Figure 34: Conversion of images shown in Figure 33 to binary images corresponding to (a) placebo and (b) active ingredient treated samples. Reprinted from McMullen et al. with permission from Society of Cosmetic Scientists and the Société Française de Cosmétologie, © 2010.[84]

c. Image Analysis of Triple-Stained Normal Human Keratinocytes (NHKs)

Often, one may wish to monitor the presence or expression of several different molecules in cell culture. One component that is almost always monitored is the cell nucleus, which is stained with DAPI, a molecular probe characterized by λ_{ex} = 358 nm and λ_{em} = 461 nm. DAPI binds to the inner groove of DNA present in cell nuclei and results in a blue emission that can be seen in the fluorescent microscope. In this particular example, there are two other stains: Nile red and AlexaFluor 488, which result in red and green fluorescence, respectively, in the cell culture. These stains are normally viewed by inserting filters in the microscope allowing for each component stain to be visualized individually. The Nile red stain penetrates lipid droplets and is used as an indication of lipid bodies present in the cell culture. As discussed in the section above, Alexa Fluor 488 is covalently attached to a secondary antibody which binds to a primary antibody. *The primary antibody interacts with the antigen*, in this case, HMG-CoA reductase. It is a regulatory enzyme in the mevalonate pathway, which eventually leads to the biosynthesis of cholesterol. Thus, HMG-CoA reductase expression correlates to normal human keratinocyte (NHK) cholesterol levels.

An example of a triple-stained NHK is provided in Figure 35. Staining of DAPI in cell cultures not only allows us to visualize the cell nuclei, but also permits facile quantification of the number of cells in a given field of view. This allows us to normalize the data obtained from the Nile red and Alexa Fluor 488 stains. A representative example of the image-processing steps and subsequent counting of cell nuclei stained with DAPI is shown in Figure 36. First, the original image is subjected to a color segmentation procedure in which a range of blue colors are selected in the image and are shown in red in Figure 36a. Then, the cell nuclei are isolated by converting the color-segmented image to a binary image. In the next step—conversion of Figures 36b and 36c—the binary image undergoes an image inversion. This step is performed for aesthetic reasons rather than necessity. In the last stage (Figure 36d), all of the nuclei in the field of view are counted.

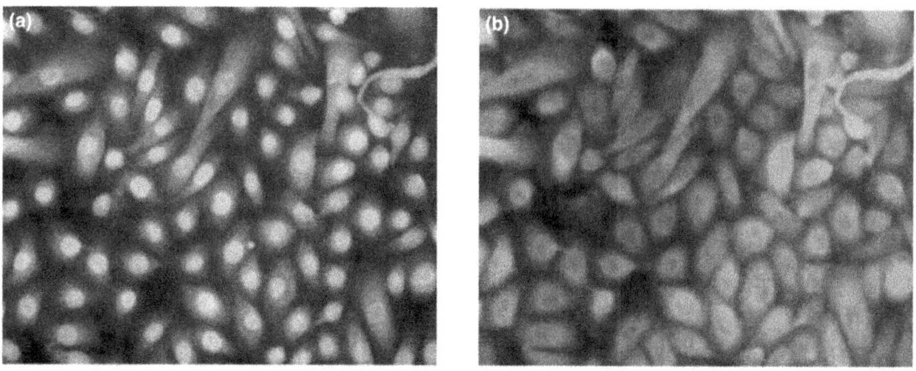

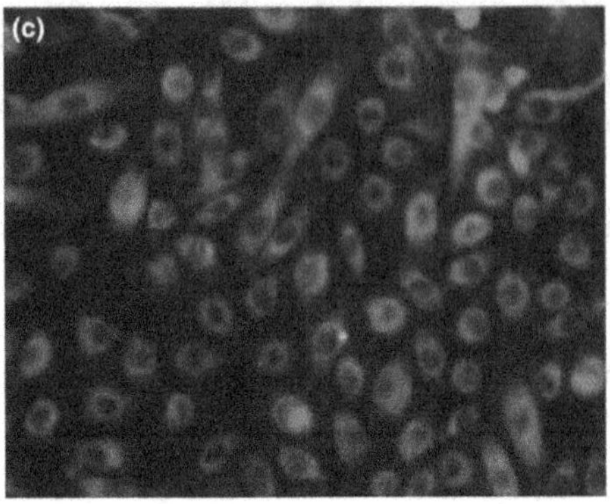

Figure 35: Triple-stained normal human keratinocytes using (a) DAPI, (b) antibody-labelled with Alexa Fluor 488 and (c) Nile red. Reprinted from McMullen et al. with permission from Society of Cosmetic Scientists and the Société Française de Cosmétologie, © 2010.[84]

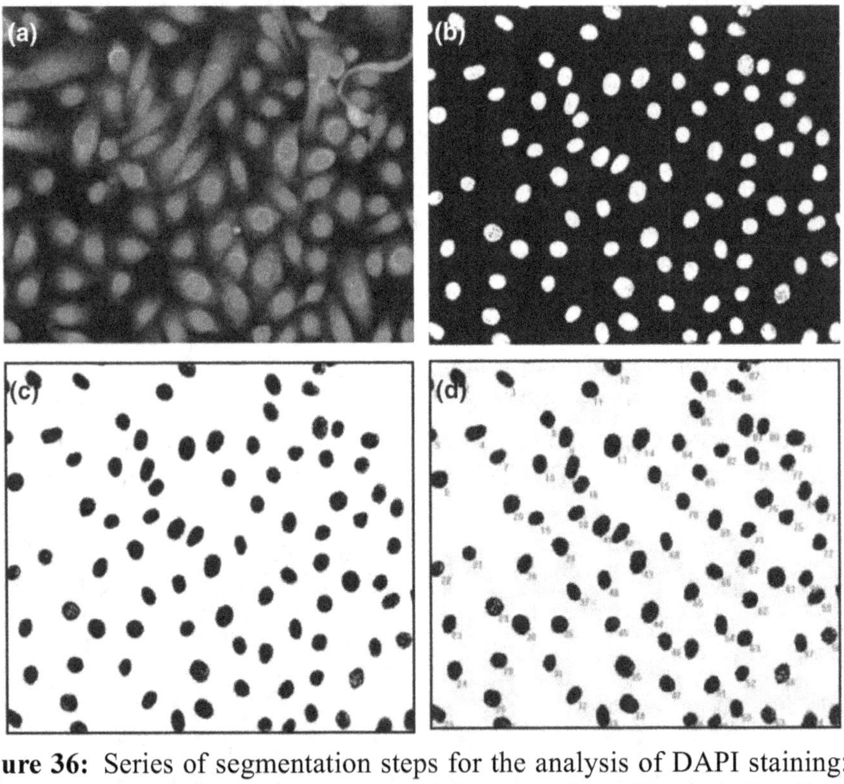

Figure 36: Series of segmentation steps for the analysis of DAPI staining: (a) color segmentation, (b) isolation of nuclei, (c) image inversion and (d) cell counting. Reprinted from McMullen et al. with permission from Society of Cosmetic Scientists and the Société Française de Cosmétologie, © 2010.[84]

The Nile red and AlexaFluor 488 fluorescence are quantified in a manner similar to that already-discussed Sections A and B. The micrographs are transformed to grayscale images followed by generation of image histograms. This step allows for the quantification of the area under the curve, which is normalized by counting the number of nuclei (DAPI fluorescence) in a given field of view. Although the data are not shown, this type of analysis is extremely useful for testing NHKs treated with active ingredients that upregulate HMG-CoA reductase (green fluorescent image) and lipids (red fluorescent image).

d. Measurement of Collagen IV Expression at the Dermal-Epidermal Junction

The dermal-epidermal junction is the boundary between the dermis and epidermis, and serves a structural function of paramount importance in binding the stratum basal layer cells with the underlying papillary dermis. Principally, it is composed of structural proteins such as laminins and collagens. From the collagen family, collagen IV is one of the most predominant members present and provides much of the structural architecture for the dermal-epidermal junction. Therefore, it is of interest to measure the amount of collagen IV present in *ex vivo* skin sections, as it is indicative of the health state of this segment of the skin. Figures 37a and 37b contain images of skin sections, stained with DAPI and a primary-secondary antibody system tagged with Alexa Fluor 488, for a placebo and active ingredient treated sample.

To prepare the images for image analysis, they were both segmented by removing all portions of the image below the dermal-epidermal junction and above the stratum corneum. The remaining viable epidermis and dermal-epidermal junction were isolated on a black background. The segmented images are shown in Figures 37c and 37d. The images were also calibrated so that distance measurements could be obtained along the length of the dermal-epidermal junction. The next image-processing step was to color segment the images by selecting the range of green colors that appear in the image because of Alexa Fluor 488 fluorescence, corresponding to the presence of collagen IV. The selected color-segmented portion of the image was then transferred to a black image background, as shown in Figure 38, resulting in a binary image. The next step would be to generate histograms of the processed images to quantify the luminosity.

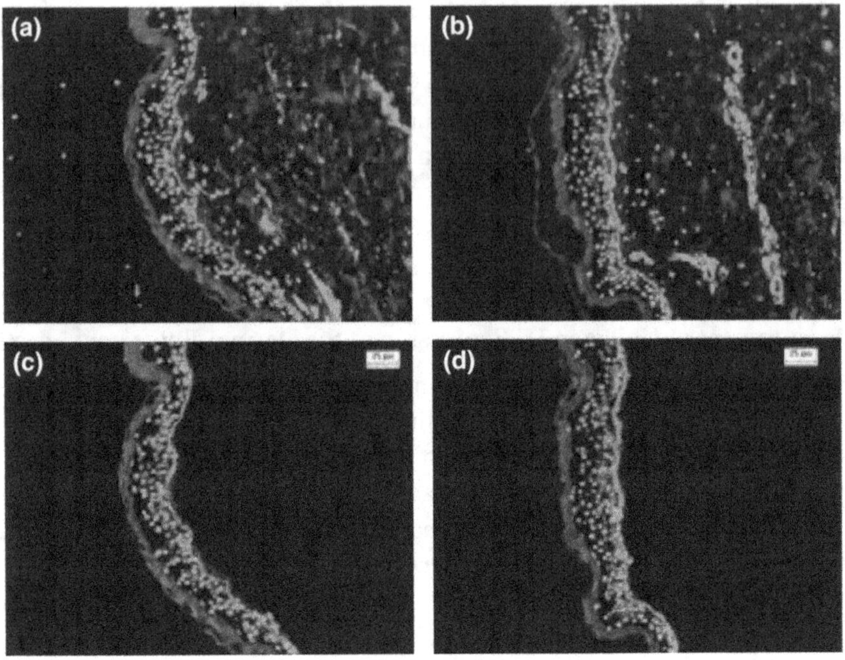

Figure 37: Fluorescent photomicrographs of thin skin sections stained with DAPI and antibody-labelled Alexa Fluor 488 to monitor collagen IV expression at the dermal–epidermal junction. Images are shown for (a) placebo and (b) active ingredient treated samples. The (c) placebo and (d) active ingredient treated sample are also shown after image segmentation and calibration. Reprinted from McMullen et al. with permission from Society of Cosmetic Scientists and the Société Française de Cosmétologie, © 2010.[84]

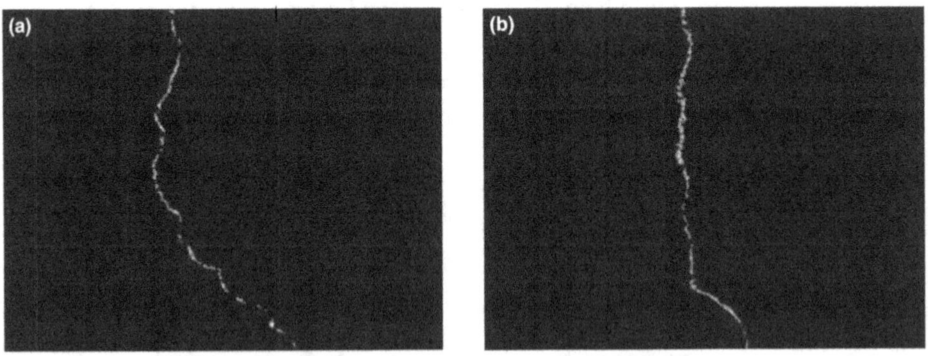

Figure 38: Color segmentation of the fluorescence that appears at the dermal–epidermal junction (as a result of collagen IV expression) in Figure 37. Reprinted from McMullen et al. with permission from Society of Cosmetic Scientists and the Société Française de Cosmétologie, © 2010.[84]

CONCLUSION

The world around us has changed so much over the last two decades. Advances in technology have changed the way that we communicate and socialize on a grand scale. Imaging science has benefited greatly due to these strides in technology. Thinking back to the late 1990s, it was still not possible to acquire a DSLR camera with resolution on parity with its film SLR counterpart. Nowadays, it is common for most laboratories and clinical centers to have a multi-spectral multi-modal image analysis system offering advanced imaging solutions in the evaluation of skin aging, melanin production, erythema, and acne vulgaris.

The development of fringe projection methods revolutionized the way we look at skin topography. Other complex instruments, such as the reflectance confocal microscope, experienced a boom in development leading to many new ways to look inside the skin. Now we can perform *in vivo* studies that provide histological-type information to clinicians and researchers. Likewise, image analysis techniques have also come a long way thanks to advances in computer software and hardware technology.

ACKNOWLEDGMENTS

The author would like to thank Dr. Guojin Zhang for her contribution of the AFM images. Also, a word of gratitude goes to Dr. Gopi Menon for engaging in intriguing discussions on the microscopy of skin and for his contributions to the TEM section of the manuscript.

REFERENCES

1. R Velthuizen et al. (2007). Quantifying skin ashing using cross-polarized imaging. In K.-P. Wilhelm, P. Elsner, E. Berardesca & H. Maibach (Eds.), *Bioengineering of the Skin*. New York: Informa Healthcare.
2. C El Gammal et al. (2007). Anatomy of the skin surface. In K.-P. Wilhelm, P. Elsner, E. Berardesca & H. Maibach (Eds.), *Bioengineering of the Skin: Skin Imaging and Analysis*. New York: Informa Healthcare.
3. S Phillips et al., Polarized light photography enhances visualization of inflammatory lesions of acne vulgaris, *J Am Acad Dermatol,* 37, 948-952 (1997).
4. R Anderson, Polarized light examination and photography of the skin, *Arch Dermatol,* 127, 1000-1005 (1991).
5. N Aspres et al., Imaging the skin, *Australas J Dermatol,* 44, 19-27 (2003).
6. R Anderson and J Parrish, The optics of human skin, *J Invest Dermatol,* 77, 13-19 (1981).

7. J Facq et al., A simple replica technique for the observation of human skin, *J Soc Cosmet Chem,* 15, 87-98 (1964).
8. V Mazzarello et al., Analysis of the microtopography of the skin by silicone replicas after repeated exposure to actinic radiation at high altitudes, *JEADV,* 15, 224-228 (2001).
9. L Yin et al., Skin premature aging induced by tobacco smoking: the objective evidence of skin replica analysis, *J Dermatol Sci,* 27 (Suppl. 1), S26-S31 (2001).
10. G Grove et al., Skin replica analysis of photodamaged skin after therapy with tretinoin emollient cream, *J Am Acad Dermatol,* 25, 231-237 (1991).
11. R Keyhani et al., Qualification of a precise and easy-to-handle sweat casting imprint method for the prediction and quantification of antiperspirant efficacy, *Int J Cosmet Sci,* 31, 183-192 (2009).
12. T Cook, Profilometry of skin—a useful tool for the substantiation of cosmetic efficacy, *J Soc Cosmet Chem,* 31, 339-359 (1980).
13. S Makki et al., Statistical analysis and three-dimensional representation of the human skin surface, *J Soc Cosmet Chem,* 35, 311-325 (1984).
14. J Welzel and H Wolff. (1997). Laser profilometry. In K.-P. Wilhelm, P. Elsner, E. Berardesca & H. Maibach (Eds.), *Bioengineering of the Skin: Skin Surface Imaging and Analysis*. Boca Raton, FL: CRC Press.
15. H Kang et al., Image analysis of the skin surface topography after repeated exposure to surfactants, *Kor J Invest Dermatol,* 1, 75-81 (1994).
16. R Ryan et al., A replica technique for the evaluation of human skin by scanning electron microscopy, *J Cutan Pathol,* 10, 262-276 (1983).
17. R McMullen et al., Influence of various environmental parameters on sweat gland activity, *J Cosmet Sci,* 64, 1-18 (2013).
18. J Lagarde et al., Skin topography measurement by interference fringe projection: a technical validation, *Skin Res Technol,* 7, 112-121 (2001).
19. T Callaghan and K-P Wilhelm, A review of ageing and an examination of clinical methods in the assessment of ageing skin. Part 2: clinical perspectives and clinical methods in the evaluation of ageing skin *Int J Cosmet Sci,* 30, 323-332 (2008).
20. S Jaspers et al., Rapid in vivo measurement of the topography of human skin by active image triangulation usuing a digital micromirror device, *Skin Res Technol,* 5, 195-207 (1999).
21. L Tchvialeva et al. (2010). Skin roughness assessment. In D. Campolo (Ed.), *New Developments in Biomedical Engineering*. Vukovar, Croatia: In-Teh.

22. J Lagarde et al., Topography and anisotropy of the skin surface with ageing, *Skin Res Technol,* 11, 110-119 (2005).
23. U Jacobi et al., In vivo determination of skin surface topography using an optical 3D device, *Skin Res Technol,* 10, 207-214 (2004).
24. M Roh et al., Sebum output as a factor contributing to the pore size of facial pores, *Cutan Biol,* 155, 890-894 (2006).
25. B Kim et al., Sebum, acne, skin elasticity, and gender difference - which is the major influencing factor for facial pores?, *Skin Res Technol,* 19(19), e45-e53 (2013).
26. S Kim et al., Pore volume is most highly correlated with the visual assessment of skin pores, *Skin Res Technol,* Mar 20. doi: 10.1111/srt.12135, 1-6 (2014).
27. E Uhoda et al., The conundrum of skin pores in dermocosmetology, *Dermatology,* 210(1), 3-7 (2005).
28. H Jo et al., Quantitative research on skin pore widening using a stereoimage optical topometer and sebutape, *Skin Res Technol,* 13, 162-168 (2007).
29. K Sugata et al., Confocal laser microscopic imaging of conspicuous facial pores in vivo: relation between the appearance and the internal structure of skin, *Skin Res Technol,* 14, 208-212 (2008).
30. J Fulton, Utilizing the ultraviolet (UV detect) camera to enhance the appearance of photodamage and other skin conditions, *Dermatol Surg,* 23, 163-169 (1997).
31. N Kollias et al., Fluorescence photography in the evaluation of hyperpigmentation in photodamaged skin, *J Am Acad Dermatol,* 36, 226-230 (1997).
32. B Gilchrest et al., Localization of melanin pigmentation in the skin with Wood's lamp, *Br J Dermatol,* 96, 245-248 (1977).
33. S Arai. (1997). Analysis of pigmentation of human skin (UV-light images). In K. Wilhelm, P. Elsner, E. Berardesca & H. Maibach (Eds.), *Bioengineering of the Skin: Skin Surface Imaging and Analysis*. Boca Raton: CRC Press.
34. Z Draelos et al., A novel ultraviolet photography technique for assessing photodamage, *J Cosmet Dermatol,* 7, 205-209 (2008).
35. L Lucchina et al., Fluorescence photography in the evaluation of acne, *J Am Acad Dermatol,* 35, 58-63 (1996).
36. S Patwardhan et al., Auto-classification of acne lesions using multimodal imaging, *J Drugs Dermatol,* 12, 746-756 (2013).
37. R McMullen et al., Spectrofluorescence of skin and hair, *Int J Cosmet Sci,* 34, 246-256 (2012).

38. R Na et al., Autofluorescence of human skin is age-related after correction for skin pigmentation and redness, *J Invest Dermatol,* 116, 536-540 (2001).
39. R Korichi et al., Quantitative assessment of properties of make-up products by video imaging: application to lipsticks, *Skin Res Technol,* 6, 222-229 (2000).
40. S Yadav et al., Luster measurements of lips treated with lipstick formulations, *J Cosmet Sci,* 62, 317-325 (2011).
41. J Ryu et al., Improving lip wrinkles: lipstick-related image analysis, *Skin Res Technol,* 11, 157-164 (2005).
42. K Miyamoto et al. (2007). Development of a digital imaging system for objective measurement of hyperpigmented spots on the face. In K.-P. Wilhelm, P. Elsner, E. Berardesca & H. Maibach (Eds.), *Bioengineering of the Skin*. New York: Informa Healthcare.
43. T Callaghan and K-P Wilhelm. (2007). Noninvasive imaging in the evaluation of cellulite. In K.-P. Wilhelm, P. Elsner, E. Berardesca & H. Maibach (Eds.), *Bioengineering of the Skin: Skin Imaging and Analysis*. New York: Informa Healthcare.
44. S Bielfeldt et al., Non-invasive evaluation techniques to quantify the efficacy of cosmetic anti-cellulite products, *Skin Res Technol,* 14, 336-346 (2008).
45. E Sattler et al., Optical coherence topography in dermatology, *J Biomed Opt,* 18, 061224 (2013).
46. M Ulrich et al., Clinical applicability of in vivo reflectance confocal microscopy in dermatology, *G Ital Dermatol Venereol,* 147, 171-178 (2012).
47. A Gerger et al., In vivo confocal laser scanning microscopy in the diagnosis of melanocytic skin tumours, *Br J Dermatol,* 160, 475-481 (2009).
48. M Ulrich and S Lange-Asschenfeldt, In vivo confocal microscopy in dermatology: from research to clinical application, *J Biomed Opt,* 18, 061212 (2013).
49. K Nehal et al., Skin imaging with reflectance confocal microscopy, *Semin Cutan Med Surg,* 27, 37-43 (2008).
50. S Gonzalez and Y Gilaberte-Calzada, In vivo reflectance-mode confocal microscopy in clinical dermatology and cosmetology, *Int J Cosmet Sci,* 30, 1-17 (2008).
51. P Calzavara-Pinton et al., Reflectance confocal microscopy for in vivo skin imaging, *Photochem Photobiol,* 84, 1421-1430 (2008).
52. *Confocal Laser Scanning Microscopy*. Jena, Germany: Carl Zeiss.
53. J Tavoloni Bragaa et al., In vivo confocal microscopy: a promising diagnostic method for cutaneous oncology, *J Clin Exp Dermatol Res,* S3:002, doi:10.4172/2155-9554 (2012).

54. R Kleinerman et al., Ultrasound in dermatology: principles and applications, *J Am Acad Dermatol,* 67, 478-487 (2012).

55. W Siems et al., Improvement in skin elasticity and dermal revitalization in the treatment of cellulite and connective tissue weakness by means of Extracorporeal Pulse Activation Therapy: EPAT, *Aesthet Surg J,* 28, 538-544 (2008).

56. J MacGregor and E Tanzi, Microfocused ultrasound for skin tightening, *Semin Cutan Med Surg,* 32, 18-25 (2013).

57. M Quan et al., Non-invasive in vivo techniques to differentiate photodamage and ageing in human skin, *Acta Derm Venereol,* 77, 416-419 (1997).

58. X Wortsman and G Jemec. (2013). *Dermatologic Ultrasound with Clinical and Histologic Correlations*. New York: Springer.

59. J Serup et al. (2006). High frequency ultrasound examination of skin: introduction and guide. In J. Serup, G. Jemec & G. Grove (Eds.), *Non-invasive Methods and the Skin* (2nd ed.). Boca Raton, FL: Taylor & Francis.

60. S Seidenari. (2006). Ultrasound B-mode imaging and in vivo structure analysis. In J. Serup, G. Jemec & G. Grove (Eds.), *High frequency ultrasound examination of skin: introduction and guide* (2nd ed.). Boca Raton, FL: Taylor & Francis.

61. M Gniadecka. (2006). Ultrasound assessment of dermal water and edema in vivo. In J. Serup, G. Jemec & G. Grove (Eds.), *Non-invasive Methods and the Skin* (2nd ed.). Boca Raton, FL: Taylor & Francis.

62. G Pellacani et al. (2006). Ultrasound assessment of skin aging. In J. Serup, G. Jemec & G. Grove (Eds.), *Non-invasive Methods and the Skin* (2nd ed.). Boca Raton, FL: Taylor & Francis.

63. X Wortsman et al. (2006). Ultrasound imaging of subcutaneous tissue and adjacent structures. In J. Serup, G. Jemec & G. Grove (Eds.), *Non-invasive Methods and the Skin* (2nd ed.). Boca Raton, FL: Taylor & Francis.

64. D Rallan and C Harlan, Ultrasound in dermatology—basic principles and applications, *Clin Exp Dermatol,* 28, 632-638 (2003).

65. B Forslind. (2006). Skin replication for light and scanning electron microscopy. In J. Serup, G. Jemec & G. Grove (Eds.), *Handbook of Non-invasive methods and the skin* (2nd ed.). Boca Raton, FL: Taylor & Francis.

66. C Garber and C Nightingale, Characterizing cosmetic effects and skin morphology by scanning electron microscopy, *J Soc Cosmet Chem,* 27, 509-531 (1976).

67. M Mihara. (1997). Scanning electron micrscopy. In K.-P. Wilhelm, P. Elsner, E. Berardesca & H. Maibach (Eds.), *Bioengineering of the Skin: Skin Surface Imaging and Analysis*. Boca Raton, FL: CRC Press.

68. J Caussin et al., Lipophilic and hydrophilic moisturizers show different actions on human skin as revealed by cryo scanning electron microscopy, *Exp Dermatol,* 16, 891-898 (2007).

69. W Montagna and P Parakkal. (1974). *The Structure and Function of Skin* (3rd ed.). New York: Academic Press.

70. K Wolff and E Wolff-Schreiner, Trends in electron microscopy of skin, *J Invest Dermatol,* 67, 39-57 (1976).

71. G Odland. (1991). Structure of the skin. In L. Goldsmith (Ed.), *Physiology, Biochemistry, and Molecular Biology of the Skin* (2nd ed.). New York: Oxford UP.

72. P Wertz, Lipids and barrier function of the skin, *Acta Derm Venereol,* Supp 208, 7-11 (2000).

73. G Menon and P Elias. (2001). The epidermal barrier and strategies for surmounting it: an overview. In U. Hengge & B. Volc-Platzer (Eds.), *The Skin and Gene Therapy*. Berlin: Springer.

74. G Menon and R Ghadially, Morphology of lipid alterations in the epidermis: a review, *Microscop Res Tech,* 37, 180-192 (1997).

75. N Kashibuchi et al., Three-dimensional analyses of individual corneocytes with atom force microscope: morphological changes related to age, location and to the pathologic skin conditions, *Skin Res Technol,* 8, 203-211 (2002).

76. R Gaikwad et al., Atomic force microscopy characterization of corneocytes: effect of moisturizer on their topology, rigidity, and friction, *Skin Res Technol,* 16, 275-282 (2010).

77. B Bhushan et al., Friction and durability of virgin and damaged skin with and without skin cream treatment using atomic force microscopy, *Beilstein J Nanotechnol,* 3, 731-746 (2012).

78. S Strassera et al., Structural investigations on native collagen type I fibrils using AFM, *Biochem Biophys Res Comm,* 354, 27-32 (2007).

79. E ten Grotenhuis et al., Phase behavior of stratum corneum lipids in mixed Langmuir-Blodgett monolayers, *Biophys J,* 71, 1389-1399 (1996).

80. L Norlén et al., Stratum corneum lipid organization as observed by atomic force, confocal and two-photon excitation fluorescence microscopy, *Int J Cosmet Sci,* 30, 391-411 (2008).

81. A Kligman and E Christophers, Preparation of isolated sheets of human stratum corneum, *Arch Dermatol,* 88, 702-705 (1963).

82. J Russ. (2002). *The Image Processing Handbook.* Boca Raton, FL: CRC Press.

83. R Wooton et al. (1995). *Image Analysis in Histology: Conventional and Confocal Microscopy.* Cambridge, UK: University Press.

84. R McMullen et al., Image analysis to quantify histological and immunofluorescent staining of *ex vivo* skin and skin cell cultures, *Int J Cosmet Sci,* 32, 143-154 (2010).

PART 11.3

BIOPHYSICAL MEASUREMENT AND EVALUATION OF SKIN ELASTICITY AND TOPOGRAPHY

Authors
Stefanie Luebberding, PhD
Nils Krueger, PhD
IRosenpark Research
Wilhelminenstraße 13
64283 Darmstadt (Germany)

ABSTRACT

The skin is the only organ of the human body that allows an assessment by sensory perception: seeing and feeling. However, the quality of this subjective assessment strongly depends upon the clinical experience of the investigator and while "one picture is worth a thousand words," it is, unfortunately, prone to bias and inter-observer variation. Further, some subclinical morphological changes and physiological processes of the skin are not visible to the naked eye or cannot be assessed by tactile senses. **Biophysical measurement systems** fill this gap, as they allow a highly objective measurement of functional and morphological skin conditions. Since cosmetic science has become a field of high-tech research and development, biophysical measurement systems are an essential part of the evaluation process to determine the efficacy of cosmeceuticals.

Nowadays, a broad range of highly specialized skin care products are available on the market for any imaginable indication and consumer need. *However, anti-aging products that target the signs of aging are still the most important category when it comes to cosmeceuticals.*

Aging of the largest organ in the body, the skin, is a complex process that comes along with the natural aging process of the human body and results in several functional and aesthetic changes of the skin.

Two main mechanisms, atrophy and changes in the architectural organization of the dermal connective tissue, are involved in lifetime alterations of the human skin. They lead to a progressive loss of elasticity and the development of facial wrinkles. These signs are considered to be the most visible changes due to aging, and are therefore strongly related to the development of numerous anti-aging treatments and cosmetic procedures. In this context, biophysical measuring methods to objectively evaluate skin topography and elasticity are of particular interest for the assessment of anti-aging skin care.

TABLE OF CONTENTS:

11.3.1 SKIN TOPOGRAPHY

The skin surface is a polygonal relief consisting of furrows, wrinkles and wavelike structure representing the three-dimensional organization of epidermis, dermis, and subcutis. It is influenced by a wide range of morphologic characteristics such as the thickness of the *stratum corneum*, the amount of collagen in the dermis, or the size and structure of subcutaneous fat cells [1; 2].

The skin surface relief is characterized by typical patterns of intersecting lines and regularly dispersed follicular and eccrine duct openings. Primary and secondary lines form a criss-cross pattern consisting of triangles and parallelograms that are particularly well marked on the back of the hand and forearms. The tertiary lines correspond to the edges of epidermal corneocytes and are, with a depth of <0.5 μm, not visible to the human eye. The quaternary lines are also exceedingly thin, forming a discrete trabecular network on the corneocyte membrane itself [3; 4].

Due to the aging process the skin relief changes strongly (Figure 1); whereas some lines become more marked which results in the development of wrinkles, other lines flatten and disappear with aging. Although, a generally accepted definition of the term "wrinkles" does not exist, they loosely can be classified in crinkles and linear rhytides [4; 5]. Whereas crinkles disappear when the skin is slightly stretched, linear rhytides will still be visible [6].

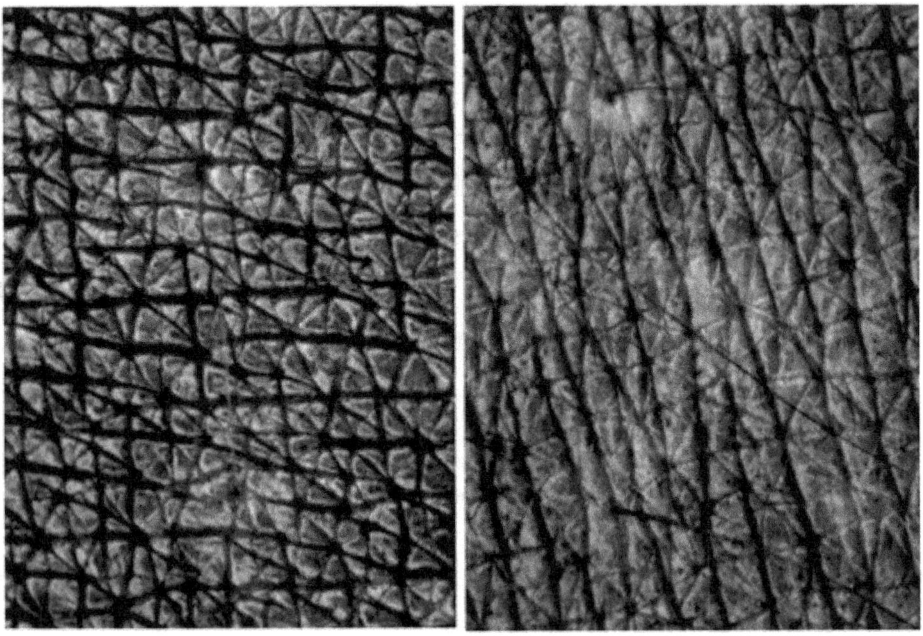

Figure 1: Skin topography, imaged by Visioscan®, **at the forearm of young (left) and older (right).**

a. Quantitative assessment of skin topography

Over the years, many quantification methods have been developed to objectify skin topography, including two-dimensional (2D) morphological analysis of skin replicas as well as fringe projection method that can be used directly without replicas [1; 7]. Recently, three-dimensional (3D) photogrammetry, also known as stereophotogrammetry, has been added to the armamentarium to noninvasively assess skin topography.

b. Replica-based methods

Profilometry [8] and shadowing method [9] represent techniques using two-dimensional analysis of replicas to evaluate skin surface topography. The most widely used material in the preparation of skin replicas is a monomeric silicone polymer (Silica®, J. & S. Davis, Hertfordshire, UK) that is mixed with a thinner and a catalyzer. Fluidly applied, it spreads onto the skin surface by virtue of its low interfacial energy. At body temperature, it quickly polymerizes to a rubbery mass without noticeable heat of reaction. As the silicone is not hard enough to allow the mechanical measurement, a hard counter-replica has to be prepared [4].

A **mechanical profilometer** is a stylus instrument that is used to measure skin surface roughness [8; 10]. The profilometry technique scans the microrelief of the skin replica with a diamond stylus moving at a constant speed horizontally across the samples. Therefore, deflections and movements of the stylus's tip are directly transformed into an electrical signal as the stylus is moved across the surface. Usually the diamond stylus has a conical shape with a diameter of 5 to 20 μm [1]. The precision of the measurement directly depends on the size of the diameter; the larger the diameter, the more imprecise the measurement, so the narrowest lines or steep increases cannot be precisely scanned [4; 11].

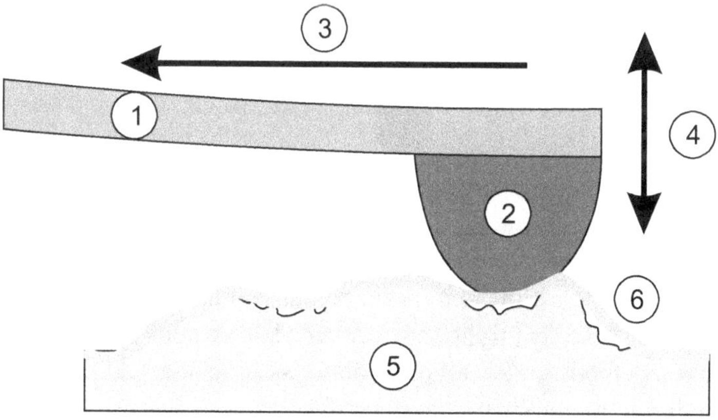

Figure 2: Schematic representation of mechanical profilometry

An advancement over mechanical profilometry is **optical laser profilometry** [12]. This noncontact technique is based on the principle of dynamic focusing: a lens focuses a spot of reflected laser light onto a photodetector, which generates a signal that is proportional to the spot's position on the detector. As the target's surface height changes, the image spot shifts due to the parallax [1].

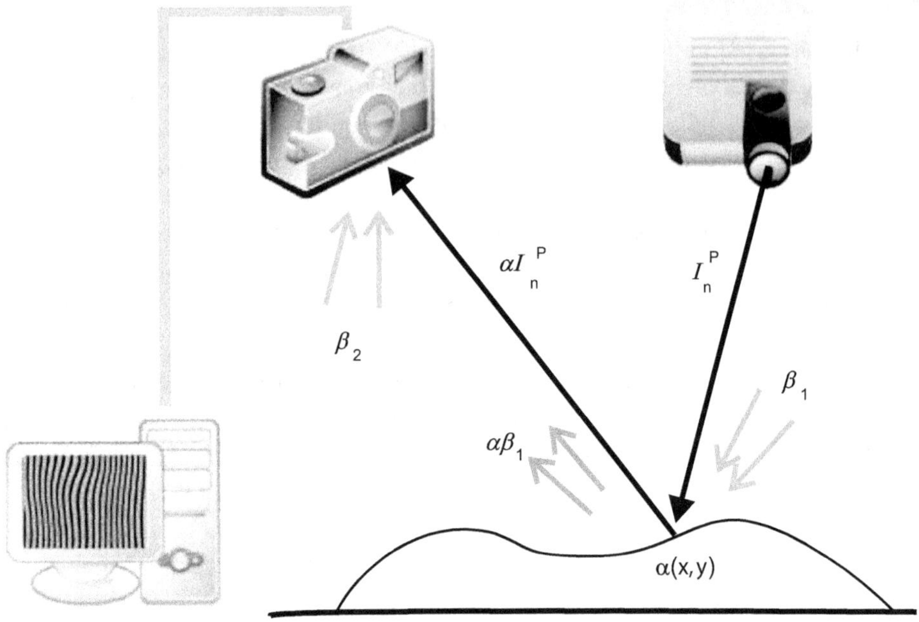

Figure 3: Schematic representation of laser profilometry

The profiles of roughness and waviness assessed by mechanical or optical profilometry are calculated by a computer software such as MapVUE® (KLA Tencor, Milpitas, USA) or Nanovea 3D (Irvine, USA). This technique generates a variety of useful surface parameters that correspond to the international standardization ISO 4284/4287. They include parameters such as Ra (mean value of roughness), Rmax (maximum single depth of roughness), Rz (mean of five measurements of depth of roughness) [1].

Profilometry techniques have the advantage of assessing skin topography with a high degree of accuracy and precision (<0.5 µm), but the scanning of skin replica is very slow [4] and large skin structures such as cellulite cannot be evaluated. Due to the mechanical load on the skin replica, material properties can be changed so that further measurements might be defective [11]. In addition, the preparation of replicas is often defective, and there is a high risk of losing accurate morphological information during the replication process [1; 9].

A more rapid method employed to assess skin topography is the **shadowing method** (also: shadowing casting method), which was developed in the early 80s. This imaging technique is contact free and is also based on the evaluation of empirical parameters generated from skin replicas [9].

The replica of the skin surface is irradiated by a parallel-beam light source with a defined incident angle. Bot, the light intensity and its incident angle, significantly influence the measurement and have to be chosen according to the depth and density of the relief [4]. The generated pattern of light and shadows is optically recorded by a camera. In order to assess the structure of the whole skin replica, the object is slowly rotated and imaged after every movement [13]. The underlying technique is based on the principle of triangulation.

The principal advantage of the shadowing method is that the imaging survey is about 15 times faster by comparison to the profilometry technique—whereas at the same time, a larger area can be assessed. It is further contact-free, so that the skin replicas are not altered during the measurement. A disadvantage of the method is that small structures can probably not be assessed precisely because large structures obliterate smaller structures [9; 14]. Also, the individual adjustment of the angle of the incident light as well as the intensity of lighting in general might contain errors [4].

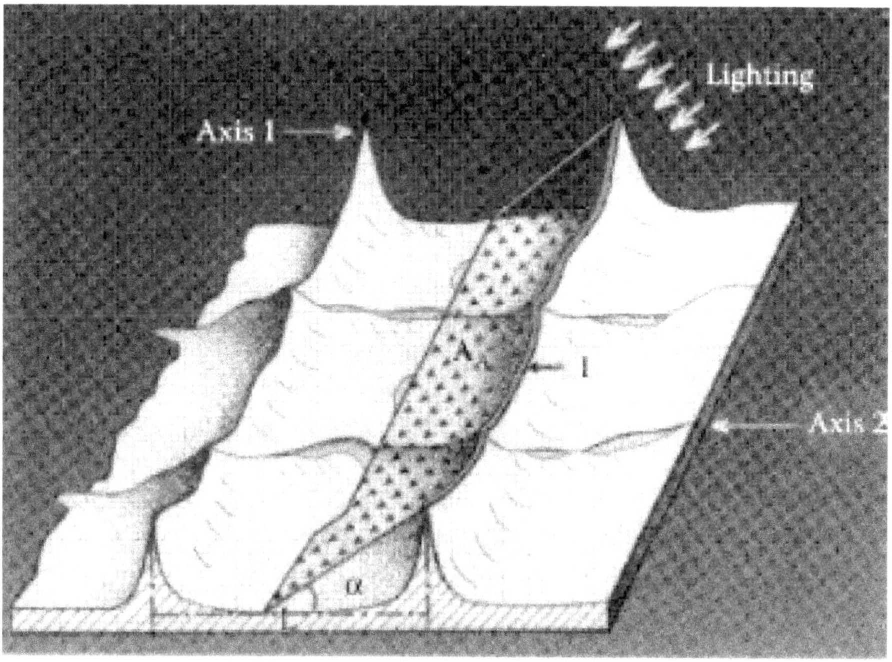

Figure 1: Working principle of the shadowing method

c. 3D Photogrammetry

Recently, digital 3D photogrammetry, also known as **stereophotogrammetry,** has become available for the noninvasive capturing of skin topography. This method is based on a group of cameras that capture two or more images of the same subject from different angles simultaneously. The digital processing of the captured images allows the three-dimensional reconstruction of the surface, which can be quantified in terms of angles, surface areas, and volume [15; 16]. For the assessment of anti-wrinkle products, the volume parameter has become one of the most important parameters as it is most suitable to show a change in overall wrinkle severity before and after a treatment. While the technique is only minimally sensitive to changes in the skin reflection, hair and other small objects on the skin surface are a common cause of artifacts and should therefore be removed carefully before images are taken.

Several devices with this technique are commercially available. The most commonly used system in cosmetic science is the VECTRA® M3 Imaging System (Canfield Scientific, USA). This system consists of three pods with two cameras and one flash each and a connected computer system. Synchronized 2D images of the subjects with 36 megapixels are captured with the six cameras within 3.5 milliseconds. The subsequent 3D reconstruction process is displayed on the monitors and takes up to several minutes. After completion, the 3D model will be mapped with 2D textures and the captured structure can be rotated in all three dimensions. The acquired 3D coordinates can be used to calculate distances between points allowing the measurement of volumetric changes [17; 18]. Several 3D models can be matched by manually selecting landmarks to provide the system with reference points [15; 16].

3D photogrammetry is capable of accurately reproducing the surface geometry of the human face, and map realistic color and texture data to the geometric shape [19; 20]. However, published studies evaluating reproducibility and accuracy of the 3D analysis show a measuring accuracy of less than 1 mm [15; 18; 20]. As age-related changes in skin topography are characterized by typical patterns in the micrometer range, stereophotogrammetry is not suitable as a measuring device for wrinkles or small volume changes yet [21]. Nevertheless, photogrammetry systems already have a great impact in the field as they are particular suitable for the clinical rating of skin statuses before and after a treatment [16; 18; 22].

d. Fringe projection method

The latest generation of 3D measuring instruments makes it possible evaluate morphological structures of human skin rapidly, precisely, and directly *in vivo*. This so-called **fringe projection method** is based on the digital projection of a striped pattern in a defined angle onto the skin *in vivo*. By analysis of the distortions of the striped pattern it is possible to reconstruct the three-dimensional structure of the skin [23–25] (Figure 4).

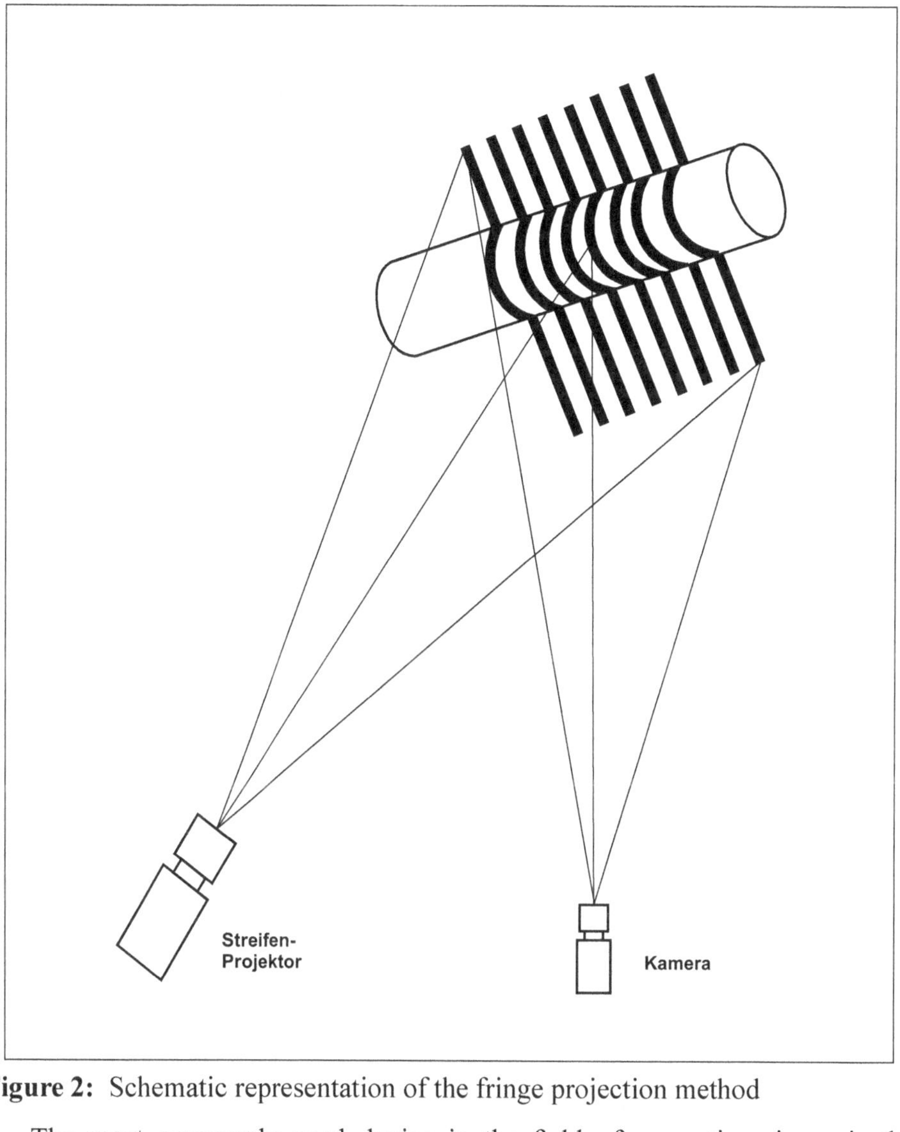

Figure 2: Schematic representation of the fringe projection method

The most commonly used device in the field of cosmetic science is the PRIMOS®-System *(Phaseshift Rapid In Vivo Measurement of the Skin)* produced by GFMesstechnik GmbH (Teltow, Germany). An alternative device based on the same principle is the 3D Breuckmann Scanner (Breuckmann GmbH, Germany).

The PRIMOS®-System consists of a digital micromirror device (DMDTM) as a projection unit, and a charge-coupled device (CCD) camera used as a recording unit (1000 × 620 pixel). The DMD consists of an array of 1024 × 768 square 16 × 16μm² mirrors. Each mirror covers one cell of a complementary metal oxide semiconductor (CMOS) static random access memory (RAM). Depending on the data in the underlying memory cell, each mirror can be titled by means of electrostatic forces either +10° (ON) or −10° (OFF). In the ON position, light is reflected through a projection lens on the surface, whereas mirrors set to the OFF position reflect the light to an absorber. This technique allows projecting a high-resolution pattern of parallel stripes on the skin surface, which is recorded by CCD video technology [26].

The PRIMOS® offers a field of view of 24 × 14 × 13 mm² [23] and measures wrinkle properties from a wrinkle depth of 40 to 50 μm [7]. The measurement of smaller folds *in vivo* is not possible due to pulsating blood flow and slightest body movements. *Skin replicas can be used for the measurement of wrinkles smaller than 40–50 μm.*

To simplify repositioning in follow-up visits the PRIMOS® system provides an overlay function. Therefore, a ghost picture representing the reference localization overlays the live picture—both pictures can be aligned with each other until the images are perfectly congruent. For data evaluation PRIMOS®-System offers also a matching function: 3D-information of both first and follow-up measurement are compared and matched to each other, so that overlapped image areas can be analyzed.

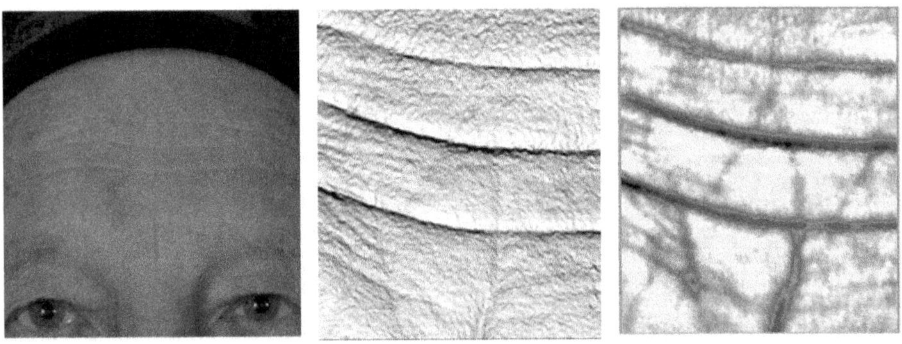

Figure 4: Example of the clinical manifestation of forehead lines of male subjects including images of 3D fringe projection method.

The biggest advantage of the fringe projection method is that the measurement is very fast and can directly be performed *in vivo* so that skin replicas become superfluous [25]. Overlay and matching function facilitate the exact repositioning to guarantee high reliability and reproducibility [21]. A disadvantage might be that the fringe projection method is not able to assess wrinkle properties less that 40–50 μm *in vivo* [7; 27].

The dedicated computer software allows the calculation of ISO 4284/4287 surface parameters. Besides, the PRIMOS software offers also a special wrinkle algorithm to assess skin wrinkles. Therefore, several parameters are particularly useful such as overall average wrinkle depth (W_d), average maximum ($maxW_d$), and maximum largest wrinkle depth (lW_d). Total wrinkle volume (W_v) and wrinkle area (aW_a, pW_a) are the most suitable parameters to assess age-related changes, especially wrinkles [27].

Table 1: Overview of PRIMOS® parameters.

Parameter	Unit
Overall average wrinkle depth (W_d)	µm
Average maximum wrinkle depth ($maxW_d$)	µm
Maximum largest wrinkle depth (lW_d)	µm
Number of wrinkles (W_n)	no
Total wrinkle volume (W_v)	mm^3
Absolute wrinkle area (aW_a)	mm^3
Percentage wrinkle area (pW_a)	%
Wrinkle shape (W_s)	arbitrary units
Wrinkle length (W_l)	µm
Arithmetic average roughness (Ra)	µm
Maximum profile height (Ry)	µm
Arithmetic average of maximum roughness (Rz)	µm

11.3.2 SKIN ELASTICITY

One important function of the human skin is to provide protection against mechanical influences. To enable such protection, the skin exhibits both flexibility and relative resistance to deformation, thus permitting movement and allowing temporary compression and distention of a part at the same time [28]. The tensile functional properties of the skin are due to structural and qualitative components of the epidermis, dermis, and subcutis [29; 30]. However, in terms of mechanical properties, the human skin can be understood as a five-layer structure.

- The **very top layer** is formed by the compact membrane of the *stratum corneum.*

- The **proximal part of the epidermis,** with its underlying desmosomes and the dermo-epidermal junction, represents the second layer.
- Papillary dermis, which is built of loose connective tissue, is the third layer.
- The strong connective tissue of the reticular dermis represents the fourth layer.
- The subcutaneous adipose tissue is the deepest layer [31].

These layers together, consisting of fibers, colloidal substance, motile liquids and a stiff epidermal layer, and their interaction at the various interfaces determine the mechanical properties of the skin [32]. Because of this complex composition of elastic solids and viscous liquids the mechanical properties of the skin are neither elastic nor viscous, but rather viscoelastic [33].

Although biophysical measuring methods have been used to assess skin elasticity for more than 30 years, it is not yet possible to assign elasticity parameters to one single structural element of the skin. Evidence is given that the elastic fibers permit the skin to return spontaneously to its initial shape after deformation [34; 35]. Thereby, not only the absolute amount of elastic fibers is relevant, but also their length and orientation. Usually elastic fibers are vertically oriented as a network and link the dermo-epidermal junction with the horizontally orientated collagen fibers. If this architectural structure is impaired due to an excessive and uncontrolled elastin proliferation, the elastic recovery capability of the skin is partly or totally lost [36]. Collagen fibers do not have any elastic properties, but rather are essential for mechanical stability and its resistance to deformation [28]. In unstretched skin collagen, collagen fibers are organized as disordered bundles. As the skin is stretched, the bundles unfold until the collagen fibers reach their maximum length. Therefore, a lack of collagen fibers, or a degenerated collagen architecture due to intrinsic and/or extrinsic skin aging or skin disease, results in a high distensibility, slackness, and a higher sensitivity regarding mechanical tension [31; 37].

Besides the role of elastin and collagen fibers, the hydration level of the epidermis and dermis also influence skin elasticity. It is known that a moistening of the epidermis with water results in an increase of distensibility and skin fatigue—but at the same time skin elasticity decreases. Also, a lack of hydration correlates in clinical evaluation with a loss of elasticity [31].

a. Quantitative assessment of skin elasticity

The noninvasive assessment of the mechanical properties of the human skin *in vivo* can be performed by distinct methods mainly characterized by the evaluation of the nature and orientation of skin deformation after an imposed force [28]. Thereby, the available techniques can be grouped into several different classes. These include: tensile with electric dynamometers [38], the torsion method [39], and impact testing (balistometrique technique) [40]. The elevation testing approach by means of the suction chamber method is actually the most frequently used tool to assess skin mechanics [28; 31].

b. Tensile Testing

Tensile testing is based on recording skin extension following the imposition of a parallel force to skin's surface [28]. Therefore, tensile testing with electric dynamometers is the oldest commercialized device for investigating mechanical properties of the skin [38]. In this procedure, based on uniaxial tension, a small disk sticks on the skin and is set into forward and backward motion by the electric dynamometers. The stretching of the skin is recorded on the *x*-axis as superimposed ellipses (Figure 7). The steepness of the slope of the ellipse gives information about the mechanical properties of the skin such as stiffness, elasticity, and viscoelasticity [41; 42].

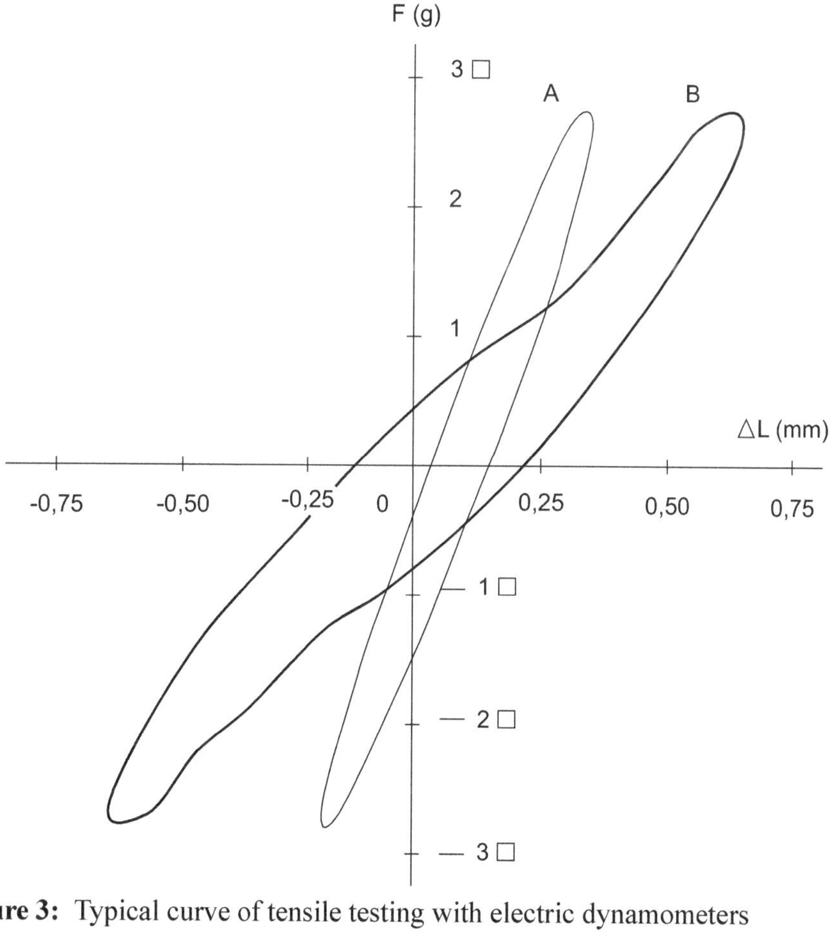

Figure 3: Typical curve of tensile testing with electric dynamometers

c. Torsion technique

The measuring probe of the torsion method consists of a central disk and a peripheral ring that is glued firmly onto the skin with double-sided adhesive tape. Due to the application of a constant torque applied by the disk to the skin, it is deformed and the degree of deformation is dependent on the mechanical properties of the skin (Figure 8) [39; 41]. Analysis of the resulting rotation angle (in degrees) of the disk versus time (seconds) provides information about the standard deformation parameters including skin elasticity, firmness, or the mechanical fatigue of the skin [43]. The assessment can be adapted by variation of number, duration, intensity, and rhythm of the twisting as well as by the dimension of the rings. To examine the mechanical properties of the epidermis a ring with a diameter of 1 mm is used, whereas rings with a higher diameter are used to include underlying skin layers [41].

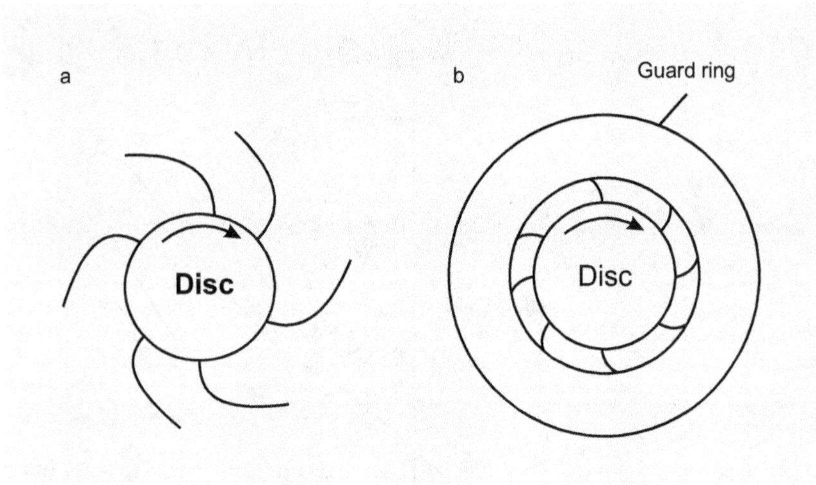

Figure 4: Schematic overview of skin deformation due to torsion method

d. Impact technique

The impact testing of the human skin, also called ballistometrique technique, was designed to approach specific tensile functions of the skin involving the deeper skin layers [28]. The balistometrique technique records the successive rebounds of a small hammer being dropped on the skin's surface with defined energy [40; 44]. The more kinetic energy is transformed into rebound, the more elastic is the surface [41]. Because of the viscoelastic properties of the human skin, parts of the rebounding energy are lost with every restitution phase, so that height and duration of the hammer decrease with every rebound. The induced rebounds are transduced into electrical signals that can be quantified and evaluated in terms of their amplitude and frequency [28]. The main parameter of the balistometrique technique is the so-called rebound-coefficient, which is calculated from the ratio between the heights of the first and second rebound. The rebound-coefficient depends mainly on skin elasticity and viscosity [28; 41].

e. Elevation Technique

Elevation technique using suction chamber devices are commonly used to determine noninvasively the mechanical properties of the skin [45–47]. The underlying principle of the suction chamber method is to assess skin extension caused by a negative pressure [31; 48–50]. Based on the measurement of the extension in comparison to the height and the duration of the vacuum, several skin elasticity parameters can be calculated. These include: skin distensibility, elasticity, or firmness [31].

Besides the Dermaflex® (Cortex Technology, Denmark), the Cutometer® (Courage & Khazaka, Germany) is the most used measuring device to assess skin elasticity in vivo. It measures the vertical deformation of the skin when it is pulled by a controlled vacuum into the probe (Figure 5). The depth of the penetration is assessed by a contact-less, optical measuring method containing of an infrared light source, a receiver and two facing prisms that project the light from sender to receiver. The intensity of the projected light depends on the penetration depth of the skin into the probe [51].

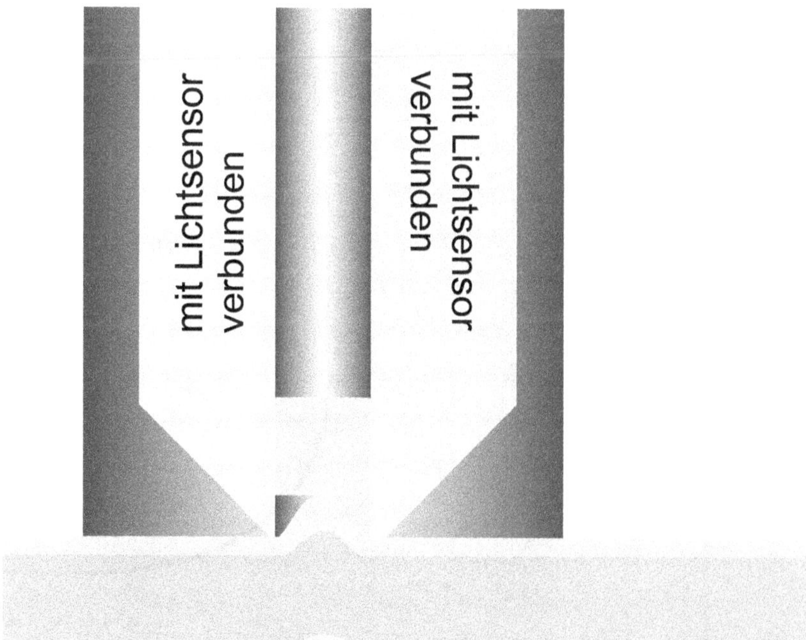

Figure 5: Schematic representation of the suction chamber method.

The Cutometer® has a measuring probe which is connected over a hose to the vacuum pump and the measuring system. The opening of the suction probe has a standard diameter of 2mm, alternatively probes with a larger diameter up to 8mm are available. While the 2mm probe is primarily suitable to assess the elasticity of the epidermis; 4 to 6 mm can be used to evaluate upper skin layers up to the papillary dermis, and the 8mm opening can be used to assess all skin layers [51]. The negative pressure can be adjusted between 20 to 500 mbar and the pressure buildup can be generated abrupt or gradual. Suction and relaxing time can vary between 0.1 and 60 seconds with a maximum repetition up to 99 times.

The suction chamber method represents the deformation of the skin in terms of the time and offers different measurement modes due to pressure variations. In scientific practice a pre-set constant negative pressure of 200 to 500 mbar is commonly used. Therefore, frequent practices are measurements with 3 to 10 cycles and suction and relaxing time of 2 to 5 seconds [33]. Elongation and retraction of the skin is presented on an external monitor already during the measurement.

A typical measuring curve consists of four phases (Figure 8). The first phase is characterized by a sharp increase, which explains the elastic extension of the skin. The second phase, representing the viscoelastic proportion of extension, is shown by flattening of the curve. Upon pressure discontinuation the curve sharply declines. This third phase represents the elastic proportion of recovery, which is followed by a flattening of the curve, which represents the viscoelastic proportion of recovery.

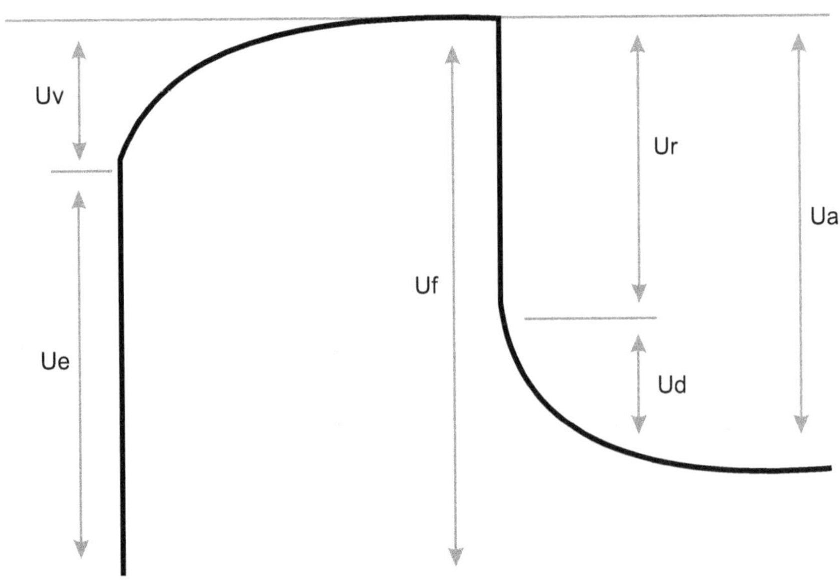

Figure 6: Skin deformation assessed by suction chamber method.

The evaluation of the stress-strain and strain-time curves obtained with the Cutometer® allows the calculation of several tensile variables representing skin's elasticity, distensibility, or recovery after deformation [28; 52] (Table 1). Parameters that are particularly suitable to assess age-related changes of the skin including the ratio of elastic recovery to distensibility (Ur /Uf), as well as the gross (Ua/Uf) and net elasticity (Ur/Ue) for evaluation of aging effects on the mechanical properties of skin [53].

Table 2: Most suitable parameters to evaluate skin aging.

Ratio of elastic recovery to distensibility	Ur/Uf
Gross elasticity	Ua/Uf
Net elasticity	Ur/Ue
Maximum recovery	Ua
Immediate recovery	Ur
Skin distensibility of the last curve	Uf5
Skin distensibility	Uf
Immediate distensibility	Ue

CONCLUSION

The use of reliable and accurate noninvasive biophysical measuring methods is an integral part of dermatology and cosmetic science nowadays. Only the objective examination of skin *in vivo* makes it possible to assess both subclinical morphological and functional changes of the skin needed for the neutral monitoring of treatment success.

However, even though the specificity and sensitivity of most biophysical measuring methods is very high, those instruments may suffer from a series of biases that can falsify the results. For instance, environmental factors such as inadequate laboratory conditions, unfavorable selection and preconditions of subjects, but also poor study design and application errors can notoriously affect most of the measurements. *Also, the interpretation of the data needs adequate expertise to understand both the technical aspects and the physiological parameters under consideration.*

In conclusion, in the era of evidence-based skin care, biophysical measuring methods have become an essential part of cosmetic science and provide new avenues for evaluation of the effectiveness of ingredients and formulations designed to develop anti-aging products. However, it should be kept in mind that even the best technology is only as precise (and accurate) as the set-up and the people using it allow it to be. Or as already the great Albert Kligman, MD, inventor of the term "cosmeceutical," used to say, "A fool with a tool is still a fool."

The authors encourage the reader to become familiar with the techniques described and proficient in their use as they represent exceedingly useful and promising techniques for development of anti-aging products and ingredients.

REFERENCES

1. Fischer TW, Wigger-Alberti W, Elsner P. Direct and non-direct measurement techniques for analysis of skin surface topography. Skin Pharmacol. Appl. Skin Physiol 1999; 12(1-2): 1–11.
2. Contet-Audonneau JL, Jeanmaire C, Pauly G. A histological study of human wrinkle structures: comparison between sun-exposed areas of the face, with or without wrinkles, and sun-protected areas. Br. J. Dermatol 1999; 140(6): 1038–1047.
3. Piérard GE, Uhoda I, Piérard-Franchimont C. From skin microrelief to wrinkles. An area ripe for investigation. J Cosmet Dermatol 2003; 2(1): 21–28.
4. Lévêque JL. EEMCO guidance for the assessment of skin topography. The European Expert Group on Efficacy Measurement of Cosmetics and other Topical Products. J Eur Acad Dermatol Venereol 1999; 12(2): 103–114.
5. Kligman AM, Zheng P, Lavker RM. The anatomy and pathogenesis of wrinkles. Br. J. Dermatol 1985; 113(1): 37–42.
6. Hatzis J. The wrinkle and its measurement—a skin surface Profilometric method. Micron 2004; 35(3): 201–19.
7. Task Force Committee for Evaluation of Anti-Aging Function. Guidelines for Evaluation of Anti-Wrinkle Products. J Jpn Cosmet Sci Soc 2007; 31(4): 423–431.
8. Grove GL, Grove MJ, Leyden JJ. Optical profilometry: an objective method for quantification of facial wrinkles. J. Am. Acad. Dermatol. 1989; 21(3 Pt 2): 631–637.
9. Corcuff P, Leveque JL. Skin surface replica image analysis of furrows and wrinkles. In: Serup J, Jemec GBE, Grove GL. Handbook of Non-Invasive Methods and the Skin, Second Edition. 2nd edition, CRC Press, Boca Raton, 2006, 89–96.

10. Makki S, Barbenel JC, Agache P. A quantitative method for the assessment of the microtopography of human skin. Acta Derm Venereol 1979; 59(4): 285–91.

11. Cook TH, Craft TJ, Brunelle RL, Norris F, Griffin WA. Quantification of the skin's topography by skin profilometry. Int J Cosmet Sci 1982; 4(5): 195–205.

12. Saur R, Schramm U, Steinhoff R, Wolff HH. Structure analysis of the skin surface using computer-assisted laser profilometry. New method for the quantitative assessment of roughness structure of the skin. Hautarzt 1991; 42(8): 499–506.

13. Corcuff P, Chatenay F, Leveque JL. A fully automated system to study skin surface patterns. Int J Cosmet Sci 1984; 6(4): 167–176.

14. Mignot J. Three-dimensional evaluation of skin surface. Micro- and macrorelief. In: Serup J, Jemec GB, Grove GL. Non-invasive methods and the skin. 2nd edition, Taylor & Francis, Boca Raton, London, New York, 2006, 179–1^93.

15. De Menezes M, Rosati R, Ferrario VF, Sforza C. Accuracy and reproducibility of a 3-dimensional stereophotogrammetric imaging system. J. Oral Maxillofac. Surg. 2010; 68(9): 2129–2135.

16. Gornick M. Digital three-dimensional photogrammetry. Accuracy and precision of facial measurements obtained from two commercially-available imaging systems. 2011;

17. Littlefield TR, Kelly KM, Cherney JC, Beals SP, Pomatto JK. Development of a new three-dimensional cranial imaging system. J Craniofac Surg 2004; 15(1): 175–181.

18. Spanholtz TA, Leitsch S, Holzbach T, Volkmer E, Engelhardt T, Giunta RE. 3-dimensional imaging systems. First experience in planning and documentation of plastic surgery procedures. Handchir Mikrochir Plast Chir 2012; 44(4): 234–239.

19. Heike CL, Upson K, Stuhaug E, Weinberg SM. 3D digital stereophotogrammetry: a practical guide to facial image acquisition. Head Face Med 2010; 618.

20. Weinberg SM, Naidoo S, Govier DP, Martin RA, Kane AA, Marazita ML. Anthropometric precision and accuracy of digital three-dimensional photogrammetry: comparing the Genex and 3dMD imaging systems with one another and with direct anthropometry. J Craniofac Surg 2006; 17(3): 477–483.

21. Luebberding S, Krueger N, Kerscher M. Life-time development of facial wrinkles of men and women: Using three-dimensional fringe projection method and Validated Assessment Scales. Submitted to Dermatolog Surg.;

22. Kau CH, Richmond S, Incrapera A, English J, Xia JJ. Three-dimensional surface acquisition systems for the study of facial morphology and their application to maxillofacial surgery. Int J Med Robot 2007; 3(2): 97–110.

23. Jaspers S. Fringe Projection for In Vivo Topometry. In: Wilhelm KP, Elsner P, Berardesca E. Bioengineering of the Skin: Skin Imaging and Analysis. 2nd edition, Informa Healthcare, Boca Raton, 2006, 137–147.

24. Friedman PM, Skover GR, Payonk G, Kauvar ANB, Geronemus RG. 3D in-vivo optical skin imaging for topographical quantitative assessment of non-ablative laser technology. Dermatol Surg 2002; 28(3): 199–204.

25. Akazaki S, Nakagawa H, Kazama H, Osanai O, Kawai M, Takema Y, Imokawa G. Age-related changes in skin wrinkles assessed by a novel three-dimensional morphometric analysis. Br. J. Dermatol 2002; 147(4): 689–695.

26. Bloemen MCT, van Gerven MS, van der Wal MBA, Verhaegen PDHM, Middelkoop E. An objective device for measuring surface roughness of skin and scars. J. Am. Acad. Dermatol. 2011; 64(4): 706–715.

27. Luebberding S, Krueger N, Kerscher M. Comparison of Validated Assessment Scales and 3D digital fringe projection method to assess lifetime development of wrinkles in men. Skin Res Technol 2013;

28. Rodrigues L. EEMCO Guidance to the in vivo Assessment of Tensile Functional Properties of the Skin. Skin Pharmacology and Physiology 2001; 14(1): 52–67.

29. Wlaschek M, Tantcheva-Poór I, Naderi L, Ma W, Schneider LA, Razi-Wolf Z, Schüller J, Scharffetter-Kochanek K. Solar UV irradiation and dermal photoaging. J. Photochem. Photobiol. B, Biol 2001; 63(1-3): 41–51.

30. Schneider LA, Wlaschek M, Scharffetter-Kochanek K. Skin aging. Clinical aspects and pathogenesis. J Dtsch Dermatol Ges 2003; 1(3): 223–32; quiz 233–4.

31. Gniadecka M, Serup J. Suction Chamber Method for Measuring Skin Mechanical Properties: The Dermaflex®. In: Serup J, Jemec G, Grove G. Non-invasive methods and skin. Taylor & Francis, Boca Raton, New York, London, 2006, 571–577.

32. Oomens CW, van Campen DH, Grootenboer HJ. A mixture approach to the mechanics of skin. J Biomech 1987; 20(9): 877–85.

33. Barel A. Suction chamber method for measurement of skin mechanics. The new digital version of the Cutometer. In: Serup J, Jemec GB, Grove GL. Non-invasive methods and the skin. 2nd edition, Taylor & Francis, Boca Raton, London, New York, 2006, 583–591.

34. Oxlund H. Changes in connective tissues during corticotrophin and corticosteroid treatment. Biomechanical and biochemical studies on muscle tendon, skin and aorta in experimental animals. Dan Med Bull 1984; 31(3): 187–206.

35. Oxlund H, Manschot J, Viidik A. The role of elastin in the mechanical properties of skin. J Biomech 1988; 21(3): 213–218.

36. Vieira ACT, Vieira WT, Michalany N, Enokihara M, Freymüller E, Cestari SCP. Elastoderma of the neck in a teenage boy. J. Am. Acad. Dermatol 2005; 53(2 Suppl 1): S147–9.

37. Kolácná L, Bakesová J, Varga F, Kostáková E, Plánka L, Necas A, Lukás D, Amler E, Pelouch V. Biochemical and biophysical aspects of collagen nanostructure in the extracellular matrix. Physiol Res 2007; 56 Suppl 1S51–60.

38. Wan Abas WA, Barbenel JC. Uniaxial tension test of human skin in vivo. J Biomed Eng 1982; 4(1): 65–71.

39. Agache P. Twistometry measurement of skin elasticity. In: Serup J, Jemec GBE. Handbook of Noninvasive Methods and the Skin. 1st edition, CRC-Press, 1995, 319–328.

40. Hargens C. Ballistometry. In: Serup J, Jemec GBE. Handbook of Non-Invasive Methods and the Skin. 1st edition, Informa Healthcare, 1995, 359–366.

41. Agache P, Varchon D. Mechanical Behaviour Assessment. In: Agache P, Humbert P. Measuring the Skin: Non-invasive Investigations, Physiology, Normal Constants. 1st edition, Springer, 2004, 446–467.

42. Cooper EP, Missel PJ, Hannon DP, Albright GB. Mechanical properties of dry, normal, and glycerol-treated skin as measured by the gas-bearing electrodynamometer. J Soc Cosmet Chem 1985; (36): 335–348.

43. Bazin R, Fanchon C. Equivalence of face and volar forearm for the testing of moisturizing and firming effect of cosmetics in hydration and biomechanical studies. Int J Cosmet Sci 2006; 28(6): 453–460.

44. Adhoute H, Berbis E, Privat Y. Ballistometric properties of aged skin. In: Leveque J-L. Aging Skin: Properties and Functional Changes. illustrated edition., Informa Healthcare, 1993, 39–48.

45. Ahn S, Kim S, Lee H, Moon S, Chang I. Correlation between a Cutometer and quantitative evaluation using Moire topography in age-related skin elasticity. Skin Res Technol 2007; 13(3): 280–284.

46. Cua AB, Wilhelm KP, Maibach HI. Elastic properties of human skin: relation to age, sex, and anatomical region. Arch. Dermatol. Res 1990; 282(5): 283–288.

47. Ryu HS, Joo YH, Kim SO, Park KC, Youn SW. Influence of age and regional differences on skin elasticity as measured by the Cutometer. Skin Res Technol 2008; 14(3): 354–8.

48. Grahame R. A method for measuring human skin elasticity in vivo with observations of the effects of age, sex and pregnancy. Clin Sci 1970; 39(2): 223–9.

49. Elsner P, Wilhelm D, Maibach HI. Mechanical properties of human forearm and vulvar skin. Br. J. Dermatol 1990; 122(5): 607–614.

50. Mine S, Fortunel NO, Pageon H, Asselineau D. Aging Alters Functionally Human Dermal Papillary Fibroblasts but Not Reticular Fibroblasts: A New View of Skin Morphogenesis and Aging. PLoS ONE. 2008; 3(12): e4066.

51. O'goshi K-I. Suction chamber method for measurements of mechanics: The Cutometer. In: Serup J, Jemec G, Grove G. Non-invasive methods and skin. Taylor & Francis, Boca Raton, New York, London, 2006, 579–582.

52. Agache PG, Monneur C, Leveque JL, De Rigal J. Mechanical properties and Young's modulus of human skin in vivo. Arch. Dermatol. Res 1980; 269(3): 221–232.

53. Krueger N, Luebberding S, Oltmer M, Streker M, Kerscher M. Age-related changes in skin mechanical properties: a quantitative evaluation of 120 female subjects. Skin Res Technol 2011; 17(2): 141–148.

GLOSSARY

Polygonal: Any closed curve consisting of a set of line segments connected such that no two segments cross. The simplest polygons are triangles (three sides), quadrilaterals (four sides), and pentagons (five sides).

Subcutis: Subcutaneous tissue (from Latin subcutaneous, meaning "beneath the skin"), also called the hypodermis, hypoderm (from Greek, meaning "beneath the skin"), or superficial fascia. The subcutis is beneath dermis which is beneath epidermis. It is used mainly for fat storage.

Eccrine glands: (/ˈɛkrən/, /ˈɛˌkraɪn/, or /ˈɛˌkrin/; from ekkrinein "secrete"; are the major sweat glands of the human body, found in virtually all skin. They produce a clear, odorless substance, consisting primarily of water and NaCl. They are active in thermoregulation and emotional sweating (induced by anxiety, fear, stress, and pain).

Trabecular: A small, often microscopic, tissue element in the form of a small beam, strut or rod, generally having a mechanical function.

Rhytide: Also known as a wrinkle, is a fold, ridge or crease in the skin. Rhytides typically appear as a result of aging processes.

Counter-replica: A positive replica of the skin created by covering the first (negative) replica with a second silicone material. Counter-replicas are often harder and more resistant to deformation.

Microrelief: Skin is characterized by a structure called micro-relief. This relief reveals a network of triangles and diamond shapes dotted with hair follicle and sebaceous gland openings.

PART 11.5

CLINICAL TESTING OF COSMETICS AND SKIN CARE PRODUCTS: METHODS AND INSTRUMENTATIONS

Author
Iqbal Sadiq, M.Phil.
Director Research and Technology
Product Investigations, Inc.
151 East Tenth Ave., Conshohocken, PA 19428, USA

ABSTRACT

In the field of skin research, visual examination and touch are no longer solely employed to assess skin conditions. The field has evolved to include instrumental methodologies to quantitatively and qualitatively assess skin properties. Principles of physics, chemistry, biology, and engineering are combined to study skin both at the surface and in-depth.

Cosmetics and Skincare products are used to enhance the look and feel of the skin and to protect the body from the elements of nature. To study the effects of cosmetics and skin care products on skin, biophysical measuring techniques can be employed in a variety of experimental models. Both dose-response and time-response studies can be performed with greater precision. For example, topical products may affect skin in a variety of ways (e.g., changes in *stratum corneum* hydration, trans-epidermal water loss, blood flow, pigment, morphology and elasticity, etc. These changes are measured by different instruments.

This chapter presents an overview of some of the commonly used, powerful techniques currently in use. The electrical impedance of skin has been shown to change with *stratum corneum* hydration and, based on this principle, a number of devices are available that are routinely used in studying *stratum corneum* hydration changes. The skin barrier can be studied by trans-epidermal water loss measuring devices. To quantify erythema on skin a number of devices based on various physical principles are in use (e.g., colorimetry, spectrophotometry, and laser doppler flowmetry).

Many imaging techniques have been developed to reveal subtle changes in skin on the surface and in depth. High-resolution digital photography with options of polarized and fluorescence imaging and videomicroscopy are useful to explore the microstructure. Some more advanced techniques such as *in vivo* laser confocal microscopy and optical coherence tomography reveal the horizontal and vertical sections of skin at various depths. Measuring skin topography parameters is useful to show smoothing of skin surface after a product application. We can now study viscoelastic properties of skin in a variety of ways using twisting, impacting, suction, and shearing devices. The list of skin measuring tools is growing . . .

TABLE OF CONTENTS

11.5.1 INTRODUCTION

The effect of skin care products that improve the structure and function of skin, as well as enhance the appearance of skin, can be studied using a number of bioengineering techniques. We no longer depend solely on clinical gradings. The idea is to get a complete picture of improvements, not just look at one or two parameters. Traditionally, visual examination and some simple evaluations have been used on large pools of subjects to show the efficacy of these products. Often the difference between the treatment and control is subtle, requiring advanced methodologies to be employed. A good collection of these skin-measuring techniques are given in *Handbook of NON-INVASIVE METHODS and the SKIN*, second edition [1]. Some skin-imaging techniques are given in *BIOENGINEERING OF THE SKIN, Skin Imaging and Analysis*, second edition [2].

Measuring *stratum corneum* hydration using electrical devices is a commonly used method. Often there is a need to use advanced methods like measuring skin hydration kinetics which are based on the property of *stratum corneum* to hold, release or accumulate water. These include sorption-desorption (S-D) and moisture accumulation test (MAT). The use of sorption-desorption method is described by Tagami et al. [3] and moisture accumulation method by Pellacani and Seidenari [4].

The barrier function of SC can be assessed by measuring the trans-epidermal water loss (TEWL) as well as by using a number of chemical probes, e.g., methyl-nicotinate, lactic acid, and balsum of Peru. Furthermore, penetration of fluorescent dyes, e.g., pyranine, can also be utilized.

Erythema can be assessed in a variety of ways. The erythema may be graded visually; however, it will depend on the particular observer, ambient light, previously seen colors as well as the mood and prejudices of the observer. Human eye is good in discriminating colors and brightness of objects when they are adjacent, but poor in grading single color or intensity. It also cannot remember a previously seen color or intensity quantitatively. The search for an objective method to assess erythema, over the last 100 years, produced a range of techniques. Topical drugs and skin care products are tested by either comparing post-treatment erythema values to pre-treatment or comparing the erythema value on the test site to the adjacent normal skin. Conversely, some products cause vasoconstriction, resulting in an apparent blanching. The pallor is caused by relatively lower amount of blood at the test site. Both redness and blanching can be graded visually as well as measured by various instrumental modalities, e.g., visual examination, various scales, graded colored paper, photoplethysmography, colorimetry, diffuse reflectance spectrophotometry, blood flow by laser doppler imager, digital color photography, thermography, etc. Subclinical erythema can be detected by reflectance spectrophotometry. Laser doppler imager is not useful for blanching assays. Blanching (by corticosteroids) can be detected very well by reflectance spectrophotometry.

Skin pigmentation can be measured by a variety of techniques, some of them common to erythema measurement, e.g., visual examination, various scales, colorimetry, reflectance spectrophotometry, optically filtered digital photography, etc. For melanin pigmentation we can also add controlled UV-photography.

Optics and advanced imaging techniques are important in showing the effects of products on skin. Filtered digital photographic techniques (cross-polarized, parallel-polarized, and fluorescence) can reveal features of skin that are not shown in standard photography. Ultraviolet light photography dramatically reveal the pigmented lesions of skin. Side-lighted videomicroscopy dramatically enhances the view of scaliness of skin, especially if blue-UV light is used for illumination. This method also shows an enhanced view of the pigmented lesion. Ultrasonography shows the skin structure (cross-section) and reveals the presence of edema. Optical Coherence Tomography (OCT) shows cross-section of skin at a much higher resolution than ultrasound. Thickness changes in SC and epidermis can be measured by Optical Coherence Tomography (OCT). Some applications of OCT on skin are given by Pagnoni et al. [5]. Confocal Scanning Laser Microscopy reveals cellular structure in various strata of skin as horizontal sections, complementing OCT's cross-sectional view. The confocal microscope can also be used to measure thickness of *stratum corneum* and epidermis. Confocal microscope images show melanin-rich areas as bright structures, particularly near basal layer. Rajadhyaksha et al. describe a confocal microscope in detail [6].

An important parameter in studying skin is topography. In the past, replicas of skin have been used to assess the surface for roughness and glyphic line structure. The replica samples have been imaged using many different angles of illumination. In some experiments we have used a narrow-angle (~ 10°) illumination by a ring light to enhance the fine surface structure. The image is digitally captured and analyzed using computer programs developed in our laboratory. The line structure is analyzed for lengths and areas. Also surface roughness is calculated. The fringe projection device has, by and large, replaced the replica method. Fringe-projection device with phase-shift procedures can reveal ultra-fine changes in skin surface roughness. This device images skin surface directly and the calculation of topography parameters are much more precise. Skin roughness and smoothness values can be calculated in a variety of ways. We have shown the disruption of surface in the photo-damaged skin compared to relatively normal skin. Detailed descriptions of the fringe projection device are given by Jasper et al. [7] and Frankowski et al. [8].

Viscoelastic properties of skin are important for a healthy skin. Skin is a complex composite made up of elastic and viscous parts. The bulk of elasticity in skin resides in the dermis with its collagen and elastic fiber matrix. The epidermis and *stratum corneum*, however, also influence the elastic properties somewhat. In general, any product that affects the hydration levels of skin or influences the dermal fiber network would show change in the viscoelastic properties of skin. To measure the elastic properties, a force (stress) is applied to the skin and then released while deformation (strain) is measured during this cycle. The *in vivo* elastic properties of the skin can be measured by several methods like ballistometry, dynamometry, torque, and suction devices.

Some *ex vivo* techniques are available to quantify features of skin, e.g., sebum output, number and size of follicular casts, and desquamation. Samples are first collected off the skin by an appropriate method and then an image is obtained under a microscope. Image analysis programs are then used for quantification.

The desquamation property of skin is commonly studied by collecting the surface scales on an adhesive disc. A more advanced method is to harvest 3D squame samples sequentially from the same site and look at the dynamics of scale-collection.

Many of the methods described above have been used to study sun-damaged skin, also referred to as photo-damage. There is great interest in treating the signs and symptoms of sun-damage. The basic science of skin intrinsic aging and photo-aging have been described by many authors [9], [10], [11], [12].

11.5.2 COSMETICS AND SKIN CARE PRODUCTS FOR HUMAN USE

Cosmetics and skin care products are used to enhance the look and feel of the skin and to protect the body from the elements of nature. Topical drugs, on the other hand, are used to prevent or treat skin diseases. Considerable overlap, however, occurs between these two fields; e.g., control and treatment of dry skin are tackled by both skin care products and skin pharmaceuticals.

The development of a skin care product starts with market research and current fashion trends; a product is then designed based on technical research and development. Before the product reaches the consumer, a number of testing and research procedures are followed at various steps. First, chemical and microbiological stability is tested. Safety tests are then performed followed by efficacy testing. Finally, usage testing is done, which is based on sensory, tactile, and visual appeal of the product.

The efficacy testing of a product on human subjects starts with hypotheses. A good hypothesis is based on current knowledge of the properties of a product and its component chemicals, and the potential effect on human skin. The experiment is designed by choosing appropriate measuring techniques and using currently acceptable principles of statistics. The size of the test panel is based on the precision and resolution of measurements. Proper controls should be used to show that the active ingredient, indeed, have produced the change.

The test product should be blinded from the subjects as well as from the evaluators to rule out any bias that may creep in. In general, a good test would have double-blinded, randomized, and placebo-controlled design. Negative and positive controls may also be added.

11.5.3 SKIN STRATA

Human skin covers the whole body, an approximate surface area of 2 m^2, varying in thickness with location as well as with age, sex, ethnicity, and dermatological conditions of health and disease.

The skin is divided into two main compartments: the outer epidermis and the inner, and much thicker, dermis. As we journey from the outermost layer of skin to the innermost, we pass through various strata of epidermis and dermis. A sketch of skin strata is shown in Figure 1.

The outermost surface is the *stratum corneum* (SC), a multilayered, keratinized surface with flattened and non-nucleated cells, post mortem. This is followed by *stratum granulosum* (SG), which is composed of one or more layers of granular cells that contain keratin fibers and either has shriveled nuclei or no nuclei. Below the SG there is a thick layer, *stratum spinosum* (SS), composed of several layers of cells with large oval nuclei and spiny processes. This is followed by *stratum basale* (SB), which is the last epidermal layer at the dermal-epidermal junction. The SB is composed of a single layer of columnar cells (basal cells), which include melanocytes and Merkel cells. The melanocytes are dendritic cells that perform melanogenesis through melanosomes. The melanin pigment is finally transferred to the keratinocytes. At the basal layer, cells divide continuously and move outwards towards the surface of the epidermis.

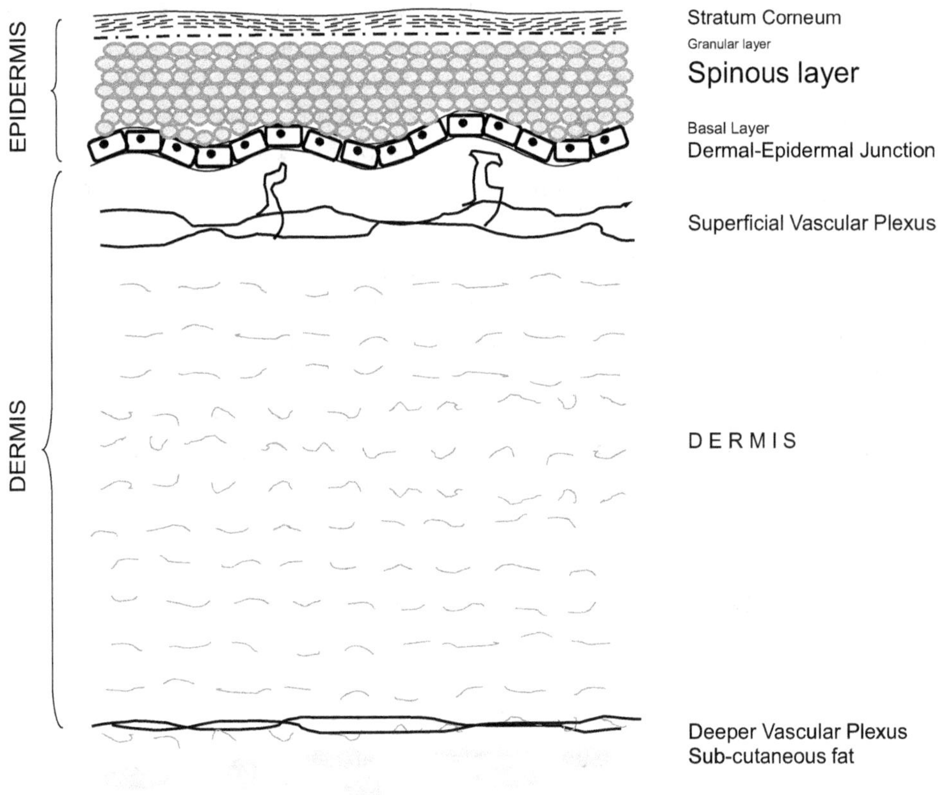

Figure 1: A general sketch showing the various strata of skin.

The dermal-epidermal junction is a wavy surface forming peaks and valleys (rete ridges). On the dermal side of this papillary surface, is the skin blood microvasculature.

The dermis forms the bulk of the skin, protecting the body from physical injury, providing pliability, elasticity, and tensile strength. The dermis is composed of bundles of fibers of various types (e.g., collagen and elastic fibers), distributed among which are blood vessels and nerves. Dispersed among these are hair follicles, sebaceous and sweat glands. A variety of cells can be found in the dermis, e.g., fibroblasts, macrophages, and mast cells. The dermis is divided into two layers, papillary dermis and reticular dermis. The cutaneous blood supply is arranged as two horizontal vascular networks, one at the dermal-subcutaneous junction and the other at the subpapillary level. From the subpapillary horizontal plexus capillary loops rise up into dermal papillae, usually one per papilla. The direction of blood flow in this network is from the arterioles to venules. Figure 2 shows the general layout of the vasculature.

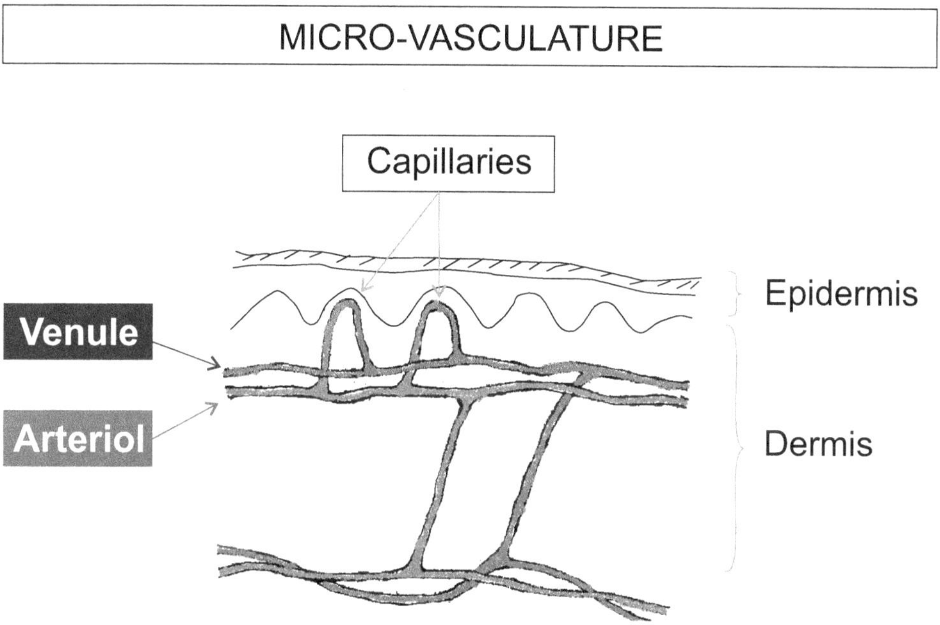

Figure 2: Microvasculature of the skin.

The main barrier to the skin is provided by *stratum corneum*. It protects skin against outside chemical insults and controls the trans-epidermal water loss (TEWL). The flattened cells of the SC, corneocytes, are continuously being renewed as a result of a process of epidermal maturation and terminal differentiation. The corneocytes are embedded in a matrix of intercellular lipids (brick and mortar model). They are also riveted together by intercellular protein structures called corneodesmosomes. There may also be ionic bonding between the corneocytes. Each corneocyte is a protein complex encapsulated within a protein shell called the cornified cell envelope. Within the corneocytes reside a number of water-soluble compounds collectively called natural moisturizing factor (NMF), which have the ability to bind water. Both the intercellular lamelar lipids and the natural moisturizing factor maintain the balance of water in a healthy *stratum corneum*. Lack of water can result in dry, brittle, cracking, and rough skin.

11.5.4 BIO-INSTRUMENTATION

a. General

in most clinical studies, evaluations are performed combining visual grading of skin attributes as well as measurements by a variety of bio-instrumentations.

Following each laboratory's "standard operating procedure" (SOP), the instruments are calibrated and tested on regular basis.

For some of the instrumental measurements, keeping the room temperature and humidity constant is critical—for example, measurement of *stratum corneum* hydration and trans-epidermal water loss. Generally, a temperature of 21° ± 1° Celsius (70° ± 1° Fahrenheit) and relative humidity of either 40% ± 5% or 50% ± 5% are required for some types of skin evaluations.

An environmental chamber is the best way to control the temperature and humidity precisely.

b. Environmental Chamber

A variety of types and sizes of environmental chambers are available. We use a closed chamber with a single entry door and with thick wall insulation for controlling the temperature and humidity. A highly precise process control unit is used for reading the values of temperature and humidity from the sensors; it also controls the ambient condition by sending pulses of hot, cold and humid air, along with cycles of dehumidification.

The mixing of hot, cold, and humid air is done outside the chamber, in a subchamber above the ceiling. The ceiling has 56,800 micro-holes, 3-mm diameter each and distributed 12 mm apart. The mixed air from above continuously filters through these micro-holes down into the chamber to provide a uniform atmosphere inside, and holds the temperature and humidity constant. In this system there is no air draft or substantial air movement inside the chamber, which is very different from an air-conditioned room where the fans blow the air into the room.

The inner dimensions of the chamber are: width 301 cm, length 355 cm, and height 213 cm. Outside the chamber there are refrigeration and heating units as well as humidity and dehumidifying units. The humidifying system consists of water mist producer (vapor injection). The water supplied to this unit comes through a two-stage laboratory water filter. The dehumidifier system consists of a large freezer coil with condenser fins, placed just outside the wall, across a screened opening.

The temperature and humidity are continuously recorded on a chart recorder. The recommended time for acclimation of subjects is between 15 and 30 minutes, but could be longer for some experiments.

11.5.5 SKIN HYDRATION

Proper level of *stratum corneum* (SC) hydration is essential for healthy skin. Lack of moisture leads to rough, dry skin and can cause a number of skin ailments.

Skin moisture can be measured in many ways but by far the most common method is to measure the electrical impedance of skin. Hydration changes in the *stratum corneum* influence the electrical capacitance and conductance of skin. Three of the most common instruments these days are: novameter, skicon, and corneometer. These are simple and easy to use instruments utilized by dermatologists to follow skin disease during treatment as well as by industry to test moisturizers and topical drugs. Figure 3 shows the three hydration probes, which are placed in contact with skin surface.

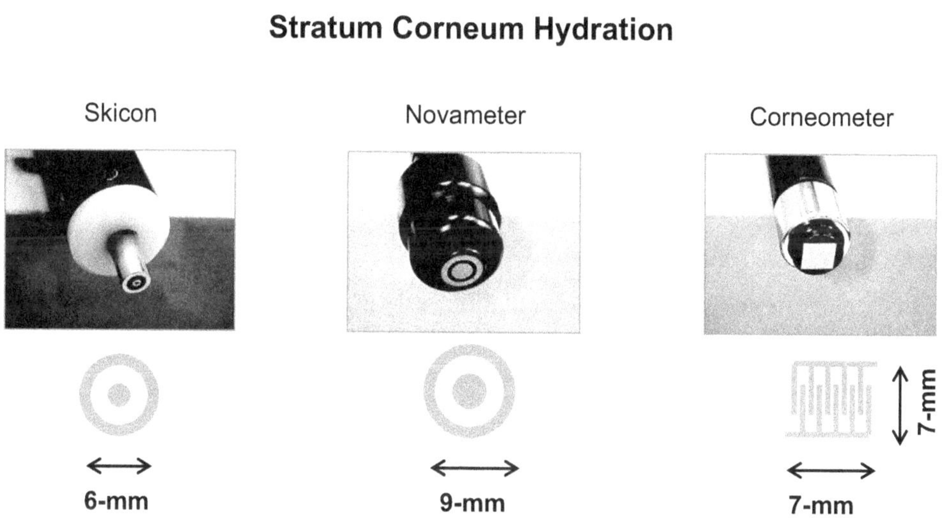

Figure 3: The hydration measuring probes of Skicon, Novameter, and Corneometer. The electrode dimensions are also shown.

a. Skicon

The Skicon (Skicon-200, I.B.S. Co. Ltd. Japan) is a conductance-measuring device with concentric circular electrodes. It uses a fixed electrical frequency of 3.5 megahertz. The measurements are given in microsiemen (μS) units and have a range of 5 to 1999.

b. Novameter

The Novameter (Model DPM9003, Nova Technologies, NH) is an impedance-measuring device with concentric circular electrodes separated by a gap of 1 mm. It uses varying electrical frequencies over a range up to 1 MHz, and the capacitance is derived from the signal-phase delay. The measurements are given in arbitrary units referred to as DPM units (DPM stands for Dermal Phase Meter). The range is 90 to 999.

c. Corneometer

Corneometer (model CM 825, Courage + Khazaka electronic GMBH, Germany) is a capacitance device, which consists of a pair of electrodes formed as an interdigital grid with small spacing between the elements. Readings are given in arbitrary units.

d. Sorption-Desorption Test

In a more sophisticated mode these instruments can be used to determine the ability of skin to be moisturized and its capacity to hold water. This is called the sorption-desorption test, in which a drop of water is applied to skin for a brief period and the dynamics of hydration is followed through a series of moisture measurements. Using this test we find the water-holding capacity, hygroscopicity, and desorption rate constant of skin in health and disease.

e. Moisture Accumulation Test

Another test is the moisture accumulation test (MAT), in which the skin is occluded with the measuring probe for a period of time and the increase in hydration is continuously recorded. Using these instruments, efficacy of moisturizers can be tested.

11.5.6 TRANS-EPIDERMAL WATER LOSS

Another important phenomenon in skin is the loss of water through epidermis, which essentially relates to the barrier function of skin. This is measured by an instrument that measures the water evaporation from a surface by detecting the partial pressure gradient of water vapors. Two pairs of sensors, measuring humidity and temperature, are arranged in a cylindrical well in such a way that one pair is farther than the other from the surface whose evaporation rate is to be measured. The schematics of this arrangement are shown in Figure 4. The reading displayed is called trans-epidermal water loss (TEWL) and is given in units of g/m^2h. In general, skin irritation, barrier disruption, and sweat output increase the TEWL. Effects of various cosmetics, toiletries, and topical drugs can be studied with this instrument. Various dermatoses can also be followed.

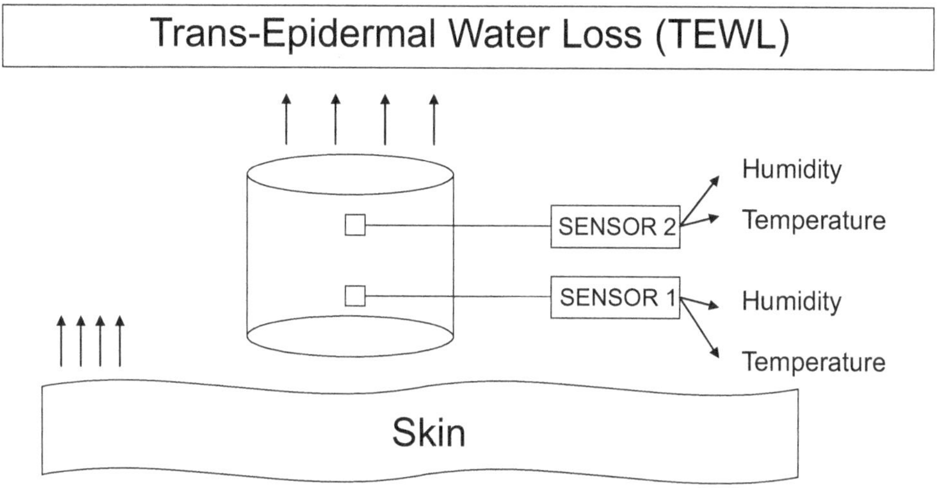

Figure 4: Measurement of Trans-Epidermal Water Loss using two pairs of humidity and temperature sensors.

a. Evaporimeter

Evaporimeter (Model EP2, Servomed, Sweden) measures TEWL in an area of 12-mm diameter circle. Measurements are done in an environmental chamber at a temperature of 70° ± 0.5°F and a relative humidity of 40 ± 5%. Readings are recorded between 45 and 60 seconds after placing the probe on the skin surface. The data can also be collected through an EP2 program. The TEWL is given in g/m^{2}h.

b. Dermalab

The Dermalab TEWL instrument (Dermalab, Cortex Technology, Denmark) has a probe diameter of 11 mm. Measurements are done in an environmental chamber at a temperature of 70° ± 0.5°F and a relative humidity of 40 ± 5%. Readings are recorded at 60 seconds post-probe contact with the skin surface. The data can also be collected through a program. The TEWL is given in g/m^{2}h.

11.5.7 SKIN BLOOD FLOW, COLOR, ERYTHEMA

The redness is caused by increased blood flow in the superficial capillaries in skin. It is important to measure erythema during treatment of skin diseases as well as during safety testing of topical products. It is also useful to test skin by provoking erythema reaction (irritation model) and then test the ability of a topical product in reducing erythema. Various instruments have been devised to measure erythema. Some are based on measuring the movement of erythrocytes and others are based on measuring the color or spectra of the light reflected off the skin. Some of the common instruments are: Laser Doppler flowmeter, colorimeter, and diffuse reflectance spectrophotometer. The inflammatory reactions of skin can be studied, e.g., due to a variety of stimuli, e.g., irritants, vasodilators, UV exposure, mechanical abrasion, topical application of products, and drugs.

a. Laser Doppler Flowmetry

The Laser Doppler Flowmeter works on the principle that light reflected off the moving erythrocytes experience a Doppler shift in frequency. The interaction of the frequency-shifted light waves with the nonshifted light waves produces a signal that is proportional to the blood flow in the capillaries. The laser Doppler imager (MoorLDI, Moor Instruments, Devon, UK), scans a laser beam on a predetermined rectangular area on the skin surface by a moving mirror that produces a raster pattern. The Doppler-shifted signal is recorded as an image of 250 × 250 pixel. The blood-flow values at each pixel are given in an arbitrary "Perfusion Unit (PU)," which is proportional to the product of "number of erythrocytes" and their "mean velocity" in a volume of tissue. Figure 5 shows the schematics of the Laser Doppler Imager. A Helium-Neon (He-Ne) Laser is used with a wavelength of 632.8 nm.

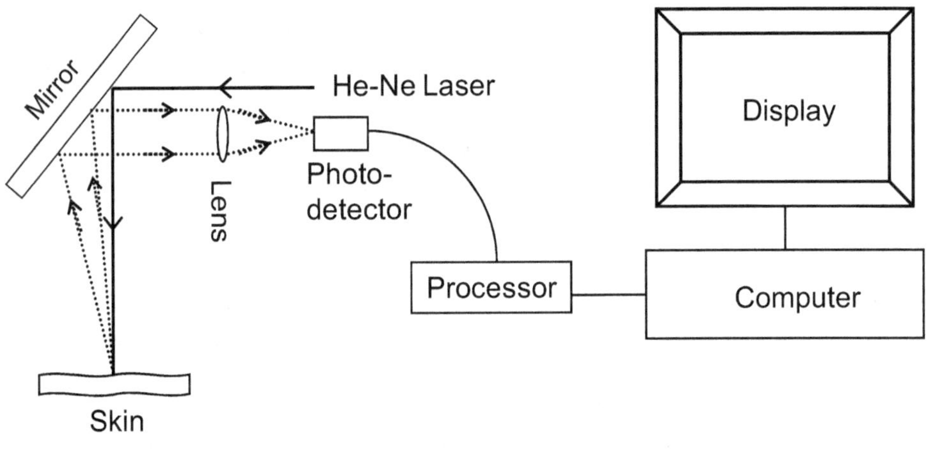

Figure 5: Schematics of the Laser Doppler Scanner.

b. Colorimetry

Chromameter measures the color of skin quantitatively. Light from a xenon flash lamp illuminates a 1-cm diameter circular area of the skin, and the reflected light is detected and analyzed for its color components and intensity. The measurement is given in L* a* b* system of colorimetric notation, where L* stands for brightness from black to white, a* describes color from green to red, and b* gives color from blue to yellow. Thus 1/L* is a measure of darkness, a* a measure of redness, and b* a measure of yellowness in relative terms. Erythema on skin is measured on a* scale and pigment on 1/L* scale. The schematics of the chromameter are shown in Figure 6.

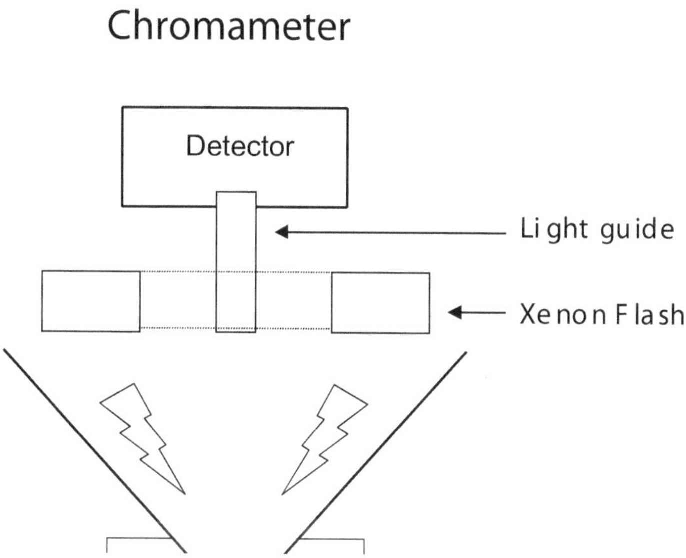

Figure 6: The probe head of the chromameter.

c. Reflectance Spectrophotometry

The spectrophotometric measurement of erythema is based on assessing the hemoglobin content of skin by measuring the specific absorbance peaks. Oxy-hemoglobin have absorbance peaks at 415, 542, and 577 nm, and deoxy-hemoglobin have peaks at 430 and 555 nm. The common end of a bifurcated fiber optic cable is placed on the skin surface, one arm is connected to a light source, and the other arm is connected to spectroscopic detector (see Figure 7). Using a tungsten-halogen light source and a spectrograph with a diode array of 1024 elements, an absorbance spectrum in the wavelength range of 400 to 800 nm is obtained.

The spectra are always referenced to a white standard. Barium sulfate and aluminum oxide are common white standards. White ceramic tile can also be used as a reference. The apparent absorbance is calculated as:

$$A(\lambda) = \mathrm{Log}_{10}\{ W(\lambda)/S(\lambda) \}$$

Where $A(\lambda)$ is the apparent absorbance, $W(\lambda)$ is the white reference spectra, and $S(\lambda)$ is the spectra from skin.

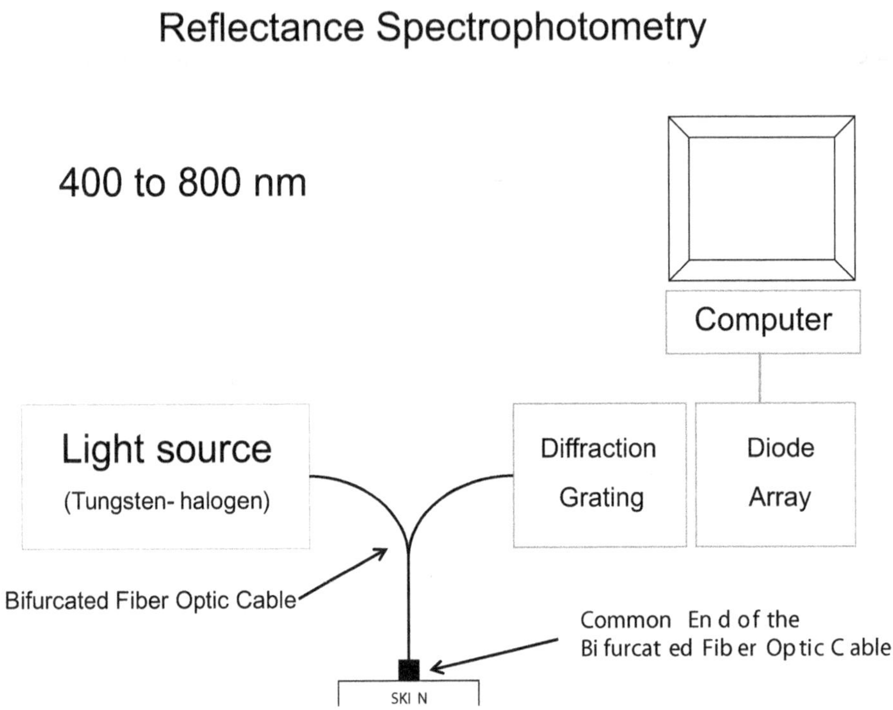

Figure 7: Reflectance Spectrophotometer with a bifurcated fiber optics cable.

Often a "dark current" is associated with the detector; a dark reference is measured as well. Placing the probe on a mat black surface and switching the light source off and then recording spectra can easily do this. In general the white reference and the dark reference is measured at the start of a measurement session. The apparent absorbance is calculated as:

$$A(\lambda) = \mathrm{Log}_{10}\{ [W(\lambda) - D(\lambda)] / [S(\lambda) - D(\lambda)] \}$$

Where $D(\lambda)$ is the dark reference.

To calculate the apparent hemoglobin content, first a straight line is mathematically fitted on the points in the wavelength range of 620 to 720 nm. This straight line is subtracted from the absorbance values of the spectra. This is done to remove the effects of melanin and scattering by other structures in the skin. An easier, but less accurate routine is to subtract the value at 630 nm. Absorbance values at 542 nm and 577 nm for oxyhemoglobin and 555 nm for deoxyhemoglobin are reported. Other quantities like total hemoglobin and melanin level can also be derived.

The choice of methodology depends on type of reaction, design of experiment, and required precision of measurement. The Laser Doppler Flowmeter measures very well the increased blood flow by irritants but gives poor results in vasoconstrictive assays using corticosteroids. Laser Doppler flowmetry can be used for continuously monitoring blood flow as well as scan large areas of skin to see the spatial distribution. The colorimeter shows the changes in red color but would not give information about specific chromophores in the skin. The diffuse reflectance spectrophotometer on the other hand shows the absorption peaks of particular chromophores, e.g., oxy-hemoglobin, deoxy-hemoglobin, and bilirubin.

11.5.8 IMAGING TECHNIQUES

a. Digital Photography

Digital photography is used in a variety of ways to assess the changes in the appearance of skin after a specific treatment regimen. Facial photography is particularly very popular.

Many photography systems are available, using different cameras, geometric arrangements, lighting systems, and optical filter systems. In general, the most frequently used photography systems are: 1) Digital Flash Photography, 2) Polarized Light Photography, 3) Fluorescence Photography, and 4) Ultraviolet Light Photography.

In case of facial photography, the camera is moved around the face to capture left face, front face and right face. Conversely, the camera position is fixed and the face is turned left or right. Generally photographs are obtained at –45, 0, +45 degree angles to the front of the face.

One of the commonly used systems is the Canfield Clinical Photography System (Canfield Imaging System, Fairfield, NJ, USA).

1. Face Photography

The photos of the left, front, and right sides of the face are obtained using a computerized photography system with a 21.1-Megapixel (5616 × 3744 pixels) Canon EOS 5D Mark II digital camera.

The camera, along with the twin flash lamps (Canfield Intelliflash), is mounted on a base that rides over an arc-movement track on the Photography-Table, see Figure 8. The camera is positioned, relative to the face, at angles: 0° (Front face), –45° (Right face), and +45° (Left face). Two strobe lights are used at the neck level to reduce the shadows under the cheeks.

The face of the subject is first positioned in front of the camera, using a chin-rest and a nose-bridge device. After the alignment, the nose-bridge device is removed. A photo of front of face (0°) is obtained. The photos of the right and left sides of the face are obtained sequentially after moving the camera –45° (Right face) and +45° (Left face).

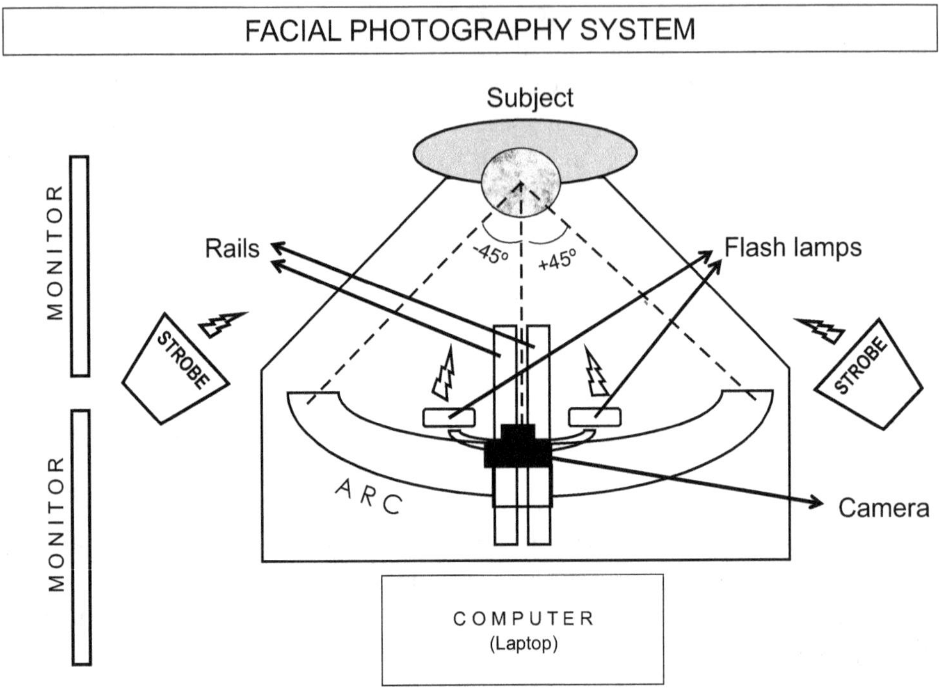

Figure 8: Top-view of the Facial Photography System.

Mirror software (Canfield Imaging Systems, NJ, USA) is used for controlling the camera and saving the captured photos in a database. Mirror "PhotoTools" is a computer program that is used for tethered capture of images from the digital camera with "Live-Preview" function. The Mirror "PhotoFile Image Management" is a database program which helps in storing, retrieving and exporting captured images, as well as applying attributes to distinguish between different sets of images. In the "Live-Preview" mode, the picture of the face is displayed on the computer screen in real time within a rectangular frame with vertical and horizontal grid lines. The face is aligned to the grid lines. After removal of the nose-bridge device, the photo is captured by clicking the "Capture" bar. The image is stored in the database. The first set of photos, e.g., at baseline, are obtained using the function called "Pre-Op." For post-treatment photos, first the appropriate baseline photo is selected, and then the "Post Op" function is selected to display the live image of the face on top of the original (baseline) image, each image with 50% transparency. The face is aligned to match the baseline image as closely as possible, and the photo is captured.

A laptop computer, DELL Latitude E6410 14, is interfaced with the camera through a USB cable. All functions of the camera are controlled by the computer.

An external flat-panel monitor is connected to the laptop computer using a VGA cable. This monitor helps during physical alignment of the face in the "live-preview" mode. Another computer is used to display baseline photos of subjects so that the position of headband and hairs can be matched, as closely as possible, in the current photo session.

2. Polarized Light Photography

The Polarized Light Photography is done using another Canfield Photography System, which has table and arch movement similar to the one described above, but different camera and flash lights. Linear polarizers are positioned on the two flash heads and on the camera lens. The lens polarizer can be rotated by 90° to achieve either cross-polarization for subsurface details or parallel polarization for enhanced surface details.

3. Fluorescence Photography

Fluorescence Photography is achieved using yet another photography system that allows visualization of porphyrin and comedonal fluorescence as well as fluorescent stains. Two filtered flash lamps emitting at a center wavelength of 417nm (visible-violet) are positioned symmetrically at the side of the camera body. A UVA-Blue cutting filter GG475 (Schott Glass) is placed in front of the camera lens. The sensitivity is set at STD (400 ISO) and two flash units are used at full power (400 watts each). F-stop is set between 22 and 8.

4. Ultraviolet Light Photography

For enhanced visualization of pigmented lesions and melanin content of skin, photography with light in the ultraviolet wavelength range (320 to 400 nm) is used. A 35-mm film camera with a 60 mm lens and a 400 W twin-flash lamp is used. Optical filters, passing Ultraviolet-A light (UVA, peak at 365 nm) and blocking visible light, are mounted on the flash lamps and in front of the camera lens. An ISO-400 black-and-white film is used to collect the image.

b. Ultrasound

A 20 MHz ultrasound machine (Cortex Tech., Denmark) is used to image a cross-section of skin. A hydrogel is applied between the skin and the ultrasound probe for coupling. The image is pseudocolored to show the ecogenic density distribution. The skin thickness is measured by the ultrasound image analysis software (Cortex Tech., Denmark).

c. Videomicroscopy

Videomicroscopy is commonly used to look at the various skin features and lesions. Two types of videomicroscopes have been utilized, one a hand-held visible light videomicroscope with changeable vertical or horizontal lighting and various magnifications, and the other a UVA-light videomicroscope with side lighting. The illumination systems are shown in Figure 9.

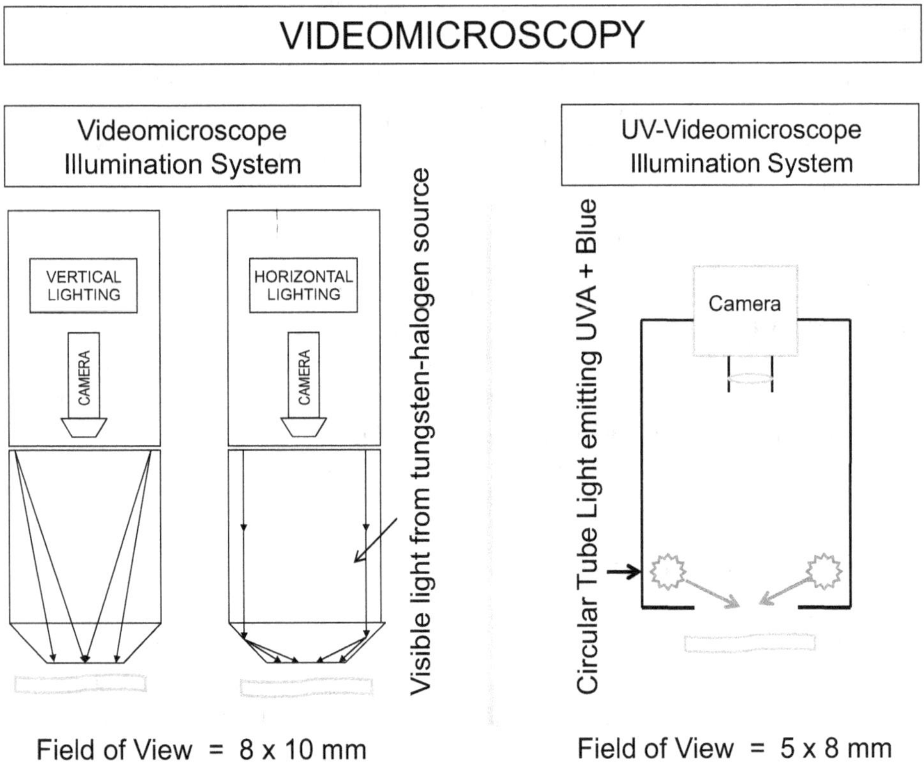

Figure 9: Visible light and UV-light videomicroscopy systems.

In-vivo microscopy of skin is done using a videomicroscope which consists of a hand-held probe, fed with light from a fiber-optic cable and connected to an image processor and a computer that displays the image live on the monitor (Hi-scope, Model KH2200 MD, Hirox, Japan). The magnifications can be selected 20-100 X (variable) and 400 X (fixed). It has the capability of varying the illumination from almost vertical to almost horizontal to the skin surface. This has made it possible to view skin at surface as well as deeper layers. In general, light falling on the skin is diffused and reflected in various proportions. Reflected light shows the surface structures; the diffused light shows color structures, e.g., pigment and erythema lesions.

Vertical illumination shows surface reflections very well, revealing the topography of skin, hairs, follicular lesions, and acne. Effects of topically applied lotions and creams on the skin can be studied in this way.

The horizontal lighting reveals the deeper levels such as pigment and capillaries in the skin, as well as the diffusing objects on the surface such as dry skin flakes. This method for illumination can be used for moisturizer efficacy studies or mildness of surfactant studies.

The theory of imaging of deeper levels by horizontal lighting is different than cross-polarized light imaging. Since for specular reflection, the angle of incidence is equal to angle of reflection, light striking a surface at a narrow angle is mainly reflected at a narrow angle; hence most of the light is reflected off the field of view. Only the portion diffused into the skin affects the image as viewed by the video sensor. Therefore, the oily shine of the skin surface is reduced, giving way to visualization of deeper levels. It may be noted that if the skin surface is too scaly, it is difficult to see the deeper layers, since the horizontal light also strongly illuminates the surface scales.

Using the videomicroscope with an appropriate illuminating system, one may follow various dermatoses and treatment regimens over a period of time, recording images along the way on the computer disk. In many cases the skin lesions can be located reasonably accurately by comparing current image with the previous one and adjusting the position and orientation of the video probe.

d. Confocal Microscopy

The confocal microscope is gaining prominence in biology, particularly the *in vivo* video rate microscope. It has great potential to complement conventional histology. In some instances the optical sectioning of confocal microscopy can replace the physical cutting of tissue for histology. It has an added advantage of looking into the skin in real time, e.g., observing the movement of erythrocytes and leukocytes through the capillaries.

Living skin can be optically sectioned by confocal microscopy from the surface downwards creating a series of horizontal images in real time without physically invading the skin. It produces high-contrast images of the cellular structure with very small depth of field (thin section), by rejecting the out-of-focus parts of the image. The optical schematics are shown in Figure 10.

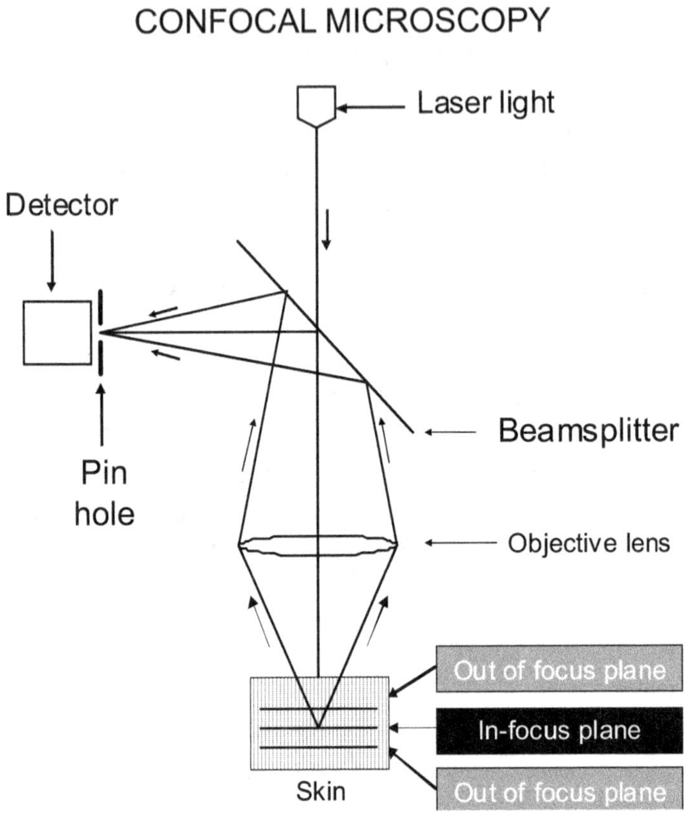

Figure 10: The Optics of the Confocal Microscope.

The confocal scanning laser microscope Vivascope1000 (Lucid, Inc. Rochester, NY) with an objective lens of 30× and 0.9 NA, scanning a field of 155 × 155 μm is used. The light source is a Gallium Arsenide (GaAs) Laser diode emitting at 830 nm. The light is detected by a Silicon Avalanche Photodiode through a pinhole of 100 μm. The scanning is achieved by a rotating mirror polygon and an oscillating mirror. The laser power is computer selectable between 0 and 20 mW. A polarization stage with adjustable angle further enhances the images. The imaging depth (z-axis) is controlled by computer in 3.6 μm steps. A horizontal resolution of 1.3 μm and a vertical resolution of 5 μm can be achieved. The objective lens is coupled to the skin surface through a circular cover glass (18 mm dia) attached to a circular ring that was affixed to the skin by a double-sided sticky tape. A variety of coupling media can be used, the most common being water. Sucrose 40%, hydrogel, and solutions of hydrogel in water (20, 25, and 50% v/v) have been used in the past for refractive index matching in a variety of situations.

A more advanced confocal microscope, Vivascope 1500 (Lucid, Inc. Rochester, NY, now called caliber I.D.), was later introduced with Z-steps of 1.6 microns, but with somewhat lower magnification. The new software can capture multiple images, as a block by x-y mapping as well as a stack in depth by z-mapping. For the z-stack the depth profile, i.e., the depth of each image of the stack, can be selected in advance. A gallium arsenide (GaAs) laser diode (830 nm) scans a field of 500 × 500 μm. The depth profiling is achieved by a computer-controlled stepper motor. The objective lens is coupled to the skin surface through a circular cover glass (18 mm dia) attached to a circular ring that affixed to the skin by a double-sided sticky tape.

e. Optical Coherence Tomography (OCT)

Optical Coherence Tomography (OCT) is a technique to record cross-sectional structures of skin. OCT is based on an optical interferometry principle, where a broadband light beam of short coherence length is split into sample and reference beams; the reflected light is coupled to produce an interference signal. The schematics of the OCT principle are shown in Figure 11.

Dermal and epidermal structures are clearly outlined. *Stratum corneum* (SC) is visualized as a bright line, sometimes thick and sometimes broken. The epidermis appears as a band with a wavy lower edge, and its thickness can be measured using the software. The geometry of isolated legions such as comedones can be visualized. The emergence of OCT as a skin-imaging tool fills the gap between the high-resolution (~ 1 micron) confocal microscopy and lower-resolution techniques like ultrasonography (~ 100 microns) and Magnetic Resonance Imaging (resolutions 50 to 300 microns).

The OCT device, SkinDex300 (GS-1 series, ISIS optronics, Mannheim, Germany), consists of an eight-channel OCT scanner and uses a 1300 nm broadband light source. It views skin 1 mm in horizontal direction and 1 mm in depth. The scanning head is optically coupled to the skin by a thin layer of gel.

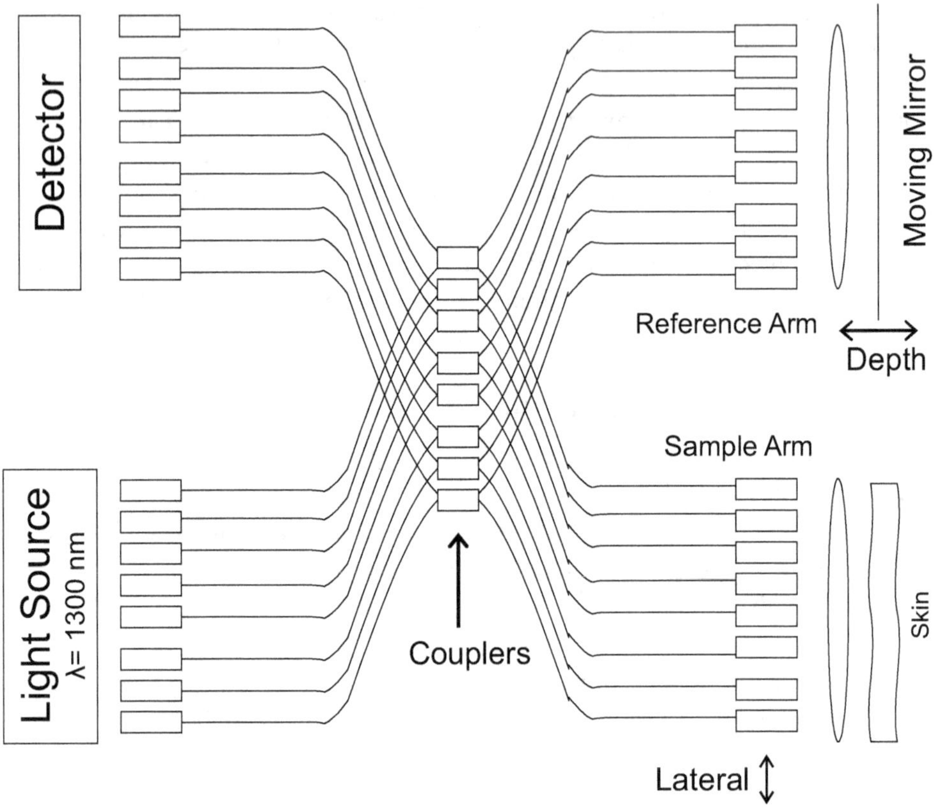

Figure 11: Schematic showing the basic principle of optical coherence tomography.

11.5.9 SKIN TOPOGRAPHY

Reduction of fine lines, wrinkles, and surface roughness, following various treatments, has been studied in the past using two main techniques: 1) Obtaining silicon rubber replica of skin, and 2) fringe projection devices. The replicas are analyzed by a number of methods, e.g., stylus surfometry, laser depth profiling, or optical shadow method. The fringe projection device projects a fringe pattern directly on the skin, and the reflected image is analyzed by the computer software.

a. Replica of Skin

The surface structure of skin has been studied extensively by many groups by obtaining a replica of skin, using a silicon rubber type compound. Skin surface texture is transferred permanently onto the replica as a negative impression, i.e., furrows will be ridges and cristae will be troughs. A number of techniques are available to analyze the replica. The image of the replica is captured through a stereomicroscope with specialized illumination, and image analysis is done by computer software. Using a narrow-angle ring light, the surface line structure is analyzed and the line lengths and areas are reported. Using a fiber-optics side lighting, roughness parameters, e.g., Rz, Ra, are calculated. Figure 12 shows the setup for microscopic imaging of replica using a side light and a ring light. Skin topography changes with age, body sites, various dermatoses, and use of topical products.

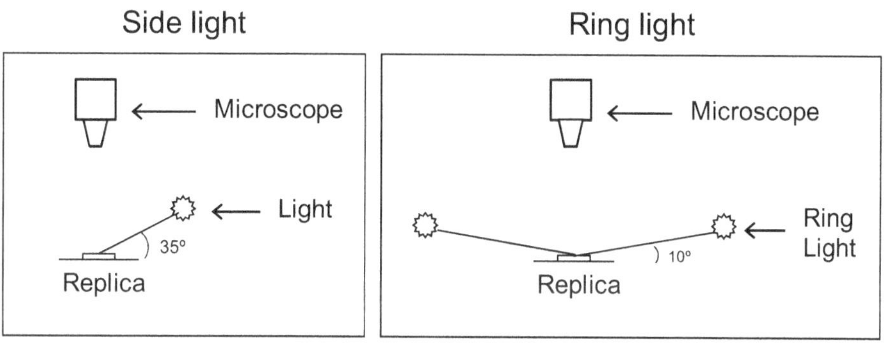

Figure 12: Imaging of Replica by Stereomicroscope with a side-light (left) and a ring-light (right).

b. Phase-shift fringe projection device

A digital micro-mirror projection device PRIMOS (Phaseshift Rapid *in vivo* Measurement of Skin, GF Messtechnik Gmbh, Teltow-Berlin, Germany) is used. This device directly measures the 3-D surface structure of skin without having to obtain a replica. Light from a tungsten-halogen lamp reflected off a digital micro-mirror projects stripes of Cos^2 type in a rectangular area of 13 mm × 18 mm on the skin surface (see Figure 13). The distortion of these stripes, due to the topography of skin surface, is captured by a videomicroscope camera. After application of phase-shift procedure and mathematical manipulation of the data by the computer, a color-coded height image of the skin surface is displayed on the computer screen. The surface height at each point of the image is precisely calculated by the software and displayed on the computer monitor on a color scale, e.g., blue is the lowest point, green is the medium height, and red a high point.

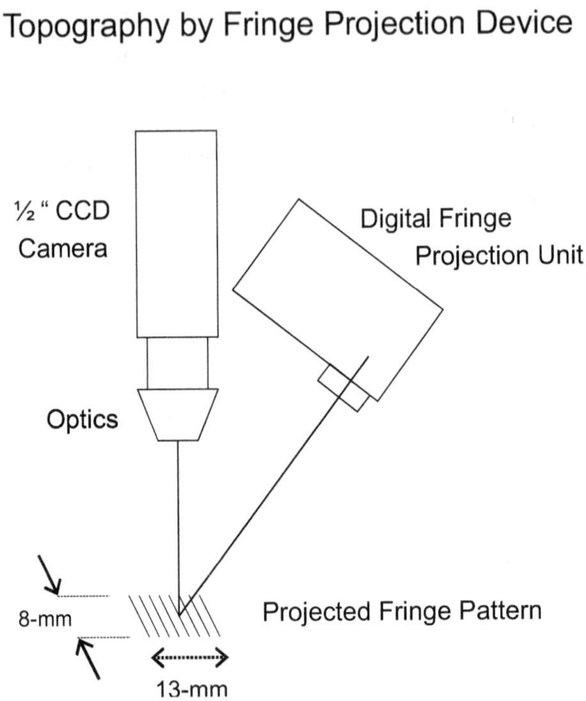

Figure 13: Schematic showing the basic design of the Fringe Projection Device.

c. Calculation of Roughness Values

First the hairs from the image are removed by a mathematical filter, then a fifth-order polynomial (n=5) is applied to the 3-D image to remove the gross contours of the skin surface. This flattening of the surface is done using the following equation:

$$Z(x,y) = \sum_{i=0}^{n}\cdot\sum_{j=0}^{n} a_{ij}.X.\left(X - \frac{X_{max}}{2}\right)^{i}\left(Y - \frac{Y_{max}}{2}\right)^{j}$$

On this processed image, 16 radial lines are marked inside a circle, each consecutive line subtending an angle of 22.5°. This is commonly called the "Star" roughness method. The roughness parameters, Rz and Ra, based on DIN4762 and DIN4788, are calculated for each of the 16 line profiles. The average value of Rz and Ra from this star formation is reported. The Rz values from baseline are compared to those obtained after treatment. Roughness parameters are derived for each line profile according to the following equations:

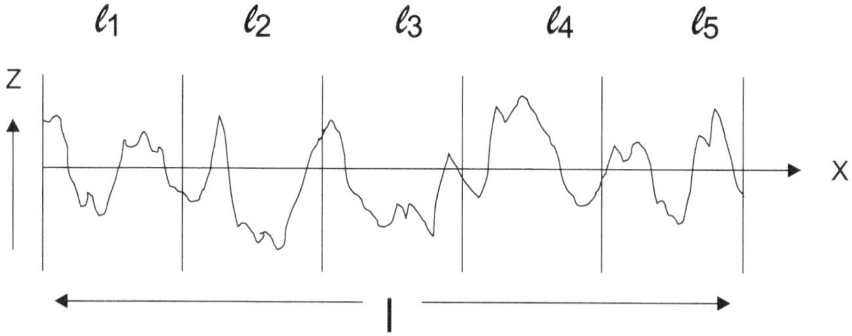

$$Rz = \frac{1}{n} z \sum_{i=1}^{i=n} Z_{max}(i) - Z_m \; l \quad \ldots \; [n = 1, 2, \ldots 5]$$

$$Ra = \frac{1}{\ell} \int_0^{\ell} (x).dx$$

d. Surface Area Calculation

In addition to the roughness parameters, Rz and Ra, the ratio of the real surface area to the area of the field of view, sometimes referred to as Rugosity, is also derived for each image. The field of view of each image is a rectangle of dimension 13mm × 18mm. The area of the theoretical plane covering the field of view is 13 mm × 18mm = 234 mm^2. Due to rough topography of the skin surface, the actual area would always be larger than 234 mm^2. The rougher the surface, the larger the area. Therefore, change in the surface area would indirectly indicate change in surface roughness.

11.5.10 VISCOELASTIC MEASUREMENTS

Skin is a complex composite made up of elastic and viscous components. To measure the elastic properties, a force (stress) is applied to the skin and then released while deformation (strain) is measured during this cycle. Some components of skin are mainly viscous and recover slowly while others recover quickly. The *in vivo* elastic properties of the skin can be measured by several methods like ballistometry, dynamometry, torque and suction devices (Figure 14).

a. Suction Device

Suction devices, e.g., Cutometer (Courage Khazaka, Germany) produces a small vacuum on the skin surface, making it rise in a small cavity. The elevation is optically detected. During a number of cycles of vacuum and release, the elevation and return of skin is measured and presented as a graph. The following elastic parameters are calculated: Extensibility, Gross Elasticity, Elastic Function, and Viscoelastic Ratio. The suction and release of skin in a single cycle is shown in Figure 15.

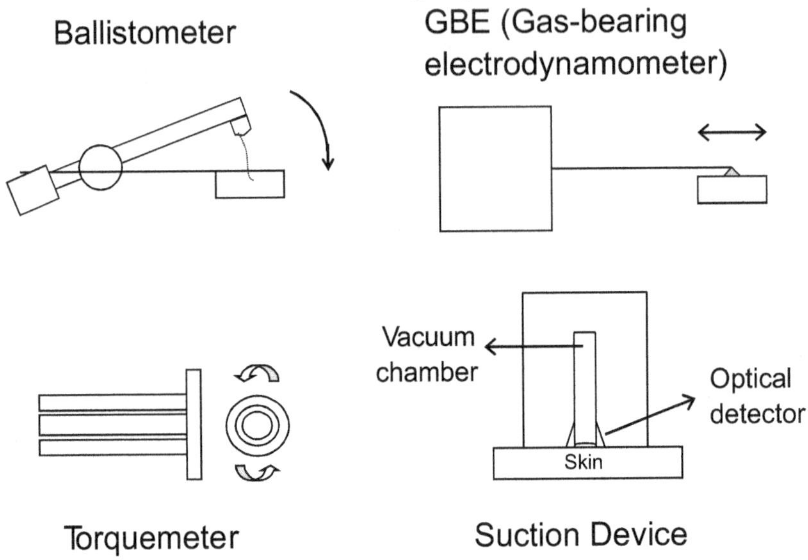

Figure 14: Sketches of some viscoelasticity measuring devices. The Ballistometer, GBE, Torquemeter, and Cutometer are based on applying force by impaction, translation, twist, and suction respectively.

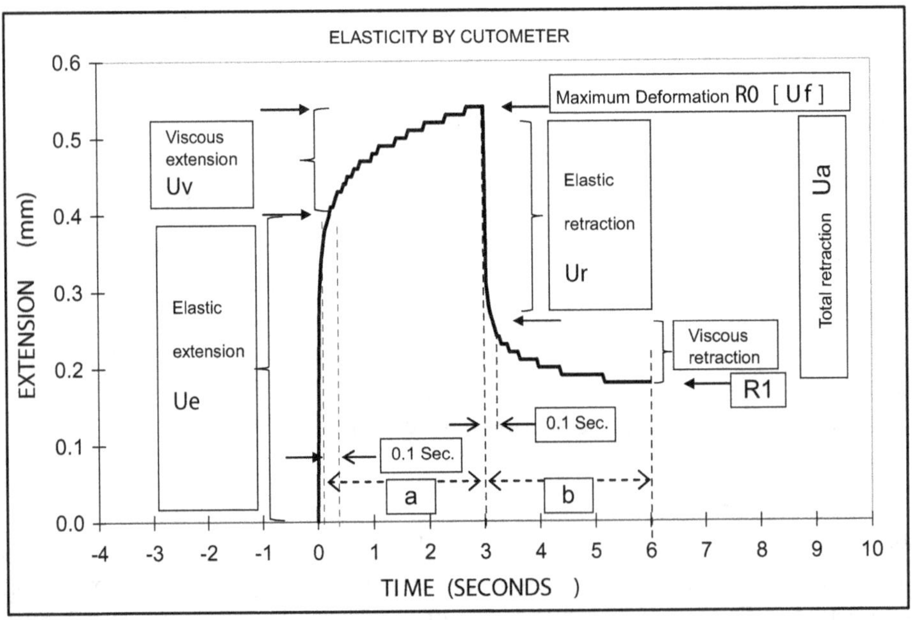

Figure 15: The parameters evaluated during the suction (3 seconds) and release (3 seconds) of skin in a single cycle by the Cutometer.

Calculation of some of the most common parameters are as follows:

1. R0 = e(a) = [Uf] Maximum Amplitude of the first cycle (Maximum Deformation). Value of extension "e" at the end of the first suction period "a."
2. R1 = e(a+b) Minimum Amplitude of the first cycle (Residual Deformation or return). Value of extension "e" at the end of first cycle (suction "a" + Release "b").
3. R2 = (R0 – R1)/R0 = [Ua/Uf] Gross Elasticity: Ratio of return to maximum extension in the first cycle.
4. R5 = [Ur / Ue] Elastic Function: Ratio of Immediate Elastic Retraction (0.1 sec. after removal of suction) to the Immediate Elastic Extension (0.1 sec. at the start of vacuum period). This refers to the Elastic component of the Gross Elasticity.
5. R6 = [Uv / Ue] Viscoelastic Ratio: Ratio of the viscous extension to the elastic extension.

There are many other ratios calculated, particularly when multiple cycles are used. Generally, three cycles of suction and release are recorded and some parameters comparing the first cycle to the third cycle are evaluated. In some experiments large number of cycles are used, e.g., 20 or 30 cycles, to show the elastic fatigue of skin.

b. Ballistometry

The ballistometer is an impacting device that lets a small spherical load fall on skin under gravity and bounce until it comes to rest. The movement is recorded electronically and displayed as a graph of diminishing peaks. The data is collected on the computer through an Analog to Digital Board and analyzed by a software program. The program detects the peaks and calculates the coefficient of restitution, which is the square root of the ratio of two adjacent peak heights. An example of ballistometry on the volar forearm vs. silicon rubber pad is shown in Figure 16.

c. Torsional Ballistometry

The torsional ballistometer (Dia-Stron, UK) is an impacting device that lets a small spherical load bounce on skin surface until it comes to rest. The movement of the ballistometer arm, which is mounted on a stainless-steel torsional wire, is recorded electronically and displayed as a graph of diminishing peaks. The data are collected on the computer. The program detects the peaks and calculates the coefficient of restitution, which is the square root of the ratio of two adjacent peak heights. The program also calculates the depth of the first indentation, and the rate of decay of the bounce peaks "Alpha" and "Area" of the bounce profile.

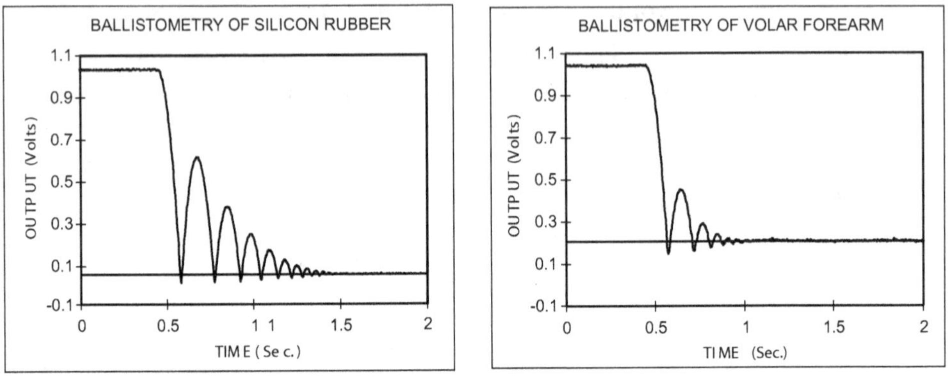

Figure 16: Graphs of diminishing peaks recorded for silicon rubber pad (left) and volar forearm of a volunteer (right).

11.5.11 SOME *EX VIVO* TECHNIQUES

a. Desquammation Measurements

A 22 mm diameter adhesive disc, D'Squame (CuDerm Corp. Dallas, TX) is used to remove a layer of *stratum corneum*. The scales collected on the disc shows the skin desquamation property and corneocyte morphology (Figure 17). The *stratum corneum* is first delipidized with a mixture of ether and acetone (1:1) for one minute. The disc is pressed with a spring-loaded pad for 30 seconds and removed.

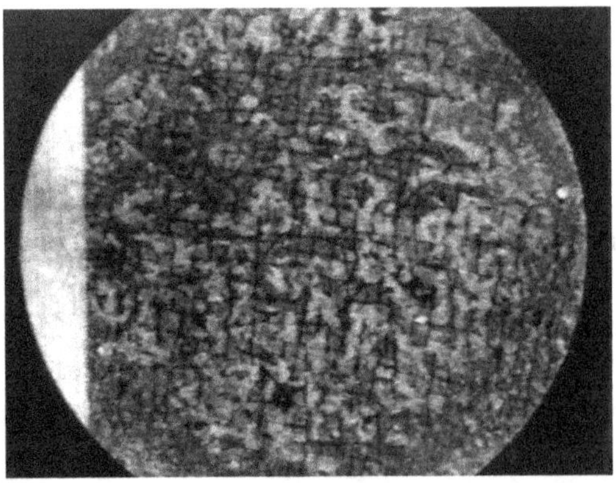

Figure 17: D-Squame sample showing scales removed from the skin.

The disc is placed on the standard black card (CuDerm Corp. TX), which is mounted under the stereomicroscope and illuminated by standardized fiber-optics light. The image is captured by a video camera and analyzed by a special computer program using Image Analysis software. Desquamation Index and percent of area covered by the scales are reported. A second D'Squame may be obtained from the same site for cytology and cell morphology.

b. Cyanoacrylate Surface Biopsy

Cyanoacrylate, a fast-setting glue, is used to harvest a layer of skin along with microcomedones and vellus hairs. One drop of cyanoacrylate adhesive (Krazy Glue) is applied to the skin within a circular paper ring of 1 cm^2 area and covered with plastic slide. After complete polymerization of the glue, which occurs in approximately five minutes, the slide is gently lifted from the surface carrying with it vellus hairs and enveloping horny material, termed "horny casts." Figure 18 shows a sample from the cheek.

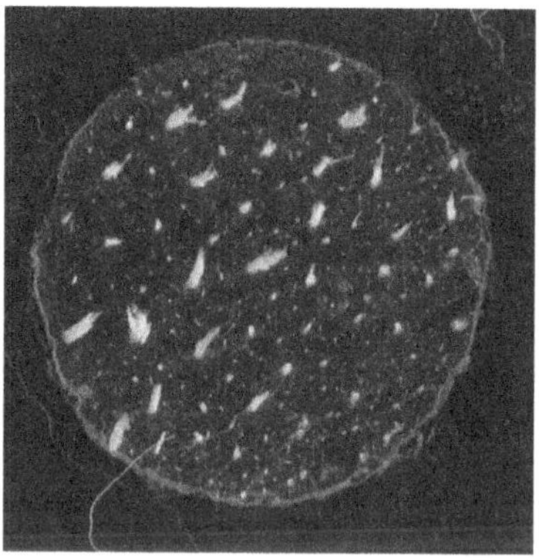

Figure 18: Cyanoacrylate surface biopsy from face showing fluorescent follicular casts.

The slide is imaged using fluorescent photographic techniques. Two filtered light sources emitting at a center wavelength of 417nm (visible-violet) are positioned symmetrically at the side of the camera body. A UVA-cutting filter (GG475) is placed in front of the camera lens. The images are then downloaded into a computer and analyzed. The number of casts and total area of casts (mm^2) are calculated.

c. Sebum Collection Assay

A porous translucent plastic film, Sebutape (CuDerm Corp., Dallas, TX), which when placed on skin collects sebum, which turns the film transparent. When the film is placed on a black card the collected sebum appears as black spots (see Figure 19). The sebum output is usually assessed on the cheeks and forehead. The site is first cleansed for 15 seconds with a nonwoven cotton pad soaked in 0.1% aqueous solution of Triton-X100, followed by swabbing with hexane for 15 seconds. The Sebutape is applied to the test site for one hour, after which it is removed and placed on the plastic film attached to the black card. The card is placed under the stereomicroscope (OPMI-1fc, Zeiss, Germany) and illuminated by standardized fiber-optics light. The image is captured by a video camera (CCD-72, DAGE-MTI, Michigan, Indiana) and stored on the computer. The count and area of sebum spots are assessed by image analysis.

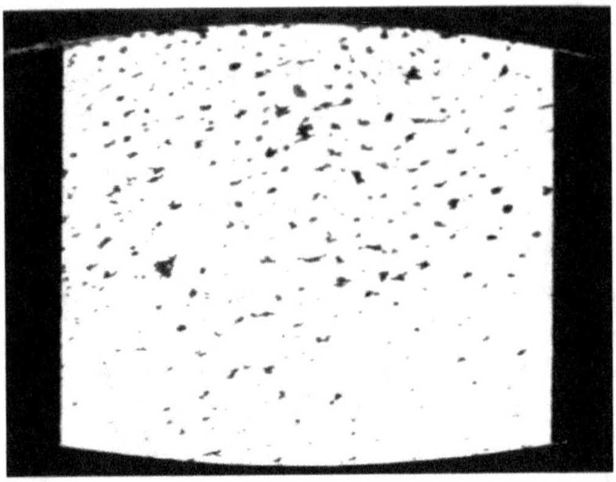

Figure 19: Sebum spots collected on the Sebutape in a one-hour period.

11.5.12 APPLICATION OF BIO-INSTRUMENTATION: SOME EXAMPLES

The three hydration measuring devices were compared in a multiple reading assay, in which eight sites were demarcated on the volar forearm and ten readings were obtained from each site using each of the devices sequentially. Each instrument measured a total of 80 readings. The normalized readings were plotted for Skicon, Novameter, and Corneometer, for site number and reading number (see Figure 20).

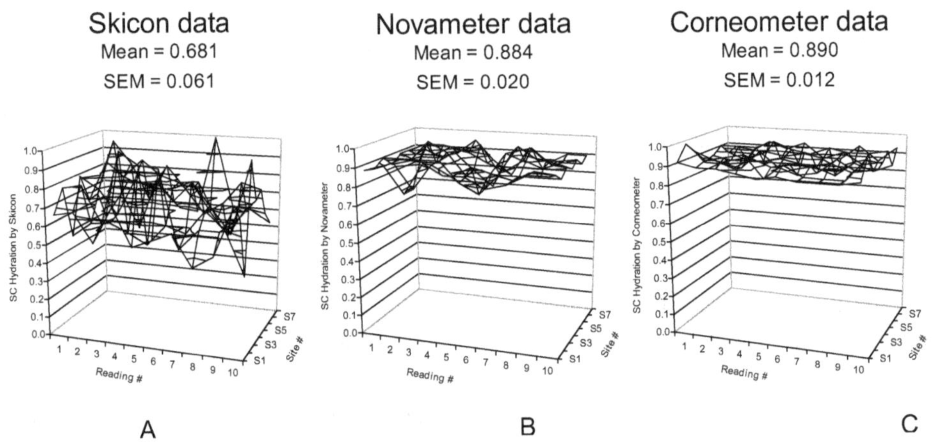

Figure 20: Plot of Hydration data from eight sites on the volar forearm using Skicon (A), Novameter (B), and Corneometer (C). Ten readings were collected from each of the eight sites. The data were normalized for each device so that hydration axis has the same scale (0 to 1).

The Standard Error of the Mean (SEM) was also calculated. Table 1 shows the data with Mean, Standard deviation (SD), and SEM.

The Standard Error of the Mean (SEM) is relatively low for all the devices, less than 10%. However, the Corneometer data show the least variance, SEM = 0.010 followed by Novameter, SEM = 0.018. The Skicon readings show relatively higher variance, SEM = 0.054.

The effect of lactic acid in changing the hydration of skin over a short period of time can be shown by measuring conductance by Skicon at various time-points post treatment. A single application of lactic acid 10% aqueous was applied to the cheek. Hydration was measured by Skicon before lactic acid application, and then after 30 min, 3 hours, 1 day, 2 days, 4 days, and 7 days. Figure 21 shows the effect of lactic acid over a period of seven days.

To demonstrate the hydration differences between "Dry" and "Normal" legs of human volunteers, Corneometer measurements were made on the legs of two dry-leg subjects and two normal-leg subjects. Ten readings were obtained from each subject, five from the left and five from the right. Mean hydration values showed statistically significant difference between dry vs. normal legs. A p-value of 0.00000000552 was obtained using a 2-Tail t-Test. Figure 22 shows the difference between dry vs. normal legs.

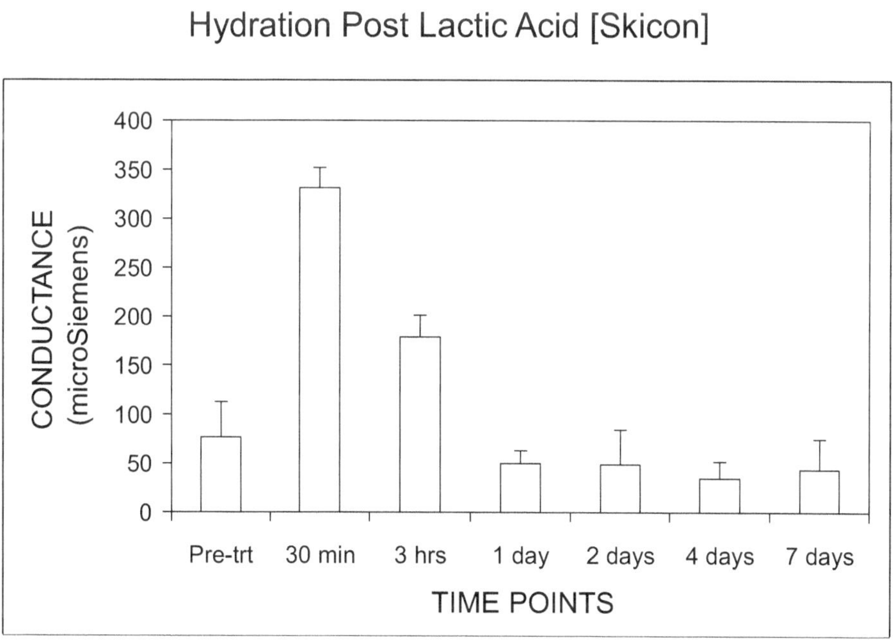

Figure 21: Single application of lactic acid 10% increases the hydration of skin significantly for a short period of time, i.e., 30 minutes and 3 hours.

TABLE 1

SITE ↓ / Reading →	SKICON 1	2	3	4	5	6	7	8	9	10		MEAN	SD	SEM
S1	60	62	48	66	48	52	56	41	47	71	>	55.10	9.539	0.055
S2	71	73	55	90	84	83	46	56	56	63	>	67.70	14.773	0.069
S3	45	52	53	49	44	54	51	63	54	33	>	49.80	7.927	0.050
S4	73	67	55	73	69	70	74	62	50	86	>	67.90	10.246	0.048
S5	59	79	72	81	74	71	72	54	54	65	>	68.10	9.712	0.045
S6	60	88	77	59	77	66	54	60	71	68	>	68.00	10.435	0.049
S7	46	59	41	67	57	67	53	41	56	54	>	54.10	9.303	0.054
S8	63	64	63	60	51	50	89	54	53	47	>	59.40	12.048	0.064
					Max>	**90**		**Min>**	**33**		**MEAN (All) >**	**61.26**	**10.498**	**0.054**

SITE ↓ / Reading →	NOVAMETER 1	2	3	4	5	6	7	8	9	10		MEAN	SD	SEM
S1	132	136	116	140	132	132	124	128	136	136	>	131.20	7.005	0.017
S2	130	136	116	136	128	136	132	128	136	134	>	131.20	6.268	0.015
S3	136	136	136	136	120	112	128	128	128	128	>	128.80	7.955	0.020
S4	128	132	148	140	122	120	142	136	138	134	>	134.00	8.794	0.021

S5	134	128	128	138	124	112	140	144	132	130	>	131.00	9.055	0.022
S6	134	140	140	136	142	120	142	132	132	134	>	135.20	6.613	0.015
S7	128	128	136	132	124	118	128	122	128	128	>	127.20	5.007	0.012
S8	130	124	128	140	124	112	136	124	132	132	>	128.20	7.800	0.019
					Max>	148		Min>	112	MEAN (All) >		130.85	7.312	0.018

CORNEOMETER

SITE ↓ / **Reading →**	**1**	**2**	**3**	**4**	**5**	**6**	**7**	**8**	**9**	**10**		**MEAN**	**SD**	**SEM**
S1	48	47	47	46	45	46	45	45	45	46	>	46.00	1.054	0.007
S2	52	48	49	50	44	48	45	45	45	51	>	47.70	2.830	0.019
S3	49	47	45	48	46	47	47	48	46	47	>	47.00	1.155	0.008
S4	45	45	44	49	45	43	44	48	45	46	>	45.40	1.838	0.013
S5	46	45	46	48	47	48	47	49	46	47	>	46.90	1.197	0.008
S6	48	48	48	50	48	47	49	48	48	49	>	48.30	0.823	0.005
S7	45	43	43	44	43	42	40	44	42	44	>	43.00	1.414	0.010
S8	46	45	48	46	48	44	44	48	44	48	>	46.10	1.792	0.012
					Max>	52		Min>	40	MEAN (All) >		46.30	1.513	0.010

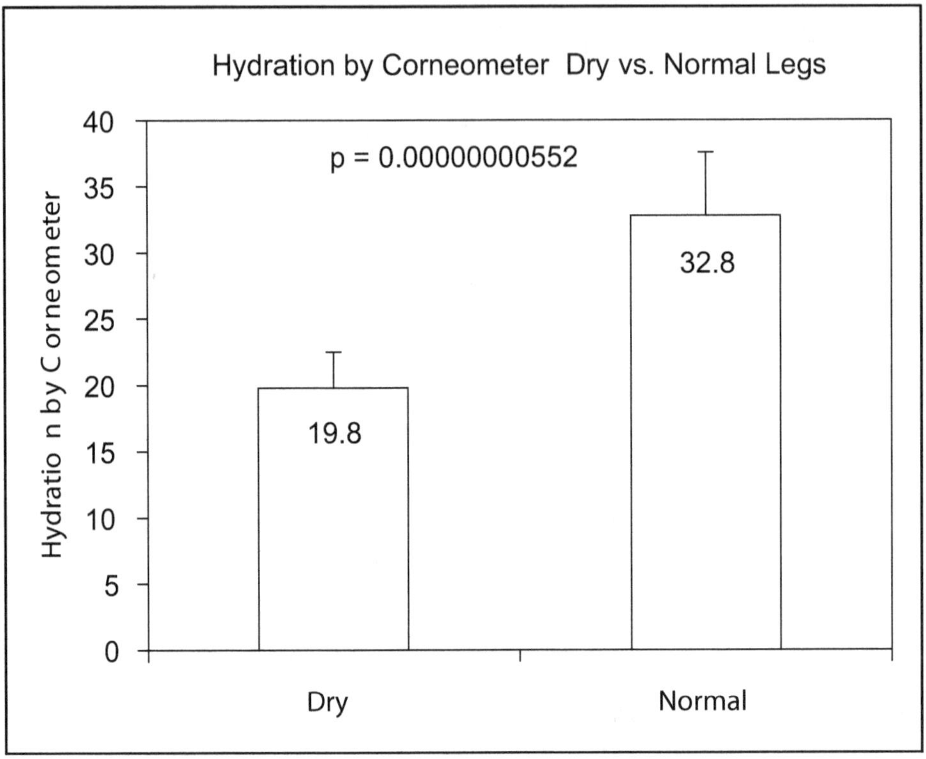

Figure 22: Hydration measurements by Corneometer on dry vs. normal legs show statistically significant difference.

Experimental irritation was induced by applying sodium lauryl sulphate (SLS) 0.5% aqueous for 24 hours. The effects were evaluated at 3 hours, 1 day, 3 days, and 7 days post-SLS patch removal by measuring Redness (a*) and Brightness (L*) by Chromameter and TEWL by Dermalab as well as visually grading erythema. Figure 23 shows these effects over a period of seven days.

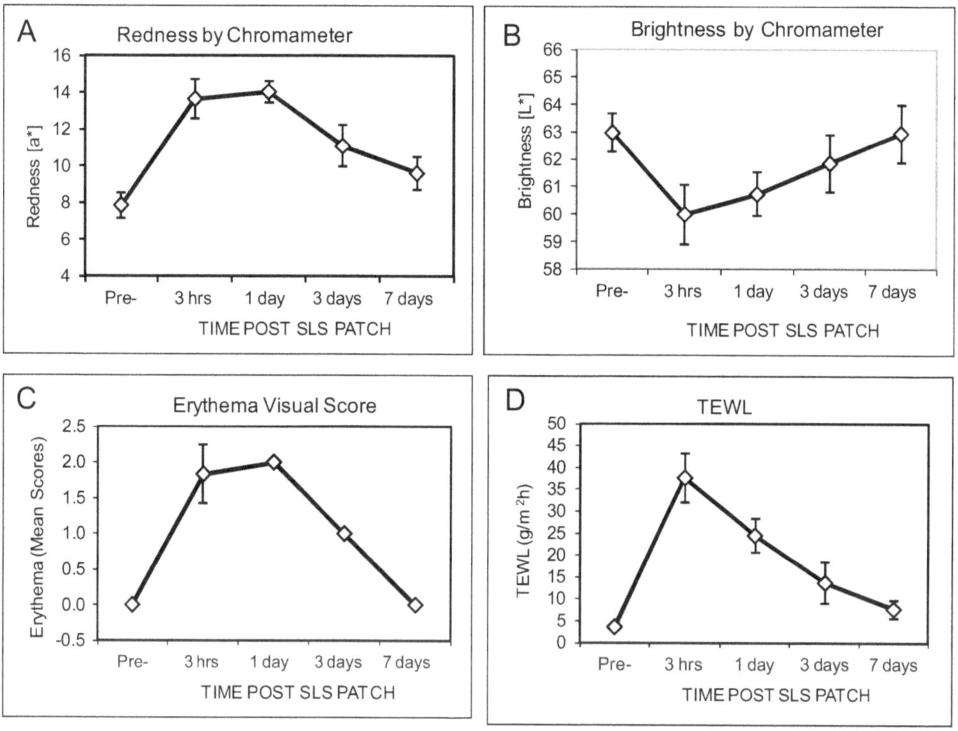

Figure 23: Evaluation of irritation produced by SLS 0.5% patch on volar forearm. Changes in Redness by Chromameter (A), Brightness by Chromameter (B), Visual erythema score (C) and TEWL (D) are shown over a period of seven days.

In another "Irritation by SLS" experiment, six SLS 0.5% patches were applied to the volar forearms, three on the left and three on the right, for 24 hours. Laser Doppler Imaging, side-lighted videomicroscopy, and UV videomicroscopy were done before SLS patch application and then at 3 hours, 1 day, 3 days, 6 days, and 16 days post-SLS patch removal.

Laser Doppler Images show strong erythema (high blood flow) on all the six sites at 3 hours and 1 day post-SLS patch removal. On day 3, erythema started to subside and on day 6, there was still some residual erythema. On day 16, erythema was completely gone. See the series of Laser Doppler Images in Figure 24.

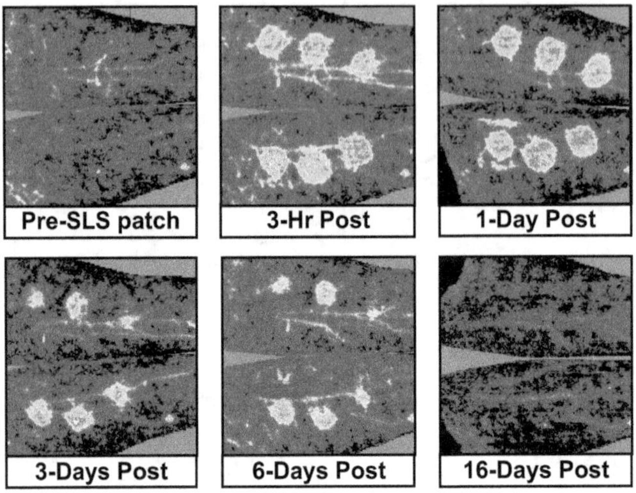

Figure 24: Laser Doppler Images of the volar forearms, pre-SLS patch applications and then 3 hours, 1 day, 3 days, 6 days, and 16 days post-SLS patch removal.

Side-lighted videomicroscopy showed marked scaliness post-SLS patch on days 3 and 6. On day 16, scaliness begin to subside. Figure 25 shows the sequence of scaliness over a period of 16 days.

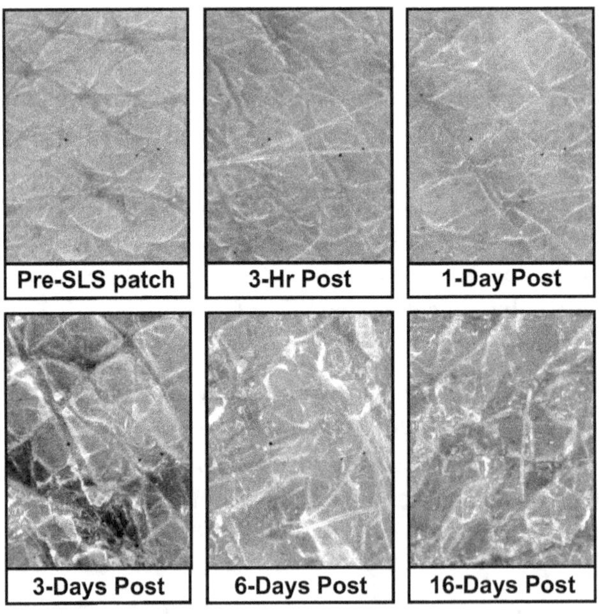

Figure 25: Side-lighted videomicroscope images of the volar forearms, pre-SLS patch applications and then 3 hours, 1 day, 3 days, 6 days, and 16 days post-SLS patch removal. Strong scaliness appears on days 3 and 6. Scaliness starts to reduce by day 16.

UV-videomicroscopy shows a trend similar to the side-lighted videomicroscopy, i.e., prominent scaliness post-SLS patch on days 3 and 6, then lower scaliness on day 16. Figure 26 shows the series of UV-videomicroscopy images.

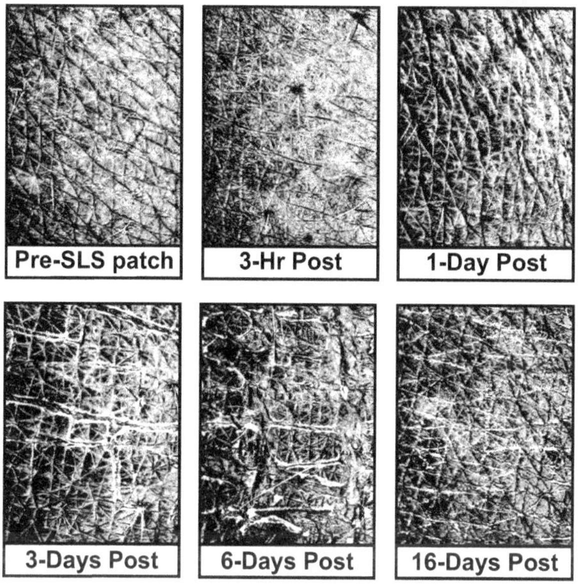

Figure 26: Series of UV-videomicroscope images showing the evolution and resolution of scaliness post-SLS patch over a period of 16 days.

Silicon rubber replicas of skin show the distortion of glyphic pattern post-SLS patch on days 3 and 6, and then recovery by day 16. Figure 27 shows the series of replica images. Replica was not obtained at "3-Hr Post" time point because replicas don't form very well if the skin surface is somewhat moist.

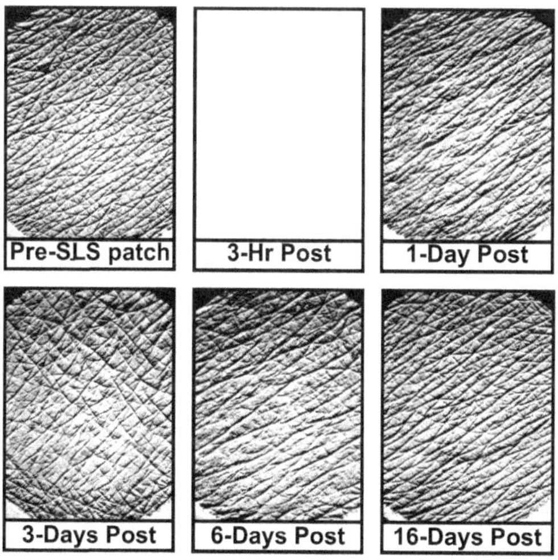

Figure 27: Series of replica images showing the distortion and recovery of glyphic pattern post-SLS patch over a period of 16 days.

To show the changes in the degree of erythema and blood flow, oral niacin (250 mg) was used by a healthy volunteer and Laser Doppler Blood Flow Imaging of the cheek was performed at several time points. The blood flow values in Perfusion Units were calculated. Skin redness values were also evaluated by a colorimeter (Chromameter "a*") as well as skin surface temperature by an infrared thermometer. Figure 28 shows the series of Laser Doppler Images obtained at baseline (before niacin) and then at 20, 40, 60, and 80 minutes post-niacin.

Laser Doppler Images show increased blood flow after orally taking niacin 250 mg, with the maximum value recorded at 40 minutes; then the value was lower at 60 minutes and finally lowered to below the pre-niacin value at 80 minutes.

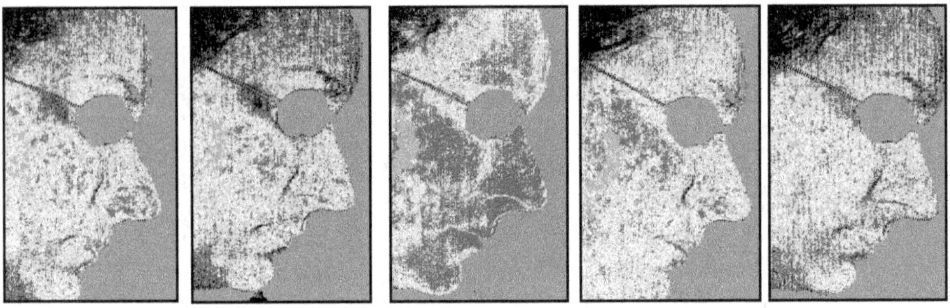

Pre- **20 min** **40 min** **60 min** **80 min**

Figure 28: Laser Doppler Images show increased blood flow after orally taking niacin 250 mg. Facial blood flow peaked at 40 minutes, then reduced somewhat at 60 minutes and finally subsided at 80 minutes.

The increase and decrease of facial blood flow and erythema is shown graphically in Figure 29, as evaluated using the Laser Doppler Imager, Chromameter, and skin surface thermometer.

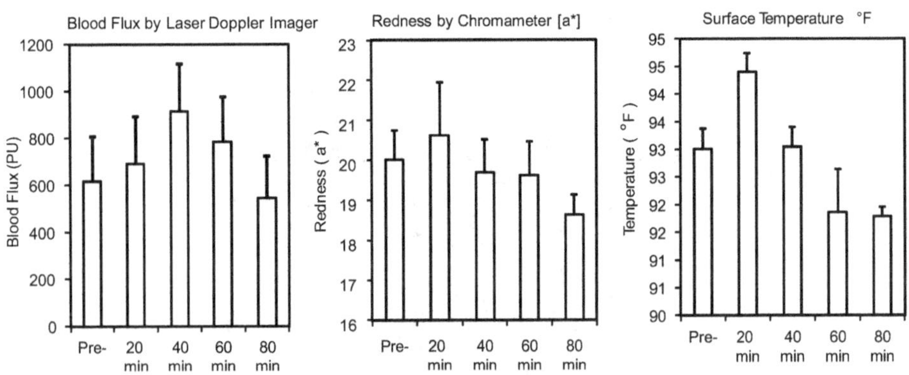

Figure 29: Measurement of skin blood flow and erythema by LDI, Chromameter, and skin surface thermometer (from left to right) over a period of 80 minutes post-niacin ingestion.

To demonstrate the erythema measuring capabilities of the Reflectance Spectrophotometer, Ultraviolet-B (UVB) light was used to generate erythema on the volar forearm. Two sites were exposed to UVB, one with minimal erythema dose (1-MED) and the other with twice the minimal erythema dose (2-MEDs). Using a Bifurbicated Fiber-Optic Reflectance Spectrophotometer, three measurements from each site were recorded. An adjacent normal skin site was also measured. A control spectrum was obtained from the upper inner arm. All spectra were referenced to a white tile. The ratio of the apparent absorbance of the control site (upper inner arm) to each of the three volar forearm sites are presented as the result. The differential spectra are shown in Figure 30. The Oxyhemoglobin peaks at 577 nm are considered as proportional to the intensities of erythema.

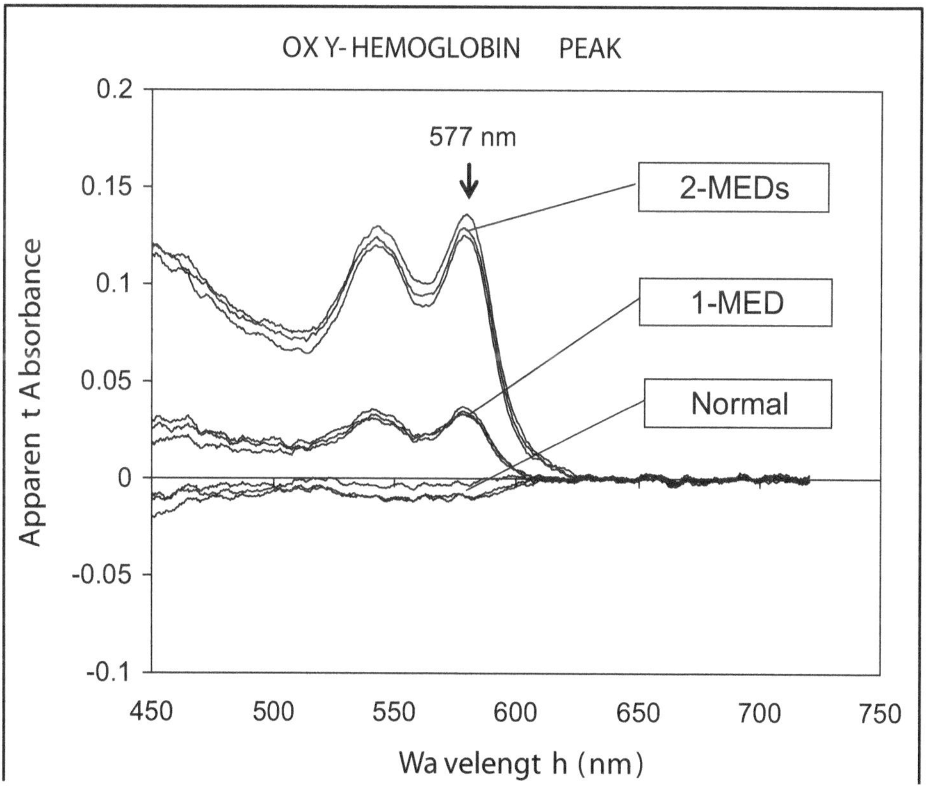

Figure 30: Reflectance Spectrophotometry showing the amplitudes of the oxyhemoglobin peaks at 577 nm after exposure of the volar forearm skin to 1-MED and 2-MEDs of UVB.

Decades of cumulative sun exposure of skin results in the gradual structural degradation and the appearance of an assortment of unwelcome signs of photo-damage, viz. dyspigmentation, wrinkles, roughness, and dull, yellowish, leathery, and lax skin. Over later years of one's life the facial skin shows these signs of sun damage. Digital photography can demonstrate the difference between an older subject with photo-damaged skin compared to a young subject with relatively less photo-damaged skin. Figure 31 shows digital photos of a 62-year-old woman compared to an 18-year-old female.

The older photo-damaged face (B) shows more wrinkles, roughness, prominent naso-labial fold and dyspigmentation compared to the young face (A). The wrinkle and roughness features are enhanced in the parallel polarized photos while the cross-polarized photos show the dyspigmentation more prominently.

Digital fluorescence photos show enhanced pigmentation and in case of the young subject follicular casts and porphyrin fluorescence on and around the nose (Figure 32). The reddish fluorescence emission is from the porphyrin produced by p-Acnes.

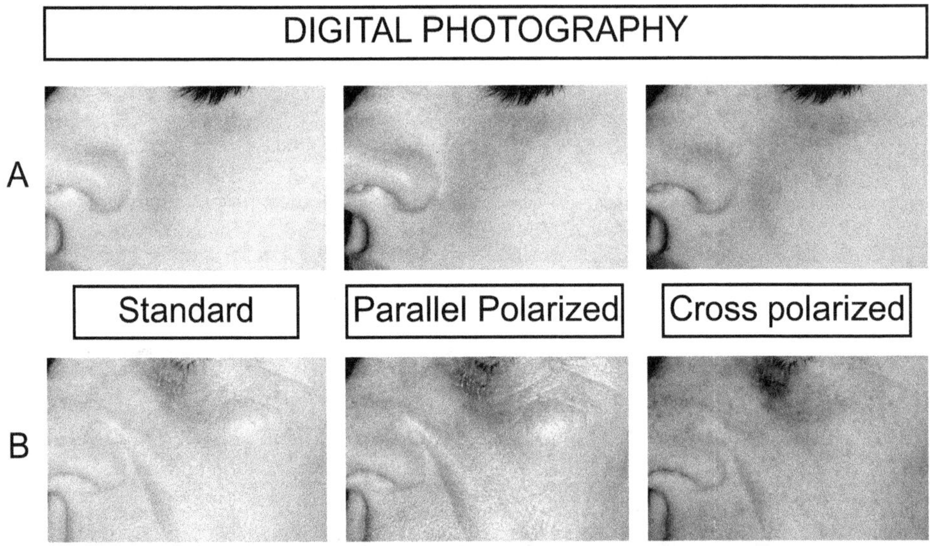

Figure 31: Facial photographs of an 18-year-old female (A) compared to a 62-year-old female (B), in "Standard," "Parallel Polarized," and "Cross-Polarized" modes. Standard flash photo shows smoother skin, less prominent pigmented spots on the face of the young female compared to rough, wrinkly, and dyspigmented facial skin of the older female. The wrinkles and roughness are shown more prominently in the parallel polarized photos. The cross-polarized photos show the dyspigmentation more prominently.

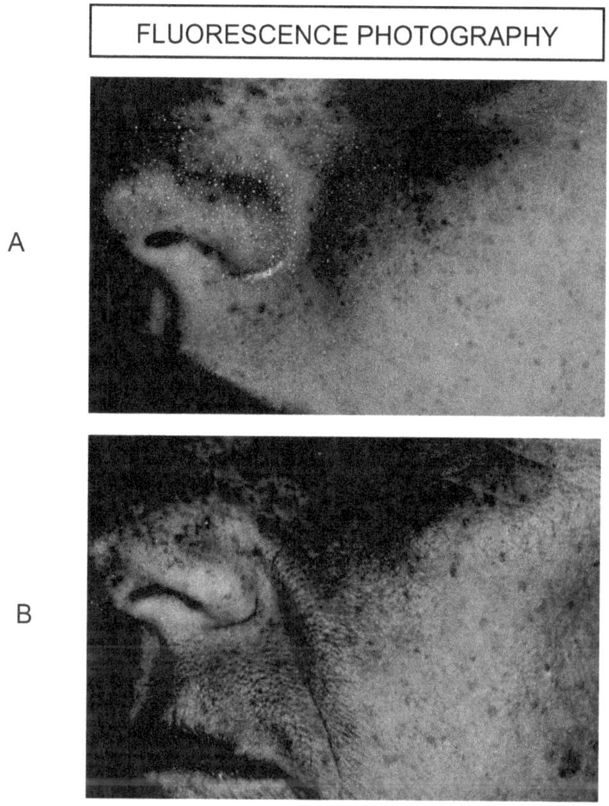

Figure 32: Fluorescence photos with the excitation wavelength centered at 417 nm show enhanced dyspigmentation, more on the older face (B) compared to the younger face (A). The young face also shows fluorescing follicular cast (yellowish spots) on the nose and surrounding area, some of them showing the presence of porphyrin (reddish spots).

In another study, the dorsal forearms of young and old subjects were compared to their respective volar forearms. The dorsal forearms are generally more exposed to sun than the volar forearms. Therefore one would expect more photo-damage on the dorsal forearm.

The studies were carried out on the mid-volar and mid-dorsal forearms of each subject, with the assumption that the dorsal forearms would suffer a greater degree of photo-damage.

To show the relative photo-damage of volar vs. dorsal surface of the fore arms, videomicroscope images of the volar and dorsal forearms of a 62-year-old subject and an 18-year-old subject were obtained at 60× setting on the Hi-Scope probe. Figure 33 shows the differences in the images.

The cumulative photo-damage over decades of sun exposure is clearly evident in the older subject (A). Loss of glyphic pattern, scaliness, and dyspigmentation are clearly evident in the dorsal surface compared to volar surface. The younger subject (B), on the other hand, shows relatively slight change in the glyphic pattern and barely any difference in pigmentation.

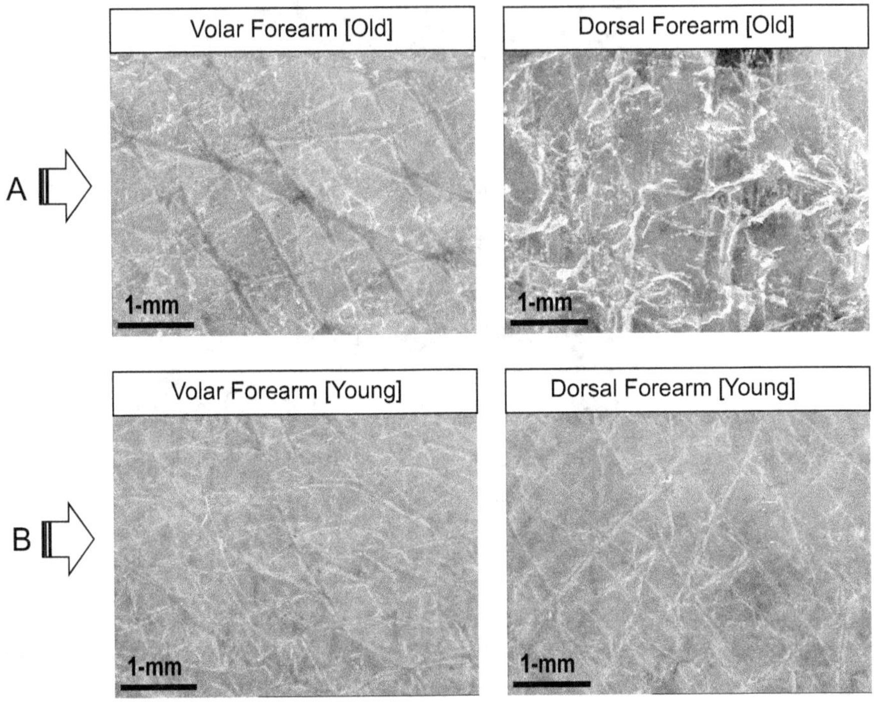

Figure 33: Videomicroscopy at 60× reveals the differences in the relative photo-damage between the volar and dorsal forearms. The younger subject (B) shows slight difference in the glyphic pattern while the older subject (A) shows gross differences. The glyphic lines are practically obliterated, obscured by overlying thick scales, a common feature of photo-damaged skin. Hyper-pigmented patches are also typical of photo-damaged skin.

Fringe projection device, pseudocolored to show three-dimentional image, shows differences in photo-damaged skin of the dorsal forearm compared to the volar forearm. Figure 34 shows the 3-D images.

A mathematical construct of the primary image, after flattening the gross contour of the skin surface but leaving the microtopography intact, is presented. The color-coded image of the surface for heights show gross differences in the volar vs. dorsal forearm of older subject (A) while the younger subject (B) show slight difference. The photo-damaged dorsal forearm of the older subject (A) shows gross distortion of the microtopography, loss of glyphic pattern, and surface details.

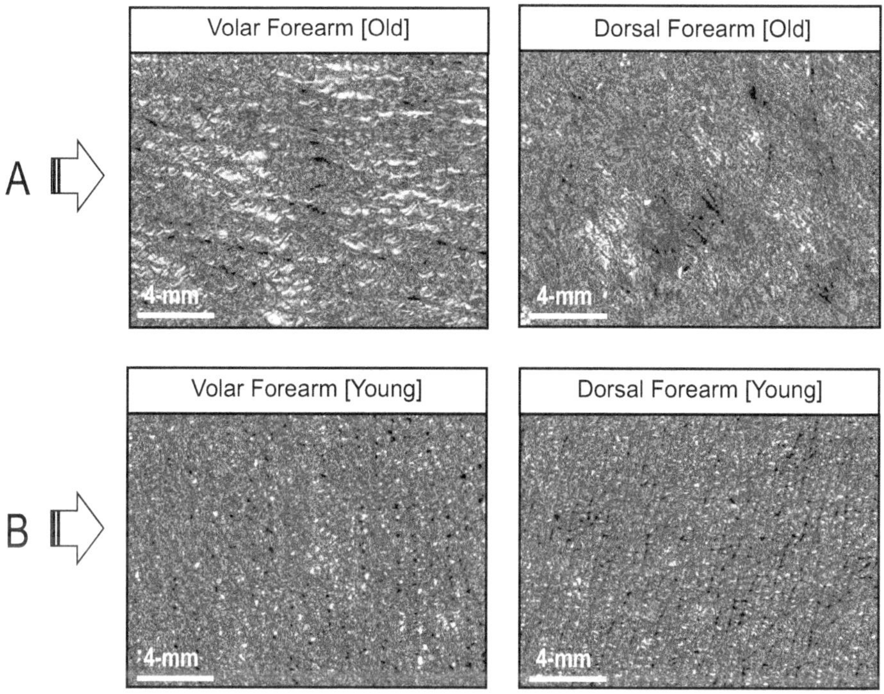

Figure 34: The color-coded 3-D images obtained with the fringe projection device show gross distortions in the microtopography of the dorsal forearm skin of the older subject (A) compared to the volar forearm. The difference between the volar and dorsal forearm of the younger subject is small.

The confocal scanning laser microscope (CSLM) images horizontal sections of skin at various depths showing the structures of tissue and cells. Figure 35 shows confocal images of normal skin (volar forearm) at various depths. In normal skin the confocal images of SC appears as a bright structure due to strong reflection. The wrinkle lines and surface structure along with some glyphic lines can be observed. The *stratum corneum* at a depth of 3.6 μm is shown in picture A. The cellular arrangement of *stratum granulosum* is shown in picture B at a depth of approximately 14.4 μm. Because of the curvature of the surface, some parts of SC are also shown at the edges. The picture C shows the *stratum spinosum* at a depth of 25.2 μm. Picture D shows the dermal-epidermal junction, with some capillary loops shown in the sub-epidermal layer, at a depth of 54.0 μm. The dermis is shown in picture E at a depth of 82.8 μm.

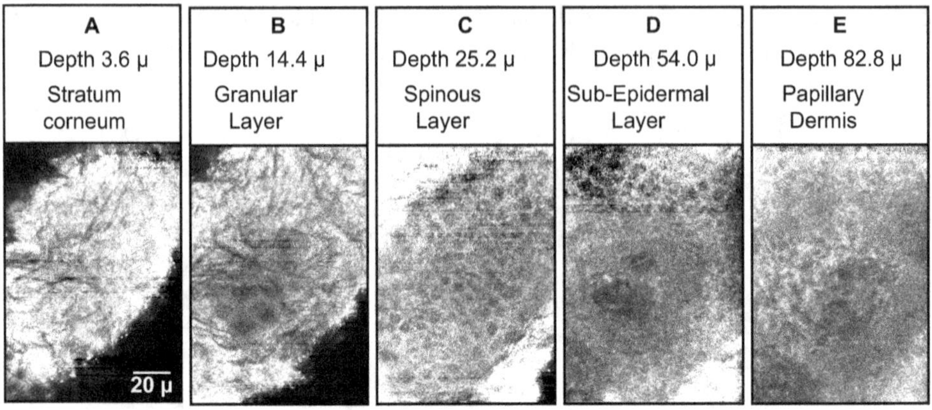

Figure 35: Horizontal sections obtained from the volar forearm by the Confocal Microscope at various depths of skin.

Confocal microscope can reveal the difference between the dark skin and light skin at the dermal-epidermal junction. The dermal-epidermal junction is a wavy surface forming conical projections. Dark-skinned individuals have thicker epidermis with more wavy dermal-epidermal junction compared to the light-skinned individuals. An example is presented in Figure 36.

The horizontal optical section of the skin obtained by a confocal microscope, at a depth of 80 microns, shows large bright circles in the dark-skinned individual compared to light-skinned individual. This is because melanin reflects 830-nm light strongly compared to other structures in skin. The dark-skinned individuals also have thicker epidermis with a wavier dermal-epidermal junction, and when a confocal microscope optically slices a horizontal section at the dermal-epidermal junction, larger circles of brighter spots are shown in the image.

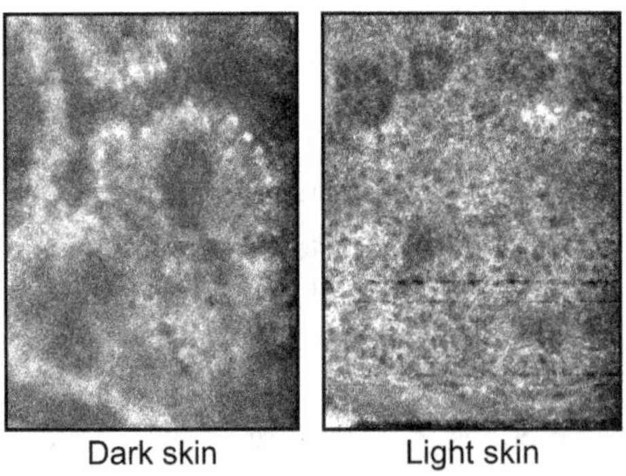

Figure 36: Confocal microscope section at the dermal-epidermal junction of a dark-skinned individual (left) compared to a light-skinned individual (right). Melanin near the basal layer is observed as bright spots as the horizontal section slices the dermal-epidermal junction.

Cross-sectional images in the depth of skin can be obtained by Optical Coherence Tomography (OCT) device. This can be a complement to Confocal Microscopy, which images horizontal sections.

The cross-sectional image slice is 1 mm deep and 1 mm in lateral direction. Dermal and epidermal structures are clearly outlined. The epidermal thickness can be measured. OCT can easily be used to study the cosmetics and skin care products that can change the epidermal thickness. *Stratum corneum* (SC) is visualized as a bright line, and its thickness cannot be measured precisely unless it is grossly swollen. The geometry of isolated legions such as comedones and seborrheic keratosis can be visualized.

As it was shown by the Confocal Microscopy, the difference between dark and light skin can also be shown by the OCT at the dermal-epidermal junction. Figure 37 shows an example of an OCT image of dorsal forearm of a dark-skinned individual compared to image of a light-skinned individual.

The dark skin shows wavier dermal-epidermal junction compared to the light skin.

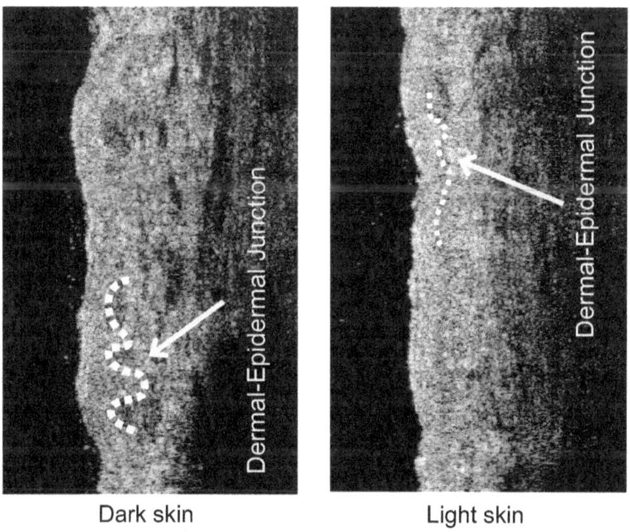

Figure 37: OCT images of dark and light skin. Dermal-epidermal junction is wavier in the dark skin.

In another example, OCT imaging showed the difference between sun-damaged skin to relatively less sun-damaged skin. Figure 38 show OCT images of the cheeks of a 60-year-old individual, with decades of cumulative sun damage, and a 20-year-old individual with relatively less sun damage. OCT image of the photo-damaged cheek of the older individual showed thinning of epidermis and flattening of the papillary junction compared to the OCT image of the young individual, which showed much thicker epidermis.

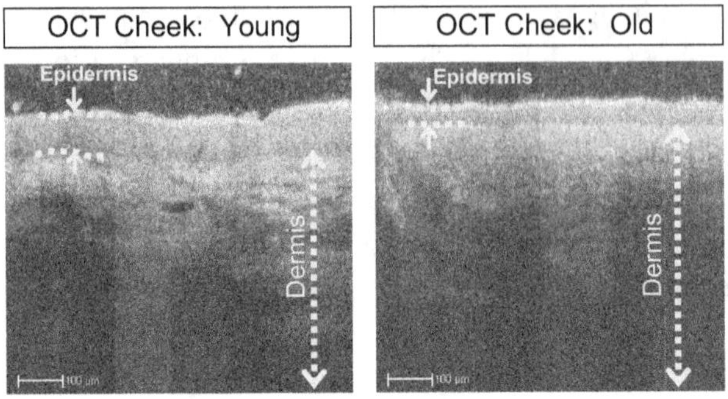

Figure 38: OCT image of the photo-damaged cheek (right) show thinning of epidermis and flattening of the papillary junction. The younger, relatively less photo-damaged skin (left) shows much thicker epidermis.

Ultrasound imaging is another method to capture cross-sectional images of the skin. The 20-megahertz ultrasound device has much lower resolution than OCT, but the images show full thickness of skin with some of the subcutaneous region as well. The epidermis appears as a line in the ultrasound image and its structure cannot be resolved. The thickness of the whole skin can be measured.

In one experiment, the reduction of cellulite on the thigh by a vibrating vacuum massaging device was shown by the ultrasound imaging. The ultrasound images were collected from the region of thigh showing cellulite, first before treatment and then after one month of daily massaging. Figure 39 shows the before-and-after images.

The image before massaging shows large pockets of cellulite fat protruding into the dermis at the base. After one month of massaging treatment the dermis is much thicker with very little fat protrusions.

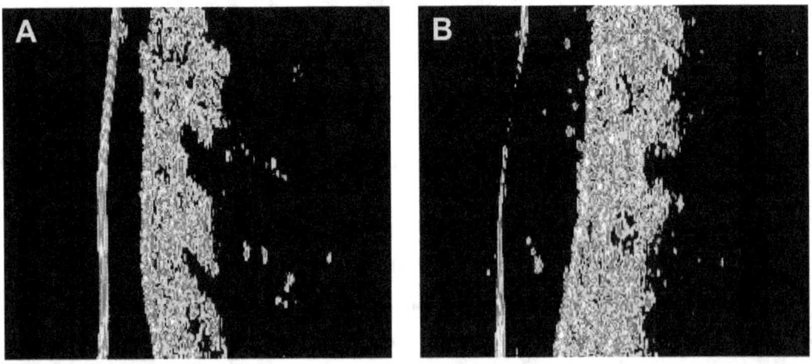

Figure 39: The effect of massaging on cellulite as revealed by ultrasound. The ultrasound images were obtained from the region of thigh showing cellulite, before treatment (A) and then after one month of daily massaging (B).

The periorbital wrinkling of face, sometimes referred to as "crow's feet," have been studied extensively in the past, particularly with regard to anti-aging treatments. Fringe projection devices have been used extensively to show the reduction of the crow's feet.

To show the ability of a fringe projection device to assess the changes in crow's feet, a "lactic acid" model was used. Lactic acid 10% aqueous when applied to crow's-feet region produces a transient effect of partially effacing the wrinkles. This effect may last for a few hours.

The digital photos obtained before and after the lactic acid treatment show the reduction of crow's-feet wrinkles clearly (see Figure 40). The 3-D imaging by the fringe projection device also shows this difference (see Figure 41).

Using the fringe projection device, a "Crow's Feet Index" was calculated based on the cross-sectional areas of wrinkles at nine different locations. This crow's-feet index showed a marked reduction at 30 minutes after the lactic acid application. Figure 42 shows this difference graphically.

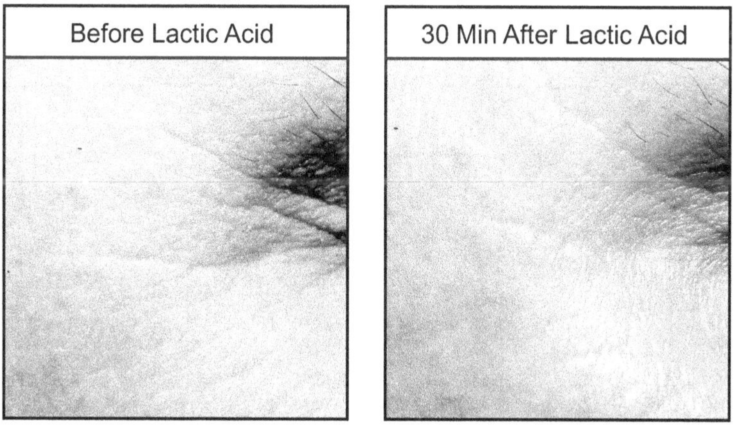

Figure 40: Digital photos of the crow's-feet wrinkle area, before lactic acid treatment (left) and 30 minutes post-lactic acid treatment (right).

Suction Device (Cutometer) is commonly used for measuring the elasticity parameters of skin. In one experiment, skin was exposed to ultraviolet light (UV) with a dose of 2-MEDs. Gross elasticity was measured by the Cutometer with a 2-mm probe at 1, 4, 7, and 14 days post-UV exposure. An adjacent Control (Ctrl) site was also measured.

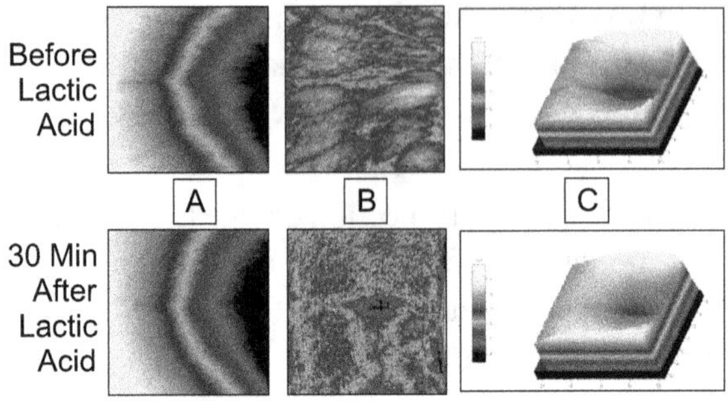

Figure 41: Fringe projection images before (top) and after (bottom) lactic acid treatment. The images are color-coded for heights. The original images (A) were processed to remove the gross contours to show flat images but with the wrinkles intact (B). The geometric 3-D images are shown in (C).

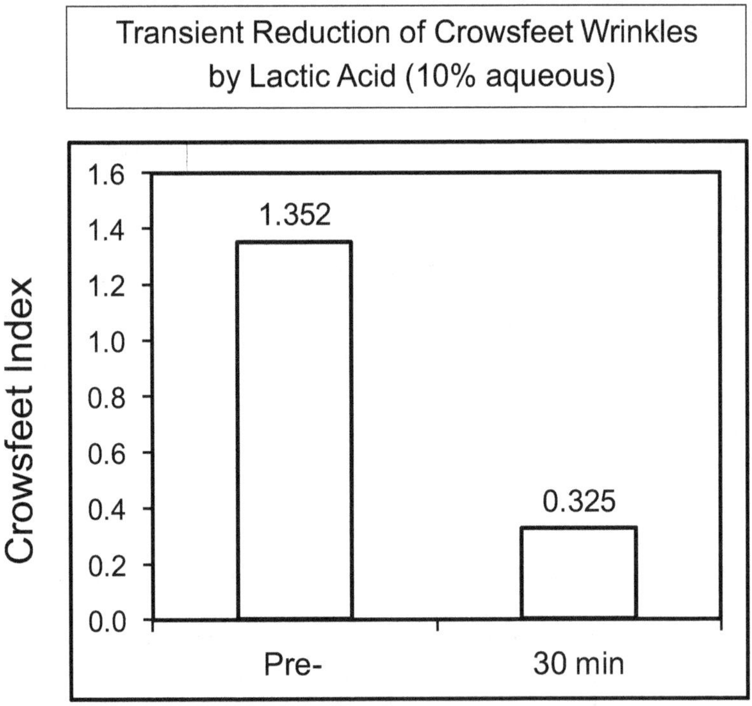

Figure 42: The Crow's-Feet Index reduced dramatically at 30 minutes after the application of lactic acid.

There was an apparent loss of gross elasticity at the UV-exposed site on Day 1, which gradually recovered by Day 14. Figure 43 shows the effect graphically. Erythema generated by UV can cause some edema on the exposed site, which may influence the elastic properties.

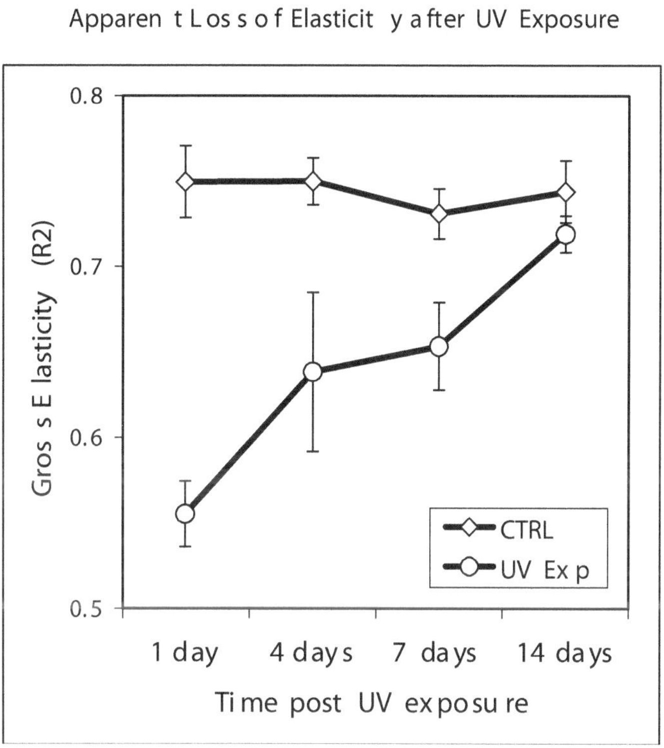

Figure 43: The UV-exposed site showed apparent loss of elasticity at day 1, followed by recovery by day 14.

CONCLUSION

The methodologies and bio-instrumentation described in this chapter can be utilized along with the traditional clinical evaluation methods to test the efficacy of cosmetics and skin care products, to present a complete picture of improvements in skin attributes.

In the field of skin research we no longer depend solely on visual examination and touch; we now have instrumental methodologies based on physics, chemistry, biology, and engineering to study skin at the surface and in depth.

Effects of cosmetics and skin care products on the skin can be studied more objectively.

In this chapter a selected number of bio-instrumentations and methodologies are described. Indeed there are many more techniques available, some of them important for scientific research.

As a result of recent advancements in science, engineering, and computer technology, many new skin-measuring techniques are evolving, and one can expect more sophisticated instrumentations and methodologies in the near future.

REFERENCES

[1] Handbook of NON-INVASIVE METHODS and the SKIN, Second Edition, Edited by Jorgen Serup, Gregor B. E. Jemec and Gary L. Grove CRC Press Taylor & Francis Group, Boca Raton, Florida, USA. (2006)

[2] BIOENGINEERING OF THE SKIN, Skin Imaging and Analysis, Second Edition. Edited by Klaus-P. Wilhelm, Enzo Berardesca, Peter Elsner and Howard I. Maibach Informa Healthcare USA Inc., New York, NY, USA. Pages 71 – 81, (2007)

[3] "Water Sorption-desorption Test of the Skin *in Vivo* for Functional Assessment of the Stratum Corneum" Hachiro Tagami, Yuko Kanamaru, Kunio Inoue, Shoko Suehisa, Fumio Inoue, Keiji Iwatsuki, Kohdo Yoshikuni and Mizuho Yamada Journal of Investigative Dermatology (1982) 78, 425–428; doi:10.1111/1523-1747.ep12507756

[4] "Water sorption-desorption test and moisture accumulation test for functional assessment of atopic skin in children". **Pellacani G, Seidenari S. Acta Derm Venereol. 2001 May;81(2):100-3.**

[5] "Optical coherence tomography in dermatology" Pagnoni, A., Knuettel, A., Welker, P., Rist, M., Stoudemayer, T., Kolbe, L., Sadiq, I. and Kligman, A.M., Skin Res. Technology **5** : 83–87 (1999).

[6] "In vivo confocal scanning laser microscopy of human skin: melanin provides strong contrast" Rajadhyaksha, M., Grossman, M., Esterowitz, D., Webb, R.H. and Anderson, R.R., J. Invest. Dermatol. Vol. **104** No. **6** (1995).

[7] "Rapid in vivo measurement of the topography of human skin by active image triangulation using a digital micromirror device" Jasper, S., Hopermann, H., Sauerman, G., Hoppe, U., Lunderstad, R and Ennen, J., Skin Res. And Technology **5** : 195–207 (1999).

[8] "Phaseshift rapid in-vivo measuring of human skin (PRIMOS) by digital fringe projection with micromirror display devices DMD" Frankowski, Gottfried; Chen, Mai; Huth, Torsten Proc. SPIE Vol. 4778, p. 66–73, Interferometry XI: Applications, Wolfgang Osten; Ed.

[9] "The nature of photoaging: Its prevention and repair Kligman" L. H. and Kligman, A. M., Photodermatology **3** : 215-227 (1986).

[10] "Aging and the skin" Kligman, A.M. and Balin, A.K., Aging of human skin in: Kligman, A.M. and Balin, A.K., (Eds), Raven Press, New York (1989).

[11] "Cutaneous Aging" Kligman, A.M. and Takase, Y. (Eds.), University of Tokyo Press (1988).

[12] "Photodamage" Gilchrest, B.A., Blackwell Science Inc. (1995).

[13] "Aging skin" Leveque, J.L. and Agashe, P.G., Marcel Dekker Inc. (1993).

www.ingramcontent.com/pod-product-compliance
Lightning Source LLC
LaVergne TN
LVHW052247200926
848481LV00002B/295